Sexual Function in the Prostate Cancer Patient

For further volumes:
http://www.springer.com/series/7635

Sexual Function in the Prostate Cancer Patient

Edited by

John P. Mulhall
Department of Urology, Cornell University Weill Medical College,
New York

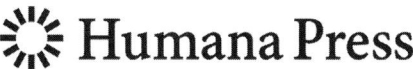 Humana Press

Editor
John P. Mulhall
Cornell University
Weill Medical College
Dept. Urology
525 East 68th St.
New York NY 10021
USA
mulhalj1@mskcc.org

ISBN 978-1-60327-554-5   e-ISBN 978-1-60327-555-2
DOI 10.1007/978-1-60327-555-2

Library of Congress Control Number: 2008942049

Printed on acid-free paper

springer.com

Foreword

Prostate cancer and sexual function have been closely intertwined since the beginning of the twentieth century, when radical perineal prostatectomy was first developed by Hugh Hampton Young as an effective therapy for localized prostate cancer. It was immediately recognized that treatment for prostate cancer came at the cost of erectile function. With the pioneering discovery by Huggins and Hodges in 1941 that prostate cancer would respond to castration or the administration of estrogens, loss of sexual function became indelibly impressed in the minds of both physicians and the public as an inevitable consequence of therapy for prostate cancer. As radiation therapy began to grow as an attractive form of treatment for prostate cancer, the relationship of treatment to sexual dysfunction became murkier. Many patients treated with radiation were elderly, their sexual function before treatment was poorly documented, and hormone therapy was used indiscriminately before and after radiation, making it difficult to elucidate the effect of radiotherapy on sexual function. The discovery by Walsh and Donker of the anatomical location of the cavernous nerves in the early 1980s and the development by Walsh of the anatomical, "nerve-sparing" radical prostatectomy brought the field into much sharper focus. Rather than sexual function being an unavoidable consequence of effective prostate cancer treatment, it became clear that fine details of surgical technique or the precise way in which the treatment for prostate cancer was delivered had a major impact on the quality of sexual function after treatment. Walsh first reported, and then many others confirmed, that it was possible for many men to recover adequate, even normal, erectile function after radical prostatectomy if a skilled procedure was done to remove the entire prostate gland while preserving the neurovascular bundles. Shortly thereafter, risk factors were identified that could predict the probability of recovery: age, quality of erectile function before the operation, and quantitative preservation of the neurovascular bundles.

The modern era of precise measurement of the effects of prostate cancer treatment on sexual function would await the development of modern outcomes research methods, especially patient-completed quality-of-life questionnaires. These have allowed more reliable and precise measurements of the effect of androgen deprivation therapy, radiation, surgery, and other treatments on sexual function.

With the availability of noninvasive forms of treatment—intracavernous injections, vasodilating agents, and oral phosphodiesterase-5 inhibitors—patients with erectile dysfunction after prostate cancer therapy had more options. With the ready availability of medical information on the Internet and in bookstores, patients' expectations rose substantially. More and more men became aware of the sexual side effects of each treatment and much more interested in finding a way to treat their cancer effectively without compromising sexual function. As a result, preservation of sexual function has become an important metric for measuring the quality of prostate cancer therapy. Even though this outcome has been reported far too casually, too often assessed only by the treating surgeons, the patients as well as referring physicians increasingly demand to know the chances that a patient will recover sexual function after therapy.

In this wonderful and timely book, Dr. John Mulhall has brought together many of the world's experts on prostate cancer and sexual function to assess in detail the state-of-the-art. These chapters offer a broad overview of the pathophysiology and treatment of sexual dysfunction in men with prostate cancer, and leave the reader with numerous pearls of wisdom about how sexual dysfunction can be assessed and prevented in the care of patients with prostate cancer.

Sexual dysfunction presents a major challenge to physicians who take on the task of treating men with prostate cancer. It is no longer good enough to cure the disease or save the patient's life. In a disease that lingers as long as prostate cancer, even when left untreated or treated palliatively, patients demand the highest possible quality-of-life compatible with the greatest length of life. They expect us to understand exactly how our treatment alters their function and to do everything we can to minimize the damage.

We now know that outcomes of cancer therapy—cancer control as well as complications and side effects—are related to the skill and experience of the individual surgeon, the dose and technique of irradiation, and the quality of care delivery systems. The best outcome requires therapy delivered with the best possible technique. For surgery, this means precise, anatomical dissection that allows preservation of the neurovascular bundles. For radiotherapy, this means precise delivery of dosage, either through brachytherapy implants or intensity-modulated radiotherapy (IMRT), to deliver maximum tumoricidal doses to the cancer with minimal collateral damage to the surrounding tissue. For systemic therapy, this means restraint in the use of androgen deprivation to situations in which the benefit clearly outweighs the side effects.

These are challenges that can be met through greater understanding of the anatomy and physiology of sexual function and through precise measurements of the effects of each therapy, not only on the cancer but also on sexual function. Dr. Mulhall and the authors of this new text have provided a valuable source of information that clearly defines the state-of-the-art today and will undoubtedly stimulate further progress in the field.

Peter T. Scardino, MD

Preface

Prostate cancer is the most common form of cancer in American men other than skin cancer. It is estimated that about 185,000 new cases of prostate cancer will be diagnosed in 2008 in the USA alone. Almost 30,000 men will die of the disease in 2008 in this country. It is the second-leading cause of cancer death in men after lung cancer. While a man has a 15% chance of being diagnosed with prostate cancer in his lifetime, only 3% die of the disease. Thus, in the modern era, the vast majority of men live for very long periods of time. Over the course of the last 20 years, numerous discoveries and refinements in management have occurred in this disease. There have been refinements in prostate biopsy technique, in imaging of prostate cancer, in surgical technique (e.g., the introduction of laparoscopic and robotic prostatectomy), in the delivery of radiation therapy, and in the treatment of advanced disease. Furthermore, the use of PSA as a screening tool has resulted in a far greater number of men being diagnosed with prostate cancer at its earliest stages. This has also translated into younger men being diagnosed with prostate cancer. Thus, a man's long-term sexual function has become an even bigger issue now given these factors.

With regard to the sexual function consequences of the treatment of prostate cancer, the field has changed dramatically over the course of the last 20 years. Many of the developments in this area have been "under the radar" and have been missed by most clinicians. Increased understanding of the pathophysiology of postprostatectomy sexual dysfunctions and post-radiation therapy erectile dysfunction, the controversial concept of penile rehabilitation, neuromodulatory drugs, and the impact of androgen deprivation therapy on sexual function are but a few of the areas in which information explosion has occurred. The purpose of this book is to give the practicing clinician, whether a urologist, radiation therapist, medical oncologist, internist, or primary care physician, a comprehensive state-of-the-art overview of sexual function changes and their treatments in the prostate cancer patient.

I am proud to say that I have been joined in this effort by the world's leading authorities in this area. I am indebted to my chairman, Dr. Peter T. Scardino, for his masterful foreword. Dr. Scardino is a surgeon–scientist who needs no introduction. He is Chairman of the Department of Surgery at Memorial Sloan-Kettering Cancer Center and has made major contributions in the treatment of and research in prostate cancer.

This book opens with a chapter on sexual dysfunctions following prostate cancer treatment. It would be remiss of us if we concentrated solely on erectile dysfunction as there are other sexual problems that are prevalent, specifically, orgasm changes, penile length changes, and the development of Peyronie's disease after radical prostatectomy. Clinical experience tells us that a man's erectile function in the months leading up to his prostate cancer treatment is different than that before his diagnosis. A chapter by Dr. David F. Penson and Dr. Christian J. Nelson highlights this, dealing with the impact of prostate cancer diagnosis on sexual function. Dr. Kevin T. McVary, a urologist, and Dr. Carol A. Podlasek, a scientist, both world authorities on the consequences of nerve injury on erectile tissue, discuss the pathophysiology of erectile function changes following radical prostatectomy using their experience with the cavernous nerve injury model as an example.

Dr. Victoria J. Croog and Dr. Michael J. Zelefsky, of the Department of Radiation Oncology at Memorial Sloan-Kettering Cancer Center, follow with a chapter of the pathophysiology of erectile dysfunction following radiation therapy. Dr. P. William McLaughlin and Dr. Gregory Merrick, both radiation oncologists, discuss the intriguing concept of erection-sparing radiation therapy and whether this is possible or not. Dr. Arthur L. Burnett II discusses the role of neuromodulatory drugs in the radical prostatectomy patient. Dr. Burnett has contributed significantly to this literature from a clinical and laboratory standpoint. It is exciting to think that, at some point in time, we may have drugs that prevent cavernous nerve injury or promote cavernous nerve regeneration at the time of surgery or even after radiation therapy.

A chapter on intraoperative maneuvers designed to minimize postoperative erectile dysfunction is written by Dr. Joseph A. Pettus and Dr. Farhang Rabbani. Dr. Rabbani, one of the world's authorities on cavernous nerve interposition grafting, gives a comprehensive and critical account of this strategy. Dr. Alexander Müller and I have contributed a chapter on the controversial topic of penile preservation and rehabilitation and present the animal and human data supporting this concept at this time. Dr. Ricardo Munarriz and Dr. Abdul Traish, a urologist and basic scientist, respectively, from Boston University, highlight the impact androgen deprivation has on male sexual function. They present elegant data that outline the severity of the impact that an agonadal state has on erectile function.

Dr. Francesco Montorsi (the founding father of the concept of penile rehabilitation) and Dr. Andrea Salonia, from Milan, Italy, discuss the use of PDE5 inhibitors in the radical prostatectomy patient population and extensively review the literature pertaining to the use of these drugs. Dr. Andrew McCullough, from New York University Medical Center, discusses intracavernosal injection therapy, while Dr. Brian R. Lane and Dr. Drogo K. Montague, from the Cleveland Clinic Foundation, discuss non-pharmacologic therapies for erectile dysfunction, including penile implant surgery, after the treatment of prostate cancer.

The penultimate chapter is written by Dr. Abraham Morgentaler, from Boston, who discusses the highly controversial subject of androgen supplementation in the prostate cancer patient. Dr. Morgentaler, the world's authority in this area, makes a cogent argument in favor of a rational approach to the use of androgens in the prostate cancer patient. The book finishes with a "crystal ball" view for the future of post-radical pelvic surgery pharmacotherapy. This chapter is written by Drs. Tony Bella and Tom F. Lue, from the University of California, San Francisco, and no one is in a better position to address this issue than they are Dr. Lue is the world's authority on stem cell therapy for erectile dysfunction.

It is my hope that you, as a clinician, will find this information useful. Furthermore, I hope that it will at the very least provoke you into thinking differently about these problems in this population and perhaps even alter how you practice.

John P. Mulhall, MD

Contents

Contributors

Anthony J. Bella, MD, FRCSC
Assistant Professor Urology and
Director of Basic Urologic Research,
Associate Scientist, Neuroscience,
University of Ottawa,
Ottawa, Canada

William O. Brant, MD
Northstar Urology,
Vail, CO, USA

Alberto Briganti, MD
Universita Vita Saluta San Raffaele,
Milan, Italy

Arthur L. Burnett II, MD
Patrick C. Walsh
Professor of Urology,
Cellular and Molecular Medicine,
The James Buchanan Brady Urological Institute,
The Johns Hopkins Hospital,
Baltimore, MD, USA

Victoria J. Croog, MD
Department of Radiation Oncology,
Memorial Sloan-Kettering Cancer Center,
New York, NY, USA

James A. Eastham, MD
Professor of Urology, Urology Service,
Memorial Sloan-Kettering Cancer Center,
New York, NY, USA

Andrea Gallina, MD
Universita Vita Saluta San Raffaele,
Milan, Italy

Bertrand Guillonneau, MD
Professor of Urology,
Head, Section of Minimally Invasive Urology,
Urology Service,
Memorial Sloan-Kettering Cancer Center,
New York, NY, USA

Brian R. Lane, MD
Cleveland Clinic,
Cleveland, OH, USA

Tom F. Lue, MD
Professor and Vice Chair Urology,
Emil Tanagho Endowed Chair in Clinical Urology,
University of California, San Francisco,
San Francisco, CA, USA

Andrew McCullough, MD
Associate Professor of Clinical Urology,
Director of Male Sexual Health,
Fertility and Microsurgery,
New York University School of Medicine,
New York, NY, USA

P. William McLaughlin, MD
University of Michigan,
Assarian Cancer Center,
Novi, MI, USA

Kevin T. McVary, MD, FACS
Professor of Urology,
Feinberg School of Medicine,
Northwestern University,
Chicago, IL, USA

Gregory Merrick, MD
Wheeling Center for Radiation Therapy,
WV, USA

Joshua Modder, MD
Department of Urology,
Feinberg School of Medicine,
Northwestern University,
Chicago, IL, USA

Drogo K. Montague, MD
Professor of Surgery,
Cleveland Clinic Lerner College of Medicine of Case Western

Reserve University,
Director, Center for Genitourinary Reconstruction,
Glickman Urological and Kidney Institute,
Cleveland Clinic,
Cleveland, OH, USA

Francesco Montorsi, MD
Universita Vita Saluta San Raffaele,
Milan, Italy

Abraham Morgentaler, MD, FACS
Director, Men's Health Boston, and
Associate Clinical Professor of Urology,
Harvard Medical School,
Boston, MA, USA

John P. Mulhall, MD
Professor of surgery, Urology Service,
Director, Male Sexual and Reproductive Medicine,
Memorial Sloan-Kettering Cancer Center,
New York, New York 10021, USA

Alexander Müller, MD
Fellow, Urology Service,
Memorial Sloan-Kettering Cancer Center,
New York, NY, USA

Ricardo Munarriz, MD
Associate Professor of Urology,
Director of the Center for Sexual Medicine,
Department of Urology, Boston University School of Medicine,
Boston, MA, USA

Christian J. Nelson, PhD
Assistant Attending,
Department of Psychiatry and Behavioral Sciences,
Memorial Sloan-Kettering Cancer Center,
New York, NY, USA

Javier Romero Otero, MD
Research Fellow in Urology,
Memorial Sloan-Kettering Cancer Center,
New York, NY, USA
Phillipe Paparel, MD
Research Fellow in Urology,
Memorial Sloan-Kettering Cancer Center,
New York, NY, USA

David F. Penson, MD
Associate Professor of Urology and Preventive Medicine,
Keck School of Medicine and Norris Cancer Center,
University of Southern California,
Los Angeles, CA, USA

Joseph A. Pettus, MD
Assistant Professor of Urology,
Wake Forest University Baptist Medical Center,
Winston-Salem, NC, USA

Carol A. Podlasek, PhD
Assistant Professor of Urology,
Feinberg School of Medicine,
Northwestern University,
Chicago, IL, USA

Farhang Rabbani, MD
Urology Service,
Memorial Sloan-Kettering Cancer Center,
New York, NY, USA

Andrea Salonia, MD
Universita Vita Saluta San Raffaele,
Milan, Italy

Raanan Tal, MD
Fellow, Urology Service,
Memorial Sloan-Kettering Cancer Center,
New York, NY, USA

Karim Touijer, MD
Urology Service,
Memorial Sloan-Kettering Cancer Center, and
Assistant Professor of Urology at Weill Cornell Medical College,
New York, NY, USA

Abdul Traish, PhD
Professor of Biochemistry,
Departments of Biochemistry and Urology,
Boston University School of Medicine,
Boston, MA, USA

Ofer Yossepowitch, MD
Department of Urology,

Memorial Sloan-Kettering Cancer Center,
New York, NY, USA

Michael J. Zelefsky, MD
Professor of Radiation Oncology,
Chief, Brachytherapy Service,
Department of Radiation Oncology,
Memorial Sloan-Kettering Cancer Center,
New York, NY, USA

Color Plates

Color Plates following p. 264

Chapter 1
Sexual Dysfunction After Radical Prostatectomy

Raanan Tal and John P. Mulhall

Abstract Prostate cancer is the most prevalent cancer among men. The most common treatment for localized prostate cancer is surgery: complete removal of the prostate, a procedure called "radical prostatectomy" (RP). With advances in prostate cancer detection, patients are diagnosed and treated earlier, at a younger age, when sexual function is an important constituent of their quality of life and well-being. Erectile dysfunction (ED) is a well-reported adverse outcome of RP; however, there are additional sexual function related sequelae that are not as often discussed with the patient, before or after surgery. Erectile dysfunction preservation has become feasible with the introduction of nerve-sparing radical prostatectomy in 1982, a surgical technique that allows removal of the prostate without transaction of the neighboring erection nerves, preventing complete loss of erections. However, "nerve-sparing" is not synonymous with "erection quality sparing" and even with excellent nerve-sparing by a highly experienced surgeon men do experience some degree of temporary or permanent decline of their erection hardness. In addition to its effect on erection quality, RP renders all patients unable to ejaculate, and consequently men are infertile after surgery. Advanced reproductive procedures are required if pregnancy is desired. Additional consequences of RP may also include changes in the nature of orgasm, penile length shortening, and penile curvature. With advances in sexual medicine research, today we have a wider knowledge of prevalence of various forms of sexual dysfunction after RP and a better understanding of the underlying mechanisms involved in their evolution. Hence, experts are able to better address sexual function issues, provide men and their partners with counsel-

From: *Current Clinical Urology* Series, *Sexual Function in the Prostate Cancer Patient*
Edited by John P. Mulhall, DOI 10.1007/978-1-60327-555-2_1,
© Humana Press, a part of Springer Science+Business Media, LLC 2009

ing, and tailor treatment individually according to patient's needs. Sexual dysfunction issues should be discussed early, preferably before surgery, despite thoughts of inappropriateness in the light of a recent cancer diagnosis, to avoid any delay in patient and partner education and treatment. Prompt rehabilitative treatment after surgery maximizes the chances of returning to full sexual function. Unaddressed sexual health concerns may have deleterious psychogenic consequences on men and their partners as individuals as well as their well-being as a couple and may include loss of self-esteem and body image, feelings of guilt and shame, and loss of self-confidence and intimacy.

The aim of this chapter, titled "Sexual Dysfunction After Radical Prostatectomy," is to provide the reader with the latest information on sexual health after RP, present emerging concepts of our understanding of its etiology and their implications for treatment.

Keywords Erectile dysfunction; Peyronie's disease; orgasmic dysfunction; penile length; incontinence.

1 Introduction

Sexual dysfunction is a well-reported adverse outcome of radical prostatectomy (RP); however, the surgeon–patient discussion is often limited only to erectile dysfunction (ED). Surgical treatment of prostate cancer is associated with significant anatomic and functional alterations that also adversely affect other components of sexual function, including absence of ejaculation, changes in orgasm, penile deformity, and alterations in penile length. Patient education regarding the possible sexual function outcomes and available therapies ideally should be carried out before surgery, to give patients and their sexual partner realistic expectations and to encourage them to raise sexual health issues and seek treatment after surgery. The concern among surgeons has been that too involved a discussion with the patient/couple may lead to patient fear and perhaps a likelihood that the patient will opt for "less-invasive" therapy such as radiation therapy. Part of such an interview should also include a brief discussion regarding the absence of data demonstrating that long-term ED rates are lower following radiation therapy compared to surgery. Post-operative follow-up should address sexual health issues, to detect and treat any impairment early in its course in an effort to avoid long-term sequelae.

2 Erectile Dysfunction

Prior to 1982 virtually all men who underwent surgical treatment for prostate cancer were incapable of achieving functional erections after surgery. Following the discovery of the anatomy of human cavernous nerves by Walsh and Donker, the first purposeful anatomic nerve-sparing RP was performed with complete recovery of sexual function within 1 year following surgery *(1)*. Nowadays, more than 25 years later, being able to recover erectile function is considered an integral part of successful "trifecta" outcome of RP, namely cancer control, urinary continence, and erectile function *(2)*. Unfortunately, nerve-sparing is not synonymous with erectile function sparing, and patients have to confront the burden of ED postoperatively. The prevalence of ED following RP varies considerably from series to series, with better results being reported from centers of excellence compared to community-based practices and from single-surgeon, single-center series compared to multi-center analyses.

2.1 Defining Erectile Function Outcomes After Radical Prostatectomy

ED prevalence has been shown to vary with the use of different definitions or whether outcomes are physician or patient reported *(3,4)*. Acquiring accurate information from patients is a challenge for a variety of reasons. The major problems in defining and reporting sexual function outcomes after RP include (i) issues with data acquisition, (ii) defining adequate erectile function, and (iii) variations in study populations. Obviously, conducting randomized, controlled study is ideal but impractical when the control is no surgery. However, this should not abrogate the investigator's responsibility to design in a prospective fashion study to answer this question. One of the primary concerns is the means of data acquisition; for example, is the data questionnaire-based or is it obtained by a third-party evaluator or the surgeon himself or herself? The latter introduces the concept of social desirability, the notion that patients will tell their surgeon what they think their surgeon wants to hear. Thus, ideally for optimum accuracy a third-party evaluator preferably utilizing a validated questionnaire should be employed. When using a questionnaire, attention should be paid to what the questionnaire actually addresses. Is it erectile function, bother or satisfaction? The gold standard questionnaire, the international index of erectile function (IIEF), is somewhat cumbersome but the questions addressing erectile function (questions 1–5 and 15) constitute the erectile function domain and while strictly speaking the IIEF is validated only for the full 15 questions, many centers utilize the EF domain as their tool of choice. The shorter sexual health inventory for men (SHIM), also known as the IIEF-5, is used frequently despite the fact that it does not have a question pertaining to the actual ability to have sexual intercourse. This question has been removed and its surrogate asks about "getting an erection firm enough for intercourse." It is recognized that there is a difference between getting an erection that one thinks is good enough for intercourse and actually accomplishing intercourse. This has been borne out in ED drug trials.

Some questionnaires assess both function and bother such as the UCLA-prostate cancer index (PCI) and the expanded prostate index composite (EPIC) *(5,6)*. In an ideal study, sexual encounter diaries (event logs) should also be used as these assess the ability to have sexual intercourse in real-time (they are completed after the encounter) and are therefore not affected by recall bias (the IIEF asks about the past 4 weeks, while the SHIM asks about the last 6 months). One of the concerns is that someone completing the SHIM will give scores for the past 1–2 months when erectile function is better than the 2 months preceding that and thus they may over-estimate their function. The event logs have the ability to demonstrate the proportion of sexual intercourse attempts that were successful which is not fully assessed by the IIEF or SHIM. It is well-appreciated that baseline erectile function is a critical predictor of erectile function recovery and that erectile function improves out to at least 24 months after RP. Thus, denoting the patients' preoperative function in some fashion (self-report, partner corroboration, or questionnaire ideally) and following this (preferably in a serial fashion) out to 24 months after surgery is ideal.

Defining adequate erectile function is more complex than it appears on the surface. What really defines adequate function? Is it a score on a questionnaire? Is it return to the ability to have intercourse? Is it return to baseline function? Does this function include the use of a PDE5 inhibitor medication? The NIH definition of ED ("the consistent inability to obtain and/or maintain an erection sufficient for satisfactory sexual relations") does not address the use of erectogenic medications, yet the urologic oncology community has accepted the need for PDE5 inhibitor use in defining adequate erectile function. Using a score on a questionnaire such as the IIEF is fraught with problems. For example, the score that defines "normalcy" on the IIEF erectile function domain is 26 (maximum 30). However, it is demonstrated in the literature that approximately 70% of men with scores between 22 and 25 considered themselves as being able to have sexual intercourse whenever they wish. At Memorial Sloan-Kettering Cancer Center we are currently using an EF domain score of 24 as a cut-off for inclusion in postprostatectomy rehabilitation studies. If patient self-report is used, should we insist on partner corroboration as clinical experience demonstrates that some men overestimate their erectile function at the time of a sexual function interview? Should we use the ability to have sexual intercourse as the definition? The problem with such a definition is that a man only requires approximately a 60% rigid erection to have the ability to have sexual intercourse. While there are centers that use this as their definition, if the patient had perfect erectile function preoperatively (100% rigid consistently) then he will have experienced a 40% reduction in his rigidity and will be using a PDE5 inhibitor to improve his erections and if he is already using a medication will be switching to another drug or strategy to ensure adequate rigidity. This is supported by the correlation of the new erection hardness score (EHS) with the IIEF scores. In men with a score of 3 (erection hard enough for intercourse but not fully hard) on the 4 point scale (a score of 4 denotes a fully rigid erection) the mean EF domain score was 18, clearly less than ideal (7). Finally, attention should be paid to the consistency of erections. If a man can have intercourse one of every ten encounters is this adequate? Clearly not. Even if one uses a score of 22 on the EF domain score, this equates to a mean per question score of 3.7, which denotes "more than half the time" and closer to "most of the time." Thus, at least a 50% success rate and more likely a 75% success rate defines adequate consistency of erection.

2.2 Erectile Function Outcomes

A summary of erectile function outcomes is presented in Table 1. Walsh et al. reported that 86% of patients were potent and 84% considered sexual bother as none or small 18 months following nerve-sparing RP *(8)*. Kundu et al. reported erectile function rate of 76 and 53% following bilateral and unilateral nerve-sparing surgeries, respectively *(9)*. According to the "Memorial Sloan-Kettering Cancer Center"

Table 1 Erectile Function After Radical Prostatectomy: Contemporary Series of Open, Laparoscopic, and Robot-Assisted Radical Prostatectomy

Author	Year	Operation type	Main outcomes
Stolzenburg *(51)*	2007	LRP–BNS	67.7% erections sufficient for intercourse
		LRP–UNS	34.1% erections sufficient for intercourse
Menon *(13)*	2007	RARP–BNS	93% intercourse rate
			51% return to baseline SHIM score without PDE5i
			22% return to baseline SHIM score with PDE5i
Zorn *(52)*	2007	RARP–BNS RARP–UNS	83% able to achieve erection for intercourse ± PDE5i
			62% able to achieve erection for intercourse ± PDE5i
Michl *(53)*	2006	ORP–BNS	54.5% able to perform sexual intercourse
		ORP–UNS	29.8% able to perform sexual intercourse
Goeman *(12)*	2006	LRP–BNS	64% able to achieve and maintain erection ± PDE5i
Rassweiler *(54)*	2006	LRP–BNS	52.5% full erections
Rassweiler *(55)*	2006	LRP–BNS	67–76% able to engage in sexual intercourse ± PDE5i
Patel *(56)*	2006	RARP BNS/UNS	78% potency ± PDE5i
Rozet *(11)*	2005	LRP–BNS	64% potency rate with PDE5i
			43% intercourse rate with PDE5i
Kundu *(9)*	2004	ORP–BNS ORP–UNS	76% have erections sufficient for penetration ± PDE5i
			53% have erections sufficient for penetration ± PDE5i
Walsh *(8)*	2000	ORP–BNS	86% able to have unassisted intercourse ± PDE5i
Rabbani *(17)*	2000	ORP – BNS ORP–UNS	55% have full or partial erections sufficient for intercourse without PDE5i
			21% have full or partial erections sufficient for intercourse without PDE5i

RARP – robot-assisted radical prostatectomy
LRP – laparoscopic radical prostatectomy
ORP – open radical prostatectomy
BNS – bilateral nerve-sparing surgery
UNS – unilateral nerve-sparing surgery
SHIM – sexual health inventory for men
PDE5i– phosphodiesterase 5 inhibitors

experience, erectile function is recovered in 70% of the cases after 2 years *(2)*. The "Prostate Cancer Outcomes Study" (PCOS) collected longitudinal quality-of-life outcomes data in men who underwent RP using the Surveillance, Epidemiology, and End Results (SEER) cancer registries of the National Cancer Institute (NCI). Data derived from the PCOS showed an inability to achieve erections sufficient for intercourse was reported in 80% of the cases, however, nerve-sparing status was not specified *(10)*.

With advances in laparoscopic surgery, RP became feasible using a laparoscopic approach with or without robotic assistance. Advantages of laparoscopic and robot-assisted surgery have been delineated, and include improved operative field visibility, decreased blood loss, early ambulation, and more rapid convalescence without compromising cancer control. To date, there is no scientific data that erectile function or urinary function outcomes are different between open and lap/robotic approaches. Despite this, claims to the contrary have been made extensively on the Internet from centers performing robotic prostatectomy. A large, randomized, controlled trial is awaited but will likely never happen. Reports on erectile function outcome following laparoscopic or robotic-assisted RP appear to present results comparable to standard open RP, however, erectile function data from the large series' reports are often limited to a small subset of patients. Rozet et al. presented a series of 600 extraperitoneal nerve-sparing RP series and report recovery of erections in 64% and ability to accomplish sexual intercourse in 43% of the cases at the relatively short median follow-up of 6 months *(11)*. Goeman et al. reported potency rates of 64% overall and 79% among men younger than 60 years, at 24 months following laparoscopic RP *(12)*. Menon et al. report 70 and 100% ability to perform intercourse at 12 and 48 months, respectively, in patients without ED preoperatively, after robotic-assisted RP. These results are significantly superior to their results of standard open nerve-sparing surgery, of 40 and 70% intercourse rates at 12 and 60 months, respectively. Despite these favorable results, in their questionnaire-based evaluation of overall sexual function, only 51% of men returned to baseline function *(13)*. To date, comparative studies of open, laparoscopic, and robotic-assisted RP failed to show a significant difference in terms of sexual function outcome *(14,15)*.

Data from the Cancer of the Prostate Strategic Urologic Research Endeavor (CaPSURE) database, a longitudinal, observational registry of men with prostate cancer, show that sexual function continues to improve at 24 months after surgery *(16)*. A study by Rabbani et al. found that recovery may occur even after 40 months, a longer duration than previously thought *(17)*. This protracted time interval, required for erectile function healing, is consistent with the mechanism involved in the etiology of post-RP ED which is primarily neural damage. While erection recovery does not uniformly occur in all cases, several predictors of recuperation have been identified including younger age at surgery, better erectile function preoperatively, erectile hemodynamic changes after surgery, and the extent of neurovascular bundle preservation *(17)*.

Awaiting recovery of neural structures, patients are advised to regain erections pharmacologically and resume sexual activity shortly after surgery. The early return to regular sexual activity may improve subjects' self body image and self-esteem and avoid a possible long-term deleterious effect of sexual activity cessation on the patient and his partner's relationship. Moreover, early treatment to achieve erection has been shown to improve long-term erectile function recovery of spontaneous erections or response to treatment by minimizing penile structural changes *(18)*. The first-line treatment option for ED following RP remains oral drugs of the phosphodiesterase 5 inhibitors' (PDE5i) group though response rates are considerably lower, compared with ED of other etiologies. In a systematic review of the literature by Montorsi and McCullough, addressing the efficacy of sildenafil citrate in the treatment of post-RP erectile dysfunction, response rate ranged 14–53%, with a combined response rate of only 35% *(19)*. In a study designed to compare the efficacy of sildenafil citrate in different etiologies, 31% of patients with post-RP ED had erections satisfactory for intercourse while response rate among men with neurogenic, arteriogenic, and psychogenic ED were 67, 70, and 78%, respectively *(20)*.

Patients who fail to respond to PDE5i's are excellent candidates for intracavernosal injection therapy with a reported response rate of 85% *(21)*. Evaluating various treatment modalities for ED post-RP, Baniel et al. found that at 1 year, 71% of subjects were using penile injection therapy and only 14% were using sildenafil *(21)*. As neuro-regeneration and penile fibrotic changes are dynamic processes, patients on injection therapy should be monitored closely for dose adjustment in the first 1–2 years after surgery. After stabilization of erectile function, if satisfactory outcome has not been reached with non-surgical treatment modalities, insertion of penile implant is an option for patients who desire the ability to have sexual intercourse, however, satisfaction rate among men who had RP appears to be lower when compared to the general penile prosthesis population *(22)*.

In summary, the prevalence of ED after RP may vary, however, it is not a rare outcome. Older patients as well as patients with preexisting ED or patients in whom nerve-sparing surgery has not been achieved are at increased risk for ED after RP. Patients should be given realistic expectations, including the relatively low chance of responding to oral agents in the first postoperative year. Intracavernosal injection therapy should be discussed early in the course of treating ED after RP.

3 Anejaculation

RP essentially disrupts the ejaculatory mechanism. Medical literature data regarding the impact of ejaculation loss following prostate cancer treatments are scarce. Anejaculation has several implications: firstly, it may interfere with subject's self-perception of his manhood and body image, then as ejaculation and orgasmic sensations are closely related, anejaculation may be associated with reduced orgasmic quality, and finally, it renders men infertile. Prostate cancer is perceived as a disease of old men, to whom infertility is no longer an issue. However, in the era of early prostate cancer detection, men are diagnosed at a younger age and have an excellent long-term recurrence-free survival rate *(23)*. At the same time, parenthood age in the general population is increasing and cancer diagnosis may actually increase the motivation for parenting *(24)*. Though advanced sperm extraction and fertilization techniques are available, the issue of anejaculation and its implication on future fertility should be discussed and not assumed to be non-relevant and semen should be cryopreserved for men desiring future fatherhood *(25)*.

The advent of intracytoplasmic sperm injection (ICSI) has allowed the application of assisted reproductive technologies to couples whose male partner can produce only tiny numbers of sperm or cannot deliver sperm in an antegrade fashion *(26–31)*. This has particular relevance to the patient who has undergone RP. Two major retrieval techniques have been reported, open and percutaneous approaches. In the standard testicular sperm extraction (TESE) technique, the procedure is performed in a blind fashion that does not identify the focal sperm-producing areas of the testis until tissue has been excised from the patient. Microdissection of testicular tubules identifies sperm-containing regions before their removal. Identification of spermatogenically active regions of the testicle is possible by direct examination of the individual seminiferous tubules. Prior to performing TESE for this indication an assessment of the testicular volumes and serum FSH levels is critical to give the patient realistic expectations about the chance of retrieving sperm. Furthermore, given that TESE sperm can only be used for IVF/ICSI an evaluation of the female partner should be conducted to ensure that her fertility potential is reasonable prior to undertaking scrotal surgery in her partner.

4   Orgasm Alterations

Despite major advances in our understanding of the erectile mechanism in the last decade, the orgasmic process remains poorly understood. Both physiological and psychogenic elements contribute to the genesis of the orgasmic phase. Ejaculatory events that include smooth muscle contraction of the accessory sex organs; buildup and release of pressure in the posterior urethra; sensation of the ejaculatory inevitability; contraction of the urethral bulb and perineum; rhythmic contractions of the pelvic floor muscles; and semen emission and ejaculation contribute to the sensation of orgasm as well as the reversal of the generalized physiological changes and sexual tension. Sensory cortical neurons perceive these events as pleasurable *(32)*. Normally, orgasm is closely coupled with ejaculation, however, after RP orgasm occurs without semen ejaculation per se, yet ejaculatory muscular activity does exist.

Though orgasmic changes receive little attention they are not uncommon and can be categorized into three areas (i) changes in orgasm, (ii) orgasmic pain (dysorgasmia), and (iii) orgasm-associated incontinence (Table 2). Schover et al., in a study of 1,236 men treated for localized prostate cancer (52% RP, 48% radiation therapy), found that 65% of the sample reported a problem with their orgasms including 31% who no longer tried to reach orgasm, 17% who tried but were unable to reach orgasm and 28% with orgasms that were disappointingly weak *(33)*. To define the type of

Table 2 Orgasmic Dysfunction After Radical Prostatectomy

Author	Year	No. of patients	Orgasmic dysfunction type and rate
Choi *(36)*	2007	475	20% orgasmic incontinence (climacturia)
Lee *(37)*	2006	42	45% orgasmic incontinence (climacturia)
Barnas *(34)*	2004	239	22% no change in orgasm intensity
			37% complete absence of orgasm
			37% decreased orgasm intensity
			4% increased orgasm intensity
			14% orgasmic pain (dysorgasmia)
Koheman *(57)*	1996	17	64% orgasmic incontinence (climacturia)
			82% decreased orgasm intensity
			14% orgasmic pain (dysorgasmia)

orgasmic dysfunction in men after RP Barnas et al. used a validated questionnaire, including questions addressing the presence or absence of orgasm, orgasm quality before and after surgery, the presence of orgasmic pain, the location of orgasmic pain, and consistency and duration of orgasmic pain. Of subjects treated surgically, 22% of patients reported no change in orgasm intensity but 37% reported a complete absence of orgasm, 37% had decreased orgasm intensity, and 4% reported a more intense orgasm after RP than before. Pain during orgasm occurred in 14% of the patients, located to the penis (63%), abdomen (9%), rectum (24%), and other areas (4%). In those respondents who had dysorgasmia, pain was reported to occur always (with every orgasm) in 33%, frequently in 13%, occasionally in 35%, and rarely in 19%. Most patients (55%) had orgasm-associated pain for less than a minute, a third reported pain for 1–5 min and pain lasting more than 5 min was reported by 12%; only 2.5% of patients complained of pain lasting more than an hour *(34)*. No consensus exists as to the etiology of orgasmic pain, however, it is postulated that bladder neck/pelvic floor spasm plays a role. Based on this assumption, a prospective, non-placebo controlled study was conducted to assess the use of tamsulosin, an alpha-adrenergic blocking agent in patients with orgasmic pain. In this study, 77% patients reported significant improvement in pain and 12% noted complete resolution of their pain with significant increase in IIEF libido score, supporting the hypothesis that orgasmic pain is related to bladder neck and/or pelvic floor muscle spasm *(35)*.

Urinary incontinence during orgasm (climacturia) is another phenomenon that may adversely affect the satisfaction with sexual activity for men following RP and their partner. Choi et al. reported that climacturia occurs in 20% following radical pelvic surgery, more often after radical prostatectomy than with radical cystectomy and it is unrelated to the type of prostatectomy performed (open or laparoscopic). It is more likely to be reported within year 1 following surgery and in men who complain of orgasmic pain and/or penile shortening *(36)*. Lee et al. reported a higher prevalence of climacturia after RP of 45%. In 68% of the cases reported it happened rarely or only occasionally, while in 21% it occurred most of the time or always.

Urine leakage quantity was only a few drops in 58% of the subjects but 16% reported a loss of more than 1 ounce and bother was none or minimal in 52%, and significant in 48%. Treatment was bladder emptying in 84% and condoms use in 11% *(37)*.

At present, there is no effective treatment to restore the nature of preoperative orgasm. Dysorgasmia can be managed symptomatically using alpha-blockers and climacturia may be managed behaviorally (fluid intake restriction and bladder emptying prior to sexual activity) or mechanically (using a rubber constriction ring or condoms, if the leakage amount is small). The mainstay of treatment is patient and partner education before surgery and supportive care afterward.

5 Peyronie's Disease

Peyronie's disease (PD) is a localized connective tissue disorder that affects the tunica albuginea of the penis. Fibrous scar tissue, which replaces the normally elastic fibers, causes a characteristic penile deformity that is most evident during erection. This pathological process can manifest as increased curvature, indentation, shortening, or an "hourglass" deformity of the penis. The diagnosis of PD is often preceded by painful erections, and can be associated with ED and palpable areas of induration (plaques) *(38)*. Despite centuries of recognition, the exact etiology of PD remains elusive. While trauma is considered to be the provocative stimulus, other contributing factors include failure of fibrin clearance; collagen alterations; genetic predisposition; autoimmune factors; free radical production; and cytogenetic aberrations *(38)*. The prevalence of PD in the general male population is reported to be 3–8%, with a higher prevalence in men with erectile dysfunction *(39,40)*. When Peyronie's penile plaques are actively sought on physical examination in men presenting for evaluation for unrelated conditions, they can be found in 9% of the cases *(41)*. Genital and/or perineal trauma, as well as lower urinary tract surgery, has been implicated as risk factors for PD *(42)*.

The prevalence of PD following radical prostatectomy has been addressed by a single paper in the literature and in this analysis of 110 men who presented with ED after RP, 45 (41%) had penile fibrotic changes, representing 11% of all men who had RP in their institute at the specified period. This incidence of PD is markedly higher than that of the general population. The clinical presentation was penile curvature in 93% and "waistband" deformity in 24%; palpable plaques were present in 31 (69%) *(43)*. The actual prevalence of PD after RP may be even higher, as this condition, manifested as penile curvature during erection, is evident only in men who achieve some degree of penile rigidity. Originally ascribed to undiagnosed preoperative PD or spongiofibrosis due to urethral catheterization, we routinely see men who had normal genital exams preoperatively who develop PD after surgery and most of our patients have PD plaques dorsally nowhere near their corpus spongiosum thus spongiofibrosis is not likely to be a major contributor. Another explanation that patients are given is that the intracavernosal injections they are using after surgery caused the tuncia fibrosis, despite the fact that there is no data to support this whatsoever. Indeed, it is not uncommon for us to see men 3 months after RP who are present in clinic for their first penile injection training session, who had no documented PD prior to RP, and who on their first injection demonstrate penile curvature never having received an injection prior to that.

While the precise process of plaque formation leading to eventual clinically evident PD following RP is still obscure, it is not unlikely that it may be related to other post-RP penile fibrotic changes, secondary to denervation and/or local ischemia *(44)*. As it is likely that non-surgical treatments of PD are more effective in the early stages of the disease, patients after RP should be routinely evaluated for existence of penile plaques, as a part of their postoperative follow-up.

6 Penile Length Alterations

Penile length changes after RP have been described (Table 3). Penile shortening, even if sexual intercourse is still feasible, once it is noticeable by the patient or his partner may adversely affect self body image, self-esteem, sense of manhood, and self-confidence. In 1999 Fraiman et al. found significant decrease in all penile dimensions after RP: decreased penile length of 8 and 9% and decreased volume of 19–22% in the flaccid and erect states, respectively. The most substantial change

Table 3 Penile Length Changes After Radical Prostatectomy

Author	Year	No. of patients	Time interval	Main outcomes
Gontero *(48)*	2007	126	1 year	1.34 cm shortening – flaccid length 2.30 cm shortening – stretched length
Briganti *(58)*	2007	33	6 months	No statistically significant length changes, both flaccid and erect states
Savoie *(47)*	2003	63	3 months	19% had 15% shortening – stretched length 1.2 cm shortening – flaccid length 1.1 cm shortening – stretched length
Munding *(46)*	2001	31	3 months	13% increased stretched length 16% no change in stretched length 71% had decreased stretched length: 23% – up to 0.5 cm 35% – 1.0–2.0 cm 13% – more than 2.0 cm
Fraiman *(45)*	1999	100	1.7–27.6 months	8% decrease in flaccid length 9% decrease in erect length Greatest change at 4–8 months

occurred between the first 4 and 8 months postoperatively *(45)*. Munding et al. found a measured decrement in penile length in 71% of men after RP, which was greater then 1 cm in 48% of the cases, 3 months postoperatively *(46)*. Similar finding were obtained in a study by Savoie et al. with a decrease in the stretched penile length in 68% of the cases and greater than 15% in 19% *(47)*. Penile length shortening has been shown to be independently associated with nerve preservation status and with postoperative erectile function outcome *(48)*.

The reasons for penile volume changes can be explained by penile anatomic-structural changes and physiological–functional changes. Anatomical fibrotic changes have been demonstrated in comparison of penile biopsies preoperatively and 2 and 12 months postoperatively that showed significantly decreased elastic fibers and smooth muscle fiber content and increased collagen content *(44)*. It is postulated that the chronic absence of erectile activity leads to a state of cavernosal hypoxia, low pO_2 tension, which favors the secretion of fibrogenic cytokines such as TGF-β_1 while during erection, the corporal smooth muscle is oxygenated and this results in the secretion of endogenous prostanoids (PGE_1), which in turn, inhibit fibrogenic cytokine production *(49)*.

In addition to anatomical changes, there are also physiological–functional alterations. It is well-recognized that even in the hands of an experienced surgeon using nerve-sparing surgery, some degree of nerve injury, commonly involving neuropraxia, is likely to occur to the cavernosal nerves. Penile relaxation is accomplished through the release of nitric oxide (NO) from cavernosal nerve endings and the generation of the second-messenger cyclic nucleotides, cGMP and cAMP and is likely to be compromised after surgery. Contractility of the smooth muscle is generally tonic and under the control of erectolytic neurotransmitters such as adrenaline. Sympathetic hyper-innervation (termed by some "competitive sprouting") refers to the concept that when autonomic nerves are injured, sympathetic fibers are biologically primed to recuperate from injury and regenerate more quickly, resulting in unantagonized sympathetic tone in the end organ *(50)*. After cavernosal nerve injury, this phenomenon results in a penile hypertonic state. Any factors that result in reduced NO secretion or increased sympathetic tone, such as nerve injury after RP, may lead to decreased relaxation or distensibility of corporal smooth muscle and may lead to loss of length. Regardless of the exact mechanism of penile length alteration, most concerning are structural changes that probably result from a combination of neural injury-associated denervation resulting in smooth muscle apoptosis, and cavernosal hypoxia-induced collagenization, as they may be the common underlying mechanism of penile shortening and long-term erectile dysfunction.

To synthesize these concepts into a working hypothesis, penile length changes can be divided into early and delayed. Early changes occur in response to the neural injury during RP: the cavernosal nerves undergo Wallerian degeneration, and in the early phase, when sympathetic nerve function is in the ascendancy the penis is a hypertonic organ, showing sympathetic overdrive. Given that the penile smooth muscle is highly contractile in response to adrenergic tone, this results in a penis that patients often refer to as "being drawn back in the body." This hypertonic state is most pronounced within the first 3–6 months after surgery. A clinical scenario supporting this is the circumcised man whose penis, soon after surgery, appears incompletely circumcised or even uncircumcised. The clue that these changes are not the result of permanent structural sequelae is that upon gentle penile stretching the penis readily elongates from its "buried" position. More concerning are delayed structural changes; these result from true irreversible structural alterations in the corporal smooth muscle. These structural changes most probably result from a combination of factors (as described above), neural injury-associated denervation apoptosis, and cavernosal hypoxia-induced collagenization in men who have a delayed return of erectile function. The difference between these changes and early hypertonicity is shown by the reduced or absent penile stretch in the group with permanent smooth muscle alterations. It is easy to appreciate how these alterations affect not only length but also girth. Finally, whether the institution of a pharmacological penile rehabilitation program early after RP can abrogate these alterations presently remains unanswered.

7 Summary

Sexual dysfunction after RP includes but is not limited to ED. ED as well as anejaculation, orgasmic dysfunction, occurrence of Peyronie's disease, and penile length shortening may adversely affect sexual function of subjects undergoing RP and their sexual partners. Patients should be educated about the foreseeable sexual consequences before surgery and close follow-up is mandatory afterward. Early diagnosis and treatment of sexual dysfunction, evaluation of its components, and prompt treatment may improve long-term outcome.

References

1. Walsh, P.C. (2007) The discovery of the cavernous nerves and development of nerve sparing radical retropubic prostatectomy. *J. Urol.* **177,** 1632.
2. Bianco, F.J., Jr., Scardino, P.T., and Eastham, J.A. (2005) Radical prostatectomy: long-term cancer control and recovery of sexual and urinary function ("trifecta"). *Urology* **66,** 83.
3. Litwin, M.S., Lubeck, D.P., Henning, J.M., et al. (1998) Differences in urologist and patient assessments of health related quality of life in men with prostate cancer: results of the CaP-SURE database. *J. Urol.* **159,** 1988.
4. Krupski, T.L., Saigal, C.S., and Litwin, M.S. (2003) Variation in continence and potency by definition. *J. Urol.* **170,** 1291.
5. Litwin, M.S., Hays, R.D., Fink, A., et al. (1998) The UCLA Prostate Cancer Index: development, reliability, and validity of a health-related quality of life measure. *Med. Care* **36,** 1002.
6. Wei, J.T., Dunn, R.L., Litwin, M.S., et al. (2000) Development and validation of the expanded prostate cancer index composite (EPIC) for comprehensive assessment of health-related quality of life in men with prostate cancer. *Urology* **56,** 899.
7. Mulhall, J.P., Goldstein, I., Bushmakin, A.G., et al. (2007) Validation of the erection hardness score. *J. Sex. Med.* **4,** 1623.
8. Walsh, P.C., Marschke, P., Ricker, D., et al. (2000) Patient-reported urinary continence and sexual function after anatomic radical prostatectomy. *Urology* **55,** 58.

9. Kundu, S.D., Roehl, K.A., Eggener, S.E., et al. (2004) Potency, continence and complications in 3,477 consecutive radical retropubic prostatectomies. *J. Urol.* **172,** 2227.

10. Hoffman, R.M., Barry, M.J., Stanford, J.L., et al. (2006) Health outcomes in older men with localized prostate cancer: results from the Prostate Cancer Outcomes Study. *Am. J. Med.* **119,** 418.

11. Rozet, F., Galiano, M., Cathelineau, X., et al. (2005) Extraperitoneal laparoscopic radical prostatectomy: a prospective evaluation of 600 cases. *J. Urol.* **174,** 908.

12. Goeman, L., Salomon, L., La De Taille, A., et al. (2006) Long-term functional and oncological results after retroperitoneal laparoscopic prostatectomy according to a prospective evaluation of 550 patients. *World J. Urol.* **24,** 281.

13. Menon, M., Shrivastava, A., Kaul, S., et al. (2007) Vattikuti Institute prostatectomy: contemporary technique and analysis of results. *Eur. Urol.* **51,** 648.

14. Anastasiadis, A.G., Salomon, L., Katz, R., et al. (2003) Radical retropubic versus laparoscopic prostatectomy: a prospective comparison of functional outcome. *Urology* **62,** 292.

15. Ball, A.J., Gambill, B., Fabrizio, M.D., et al., (2006) Prospective longitudinal comparative study of early health-related quality-of-life outcomes in patients undergoing surgical treatment for localized prostate cancer: a short-term evaluation of five approaches from a single institution. *J. Endourol.* **20,** 723.

16. Litwin, M.S., Flanders, S.C., Pasta, D.J., et al. (1999) Sexual function and bother after radical prostatectomy or radiation for prostate cancer: multivariate quality-of-life analysis from CaPSURE. Cancer of the Prostate Strategic Urologic Research Endeavor. *Urology* **54,** 503.

17. Rabbani, F., Stapleton, A.M., Kattan, M.W., et al. (2000) Factors predicting recovery of erections after radical prostatectomy. *J. Urol.* **164,** 1929.

18. Mulhall, J., Land, S., Parker, M., et al. (2005) The use of an erectogenic pharmacotherapy regimen following radical prostatectomy improves recovery of spontaneous erectile function. *J. Sex. Med.* **2,** 532.

19. Montorsi, F., and McCullough, A. (2005) Efficacy of sildenafil citrate in men with erectile dysfunction following radical prostatectomy: a systematic review of clinical data. *J. Sex. Med.* **2,** 658.

20. McMahon, C.G., Samali, R., and Johnson, H. (2000) Efficacy, safety and patient acceptance of sildenafil citrate as treatment for erectile dysfunction. *J. Urol.* **164,** 1192.

21. Baniel, J., Israilov, S., Segenreich, E., et al. (2001) Comparative evaluation of treatments for erectile dysfunction in patients with prostate cancer after radical retropubic prostatectomy. *BJU Int.* **88,** 58.

22. Akin-Olugbade, O., Parker, M., Guhring, P., et al. (2006) Determinants of patient satisfaction following penile prosthesis surgery. *J. Sex. Med.* **3,** 743.

23. Ung, J.O., Richie, J.P., Chen, M.H., et al. (2002) Evolution of the presentation and pathologic and biochemical outcomes after radical prostatectomy for patients with clinically localized prostate cancer diagnosed during the PSA era. *Urology* **60,** 458.

24. Schover, L.R. (2005) Motivation for parenthood after cancer: a review. *J. Natl. Cancer Inst. Monogr.* 2.

25. Knoester, P.A., Leonard, M., Wood, D.P., et al. (2007) Fertility issues for men with newly diagnosed prostate cancer. *Urology* **69,** 123.

26. Van Steirteghem, A.C., Nagy, Z., Joris, H., et al. (1993) High fertilization and implantation rates after intracytoplasmic sperm injection. *Hum. Reprod.* **8,** 1061.

27. Van Steirteghem, A., Nagy, Z., Liu, J., et al. (1994) Intracytoplasmic sperm injection. *Baillieres Clin. Obstet. Gynaecol.* **8,** 85.

28. Van Steirteghem, A., Devroey, P., and Liebaers, I. (2002) Intracytoplasmic sperm injection. *Mol. Cell Endocrinol.* **186,** 199.

29. Bonduelle, M., Camus, M., De Vos, A., et al. (1999) Seven years of intracytoplasmic sperm injection and follow-up of 1987 subsequent children. *Hum. Reprod.* **14**(Suppl 1), 243.

30. Palermo, G., Joris, H., Devroey, P., et al. (1992) Pregnancies after intracytoplasmic injection of single spermatozoon into an oocyte. *Lancet* **340,** 17.

31. Palermo, G.D., Schlegel, P.N., Sills, E.S., et al. (1998) Births after intracytoplasmic injection of sperm obtained by testicular extraction from men with nonmosaic Klinefelter's syndrome. *N. Engl. J. Med.* **338,** 588.

32. Kandeel, F.R., Koussa, V.K., and Swerdloff, R.S. (2001) Male sexual function and its disorders: physiology, pathophysiology, clinical investigation, and treatment. *Endocr. Rev.* **22,** 342.

33. Schover, L.R., Fouladi, R.T., Warneke, C.L., et al. (2002) Defining sexual outcomes after treatment for localized prostate carcinoma. *Cancer* **95,** 1773.

34. Barnas, J.L., Pierpaoli, S., Ladd, P., et al. (2004) The prevalence and nature of orgasmic dysfunction after radical prostatectomy. *BJU Int.* **94,** 603.

35. Barnas, J., Parker, M., Guhring, P., et al. (2005) The utility of tamsulosin in the management of orgasm-associated pain: a pilot analysis. *Eur. Urol.* **47,** 361.

36. Choi, J.M., Nelson, C.J., Stasi, J., et al. (2007) Orgasm associated incontinence (climacturia) following radical pelvic surgery: rates of occurrence and predictors. *J. Urol.* **177,** 2223.

37. Lee, J., Hersey, K., Lee, C.T., et al. (2006) Climacturia following radical prostatectomy: prevalence and risk factors. *J. Urol.* **176,** 2562.

38. Smith, C.J., McMahon, C., and Shabsigh, R. (2005) Peyronie's disease: the epidemiology, aetiology and clinical evaluation of deformity. *BJU Int.* **95,** 729.

39. Sommer, F., Schwarzer, U., Wassmer, G., et al. (2002) Epidemiology of Peyronie's disease. *Int J Impot Res.* **14,** 379.

40. El-Sakka, A.I. (2006) Prevalence of Peyronie's disease among patients with erectile dysfunction. *Eur Urol.* **49,** 564.

41. Mulhall, J.P., Creech, S.D., Boorjian, S.A., et al. (2004) Subjective and objective analysis of the prevalence of Peyronie's disease in a population of men presenting for prostate cancer screening. *J. Urol.* **171,** 2350.

42. Bjekic, M.D., Vlajinac, H.D., Sipetic, S.B., et al. (2006) Risk factors for Peyronie's disease: a case-control study. *BJU Int.* **97,** 570.

43. Ciancio, S.J., and Kim, E.D. (2000) Penile fibrotic changes after radical retropubic prostatectomy. *BJU Int.* **85,** 101.

44. Iacono, F., Giannella, R., Somma, P., et al. (2005) Histological alterations in cavernous tissue after radical prostatectomy. *J. Urol.* **173,** 1673.

45. Fraiman, M.C., Lepor, H., and McCullough, A.R. (1999) Changes in penile morphometrics in men with erectile dysfunction after nerve-sparing radical retropubic prostatectomy. *Mol. Urol.* **3,** 109.

46. Munding, M.D., Wessells, H.B., and Dalkin, B.L. (2001) Pilot study of changes in stretched penile length 3 months after radical retropubic prostatectomy. *Urology* **58,** 567.

47. Savoie, M., Kim, S.S., and Soloway, M.S. (2003) A prospective study measuring penile length in men treated with radical prostatectomy for prostate cancer. *J. Urol.* **169,** 1462.

48. Gontero, P., Galzerano, M., Bartoletti, R., et al. (2007) New insights into the pathogenesis of penile shortening after radical prostatectomy and the role of postoperative sexual function. *J. Urol.* **178,** 602.

49. Moreland, R.B. (1998) Is there a role of hypoxemia in penile fibrosis: a viewpoint presented to the Society for the Study of Impotence. *Int. J. Impot. Res.* **10,** 113.

50. Zhou, S., Chen, L.S., Miyauchi, Y., et al. (2004) Mechanisms of cardiac nerve sprouting after myocardial infarction in dogs. *Circ. Res.* **95,** 76.

51. Stolzenburg, J.U., Rabenalt, R., Do, M., et al. (2007) Endoscopic extraperitoneal radical prostatectomy: the University of Leipzig experience of 1,300 cases. *World J. Urol.* **25,** 45.

52. Zorn, K.C., Gofrit, O.N., Orvieto, M.A., et al. (2007) Robotic-assisted laparoscopic prostatectomy: functional and pathologic outcomes with interfascial nerve preservation. *Eur. Urol.* **51,** 755.

53. Michl, U.H., Friedrich, M.G., Graefen, M., et al. (2006) Prediction of postoperative sexual function after nerve sparing radical retropubic prostatectomy. *J. Urol.* **176,** 227.

54. Rassweiler, J., Stolzenburg, J., Sulser, T., et al. (2006) Laparoscopic radical prostatectomy – the experience of the German Laparoscopic Working Group. *Eur. Urol.* **49,** 113.

55. Rassweiler, J., Wagner, A.A., Moazin, M., et al. (2006) Anatomic nerve-sparing laparoscopic radical prostatectomy: comparison of retrograde and antegrade techniques. *Urology* **68,** 587.
56. Patel, V.R., Thaly, R., and Shah, K. (2007) Robotic radical prostatectomy: outcomes of 500 cases. *BJU Int.* **99,** 1109.
57. Koeman, M., van Driel, M.F., Schultz, W.C., et al. (1996) Orgasm after radical prostatectomy. *Br. J. Urol.* **77,** 861.
58. Briganti, A., Fabbri, F., Salonia, A., et al. (2007) Preserved postoperative penile size correlates well with maintained erectile function after bilateral nerve-sparing radical retropubic prostatectomy. *Eur. Urol.* **52,** 702.

Chapter 2
The Impact of Prostate Cancer Diagnosis and Post-treatment Sexual Dysfunction on Quality of Life

David F. Penson and Christian J. Nelson

Abstract There is little doubt that prostate cancer is a significant public health burden. The malignancy continues to be the most common solid tumor among American men and the second leading cause of cancer death *(1)*. However, not all prostate malignancies are deadly and, in fact, a significant number of newly detected prostate tumors are "overdiagnosed" *(2)*. In other words, had the patient never been screened for prostate cancer, he never would have known he had the disease and, more importantly, he never would have suffered any clinical sequelae from the tumor. This observation, coupled with the fact that, to date, there are no adequately sized randomized clinical trials documenting that one active therapy is superior to another in terms of overall or disease-specific survival, has caused patients and providers to strongly consider quality of life when choosing therapy for prostate cancer. In fact, some studies have shown that survivors value quality of life to a much greater degree than the impact of treatment on survival when choosing therapy for localized prostate cancer *(3)*. To this end, it is critical to understand both the effect of the diagnosis of prostate cancer on quality of life and also the impact of sexual dysfunction on quality of life in men with this disease. The goal of this chapter is to review the effect of prostate cancer diagnosis and post-treatment sexual dysfunction on quality of life.

Keywords Prostate cancer; sexual dysfunction; quality of life.

From: *Current Clinical Urology* Series, *Sexual Function in the Prostate Cancer Patient*
Edited by John P. Mulhall, DOI 10.1007/978-1-60327-555-2_2,
© Humana Press, a part of Springer Science+Business Media, LLC 2009

1   Assessing Quality of Life in Prostate Cancer Survivors

In order to assess the effect of prostate cancer and sexual dysfunction on quality of life, we must be able to measure this rather nebulous entity. To aid in this endeavor, we use a variable from the field of health services research, health-related quality of life (HRQOL). HRQOL includes both objective evaluation of patients' functional status and their perceptions of their own health and its impact on their existence *(4)*. It should be noted that these surveys usually measure different aspects, or domains, of HRQOL, thus providing a more comprehensive portrait of the survivorship experience. For the most part, these domains can be broken into two categories: generic and disease-specific. Generic domains address the aspects of HRQOL that are common to all patients, regardless of their disease process. Examples of generic HRQOL domains include general physical, emotional or social functioning, general health perceptions, and overall vitality. Disease-specific domains focus on the impact of particular organic dysfunctions associated with the disease that may affect HRQOL. Prostate cancer-specific domains include nausea, bony pain, anxiety regarding cancer recurrence, urinary or sexual dysfunction, etc. In this chapter, we will focus almost exclusively on the sexual domains.

Many physicians mistakenly believe that they can accurately assess a patient's quality of life from the clinical interaction. Studies have shown, however, that this is not the case. In a study from CaPSURE, a longitudinal observational disease registry of men with prostate cancer, patient-reported health-related quality of life in 2,252 prostate cancer survivors was compared to physicians' estimates of the patients' quality of life. Seventy-five percent of patients reported fatigue, while only 10% of their physicians believed that the patient experienced this symptom. Furthermore, 97% of patients reported some degree of sexual dysfunction, while only 52% of their physicians reported that the patient had this problem *(5)*. This study underscores the importance of collecting quality of life information directly from the patient. HRQOL is, therefore, measured by directly questioning the patient using surveys (also known as instruments). These questionnaires can be administered in a standardized fashion by an objective third-party interviewer, or they can be self-administered by the patient. The instruments are developed using the principles of psychometric test theory and are rigorously tested and reviewed prior to use to insure that collected data are both valid and reliable. In the past decade, several validated and reliable questionnaires have been developed that are specifically designed to measure HRQOL in men with prostate cancer. These surveys have been used to compare the effect of various treatments on quality of life, allowing us to reach meaningful conclusions that may be helpful in assisting patients when choosing therapy for their disease.

Given the unique effect of sexual function on a man's gender identify and sense of self, there are two key points that must be considered when assessing the relationship of sexual dysfunction and HRQOL in prostate cancer. Firstly, it is probably important that HRQOL assessments be targeted to the patient's current or very recent sexual function status. In other words, studies that query the patient about his pre-treatment sexual function 6–12 months earlier may produce questionable results, as patients tend to exaggerate their earlier potency. To illustrate this point, Litwin and McGuigan *(6)* assessed HRQOL in 107 men immediately prior to RP. At an average of 21 months following surgery, they asked the same patients to recall their pre-operative quality of life. They found that patients overestimated their baseline HRQOL in the urinary and sexual function domains by 13 and 27%, respectively. In contrast to this, Legler and colleagues *(7)* compared responses to a pre-treatment HRQOL survey in 133 men in the Prostate Cancer Outcomes Study (PCOS) to recall function in these same patients 6 months later. Specifically in the sexual function domain, the correlation coefficient comparing pre-treatment scores to 6-month scores was 0.69, indicating reasonable agreement between the two scores. In summary, while there may be less recall bias than one might think, it is always better to collect HRQOL information in a prospective, longitudinal setting whenever possible.

The second unique consideration when assessing the effect of sexual dysfunction on HRQOL is the importance of collecting both function and bother information. Function refers to the degree of symptoms that a patient experiences. If one questions a patient regarding the number of attempts at intercourse over the past week or the presence of morning erections, function is being addressed. Alternatively, if one queries the patient concerning the degree of problems that he has experienced due to his sexual dysfunction, bother is being measured. Gill and Feinstein *(8)* performed an extensive review of the literature and determined that the vast majority of HRQOL instruments only assess function. While this may be adequate in certain medical conditions, it is particularly problematic when assessing the effect of ED on quality of life, as function and bother do not necessarily correlate, as will be discussed later in the chapter.

2   The Effect of Prostate Cancer Diagnosis on Generic Quality of Life

It is well-understood that men with prostate cancer face disease-specific HRQOL concerns that include urinary, bowel, and sexual dysfunctions *(9,10)*. In addition to these physical aspects of HRQOL, mental health concerns also play an important role and can have a major impact on HRQOL. It is not surprising that many patients experience high levels of distress when coping with cancer. To this end, one might expect that the diagnosis of prostate cancer in and of itself may have an effect on generic or disease-specific HRQOL. A review of the available literature, however, indicates that this is not the case.

In the disease-specific domains, there is no substantial evidence that the diagnosis of prostate cancer itself leads to HRQOL changes. In 2007, the vast majority of prostate cancer survivors are diagnosed with localized disease and, therefore, have minimal or no symptoms *(11)*. Therefore, one would not expect significant HRQOL changes immediately following a new diagnosis. However, there is no adequately sized completed study that has assessed men during pre-screening/diagnosis and then followed them through their disease course. As such, the available evidence on the impact of prostate cancer diagnosis on QOL comes from the studies that have assessed men post-diagnosis and pre-treatment, or studies that included an active surveillance cohort.

The available evidence suggests that urinary, bowel, or sexual functions are not directly affected by diagnosis or by the onset of the disease. In a study of 214 men with prostate cancer who were compared to 273 age-matched controls, Litwin et al. *(12)* found no difference in urinary function or bowel function of men with prostate cancer who elected observation only versus the age-matched controls These results are supported by the results from Lubeck and colleagues *(13)* who conducted longitudinal assessments of 692 men with prostate cancer. In this study, men in the observation only group *(n=87)* reported few urinary or bowel difficulties at the time of diagnosis, 1 year post-diagnosis, or 2 years post-diagnosis. Hoffman and colleagues *(14)* analyzed the HRQOL responses of 293 men from the New Mexico component of the PCOS cohort and compared them to 618 healthy controls matched on age and ethnicity. The unique characteristic of the PCOS cohort in general and the New Mexico component specifically is that the study is population-based (meaning that all men in a geographic region who had the disease were included in the study regardless of where they received treatment, minimizing selection bias) and that the study is the longest and largest longitudinal study of its kind, making it a singular resource for addressing questions regarding quality of life in prostate cancer. In the New Mexico study, the PCOS researchers found that the prostate cancer patients reported significantly better baseline urinary control and less urinary bother. No significant differences were noted in the sexual or bowel domains at baseline. Similarly, Bacon et al. *(10)* compared general HRQOL in 783 men with incident prostate cancer to 1,928 age-matched healthy controls. They found that the men with localized prostate cancer actually reported significantly better physical function and less bodily pain (both $p < 0.0002$) than the healthy controls but had worse general health, vitality, social function, and role limitations due to physical and emotional problems (all p values < 0.004). The observation from the Hoffman *(14)* and Bacon *(10)* studies that men with newly diagnosed prostate cancer appear to have better baseline HRQOL in certain domains is likely due to a "healthy screenee" bias. In other words, healthier and more robust men are more likely to undergo prostate cancer screening, which results in these men having better baseline function than age-matched controls. This "healthy screenee" bias has also been observed in the SEER-Medicare dataset *(15)*. Taken as a whole, these studies appear to indicate that a new diagnosis of prostate cancer does not appear to have a deleterious effect on disease-specific HRQOL.

Although the results above seem to indicate otherwise, there are some authors who argue that sexual function may be impacted by diagnosis or to some extent be linked to the nature of the disease *(9)*. These authors point to the results from a handful of comparison studies that indicate that men diagnosed with prostate cancer and who opted for watchful waiting report reduced sexual function when compared to age-matched controls. In a comparison group design, Helgason et al. *(16)* assessed 342 men with prostate cancer and 314 health age-matched controls. The 139 men in the observation group reported more sexual dysfunction and more distress over this dysfunction than did the men in the control group. In the Litwin et al. *(12)* study, the observation group also reported lower sexual function than the age-matched controls. There are two points to bear in mind when considering these results. Firstly, patients who elect observation often have more co-morbid disease *(17)*. Neither of these studies controlled for co-morbidities and, therefore, selection bias may be responsible for the findings. The other point to remember when considering these reports is that the time since diagnosis of the observation groups ranged from 2 to 5 years suggesting that these symptoms may be related to disease sequela as opposed to a reaction to diagnosis *(9)*. Given these points, it is likely that the diagnosis of prostate cancer itself has little or no effect on disease-specific HRQOL.

In terms of the generic HRQOL domains, there is no evidence that the diagnosis of prostate cancer affects these domains. In the studies previously cited, there were no differences found in the generic domains of the SF-36 in men diagnosed with prostate cancer when compared to age-matched controls. In fact, it appears that the various prostate cancer treatments have little effect on long-term generic HRQOL outcomes either. Penson et al. *(18)* studied 2,693 men newly diagnosed with localized prostate cancer in the PCOS cohort who had baseline (diagnosis) and 2-year HRQOL data. No differences in 2-year general HRQOL outcomes were noted among the various treatments for localized prostate cancer. Potosky et al. *(19)* observed similar findings at 5 years. In the 2-year study, Penson et al. *(18)* noted that men with sexual and urinary dysfunctions had significantly worse outcomes in the bodily pain, mental health, role limitation, vitality, and overall health status domains of general HRQOL, when controlling for baseline function, treatment and 27 other co-variates, indicating that impotence and incontinence negatively impact HRQOL. This underscores the need to understand the incidence of erectile dysfunction following prostate cancer treatment and its effect on HRQOL. We will explore this further later in this chapter.

3   The Psychological Effect of a New Prostate Cancer Diagnosis

Although the diagnosis of prostate cancer itself does not appear to directly affect generic HRQOL, this is not to say it has no effect at all. In fact, the diagnosis of prostate cancer likely has a significant effect on the psychological functioning of the patient, which in turn will affect quality of life. It may be that generic HRQOL instruments, such as the SF-36 *(20)* or the FACT-G *(21)* simply are not precise enough to capture this impact. To this end, other more psychologically oriented instruments may be more useful for measuring this effect.

There is little doubt that the diagnosis of cancer may bring with it significant distress *(22,23)*. The number of cancer patients who report clinically significant distress has been estimated to range from 34 to 46% *(22)*. An elevation in distress and anxiety is considered normal and expected as patients and their families attempt to understand the diagnosis and consider options for treatment. In general, the trajectory is such that this distress peaks at diagnosis and treatment decision, and then for many patients, tends to dissipate to normal or subthreshold levels as patients and their families accommodate to the cancer diagnosis and treatment implications *(24)*. This is especially true for patients diagnosed with treatable disease, and specifically demonstrated in studies of men with early stage prostate cancer *(24–28)*.

When men with prostate cancer do experience distress, the literature suggests that these men primarily manifest their distress in anxiety and depression with the focus primarily on anxiety. For example, in a study of 121 both early and late prostate cancer patients who were on average 4 years post-diagnosis, Roth and colleagues *(29)* found that 33% of these men scored at or above the anxiety cut-off score of the Hospital Anxiety and Depression Scale (HADS) *(30)*, while a lower (although still clinically elevated) 15% of men scored at or above the cut-off score for depression on the HADS. These results are confirmed in another cross-sectional study conducted by Balderson and Towell *(31)* who surveyed 94 men in the United Kingdom with various stages of prostate cancer. These men were on average 2–3 years post-diagnosis. These researchers found that overall 38% of the men were experiencing distress as measured by the HADS, and this sample exhibited a higher mean anxiety score (7.17) as compared to a mean depression score (5.09). These results have directed the research investigating the psychological impact of prostate cancer to focus more closely on anxiety as opposed to depression.

Over the past 10 years, a handful of studies have assessed distress and anxiety at diagnosis, providing preliminary evidence of the impact of prostate cancer diagnosis on the psychological state of the patient. Nordin et al. *(32)* assessed 118 Swedish prostate cancer patients with the Hospital Anxiety and Depression Scale. At diagnosis, 12% of the patients reported scores at or above the cut-off for anxiety and the same percentage scored significantly for depression. As expected, these rates were higher for those diagnosed with advanced disease as compared to localized disease. Of those diagnosed with advanced disease, 18% reported anxiety and 15% reported depressive symptoms. This is in contrast to localized disease where 9% reported anxiety and 10% reported depression. In a study of 88 men with newly diagnosed clinically localized prostate cancer, Bisson et al. *(33)* reported that 22% of men had meaningful levels of anxiety as measured with the HADS, and 5% reported significant depressive symptoms. In a recent study, Korfage et al. *(27)* studied 299 men with newly diagnosed localized prostate cancer from the Netherlands. These men were assessed with the state subscale of the State Trait Anxiety Inventory. The use of this scale confirmed the high rates of anxiety reported with the HADS in previous studies as 28% of men reported scores of anxiety above the cut-off score of the STAI-state.

Although none of these studies assessed men before the diagnosis of prostate cancer, these rates of distress and anxiety are generally considered elevated and indicate that the diagnosis of prostate cancer increases distress in these men. This conclusion is supported by a recent article published by Korfage et al. *(26)* who assessed 3,800 men pre-screening with the mental health subscale of the SF-36 Quality of Life measure. The authors then followed these men longitudinally and 52 men were diagnosed with prostate cancer as a result of the screening. These researchers re-administered the questionnaire to these 52 diagnosed men before initial treatment and then 6 months following treatment. The SF-36 mental health subscale does not produce "caseness" (i.e., the percentage of men scoring above a cut-off), but these authors did find a significant decrease in men's mental health scores (indicating a decline in mental health functioning) from the pre-screening assessment to the assessment just before initial treatment. This scale specifically assesses mental health items such as feeling nervous, down, and depressed. At the assessment 6 months after treatment, the mental health scores had elevated to the point of no significant difference between baseline scores as compared to the 6-month follow-up score. In summary, while there appears to be little long-term psychological effect of prostate cancer in men with localized disease, patients not surprisingly experience significant psychological distress and anxiety in the period immediately following diagnosis.

4 The Effect of Post-treatment Sexual Dysfunction on Quality of Life

Sexual dysfunction can occur after all treatments for prostate cancer usually as a result of nerve or vascular injury (in the case of surgery or radiation) or endocrinologic abnormalities (following hormone ablation therapy). Although numerous different forms of sexual dysfunction can occur following treatment, including erectile dysfunction, ejaculatory dysfunction, and libido disturbances, we will focus primarily on erectile dysfunction (ED), as it is the best studied of the sexual dysfunctions that occur after treatment for prostate cancer. Given the earlier observation from the PCOS study that erectile dysfunction is independently associated with worse generic HRQOL 2 years following the diagnosis of prostate cancer *(18)*, it is important to understand the incidence of dysfunction and its effect on disease-specific HRQOL after each commonly used therapy for prostate cancer.

4.1 Radical Prostatectomy

Impotence occurs fairly commonly after radical prostatectomy *(34)*. Erectile dysfunction following surgery rates are likely related to a number of factors, including pre-operative function *(35)*, stage of the cancer *(36)*, age of health of the patient *(35)*, and potentially the operating surgeon *(37)*. To this end, while reports from single high-volume centers likely represent optimal outcomes, it is better to review data from multi-center studies and population-based projects. To date, the largest population-based report of longitudinal outcomes following radical prostatectomy comes from the PCOS *(38)*. Penson et al. *(39)* studied outcomes in the 1,213 men in PCOS who underwent radical prostatectomy for localized prostate cancer and were followed for 5 years. At baseline, 81% of patients reported erections firm enough for intercourse. This high-baseline potency rate is likely due to a combination of factors, including a "healthy screenee" bias and selection bias, as sicker men are less likely to be offered surgery. Six months following diagnosis (and surgery), only 9% of patients report erections firm enough for intercourse. This improved to 17% at 12 months, 22% at 2 years and 28% at 5 years. It is interesting to consider the proportion of patients reporting that their sexual dysfunction was a moderate to big problem in this study. At baseline, 20% of patients reported that their sexual dys-function was a moderate to big problem, corresponding nicely to a 19% ED rate. At 6 months, 70% report that it was a moderate to big problem, which is less than the 91% who report that their erections were not firm enough for intercourse. While the degree of ED improved somewhat at years 1, 2, and 5, it is interesting to note that the amount of bother that the dysfunction caused improves with time. At 12 months, 61% stated it was a moderate to big problem; at 24 months, 54%, and at 60 months, 46%. This underscores the fact that function and bother do not correlate in the sexual domains in prostate cancer patients.

Other authors have noted a similar relationship between sexual function and bother following radical prostatectomy. Bates et al. *(40)* assessed HRQOL in 83 men who underwent radical retropubic prostatectomy using the ICS-male question-naire. Of the 74 men who reported pre-operative potency, 44 (59%) were completely impotent. However, 45% of these impotent men reported that this was not a problem and 20% reported it was only a "bit of a problem." It should be noted that this find-ing is not limited to the post-prostatectomy setting. In a study of 528 men, including 214 men with localized prostate cancer who underwent either surgery, radiotherapy, or watchful waiting, and 273 controls, level of sexual function was compared to degree of bother experienced *(12)*. Although there was reasonable correlation (90% of men with good or very good sexual function experienced none, or very little bother, while 78% with poor or very poor sexual function experienced great bother from their condition), there were still a considerable number of patients in whom function and bother did not agree.

It is interesting to consider why some patients experience significant erectile dys-function yet report little or no bother from their condition. One possible explana-tion for the discordance between function and bother in prostate cancer patients is the psychological ability for patients to "rationalize away" their ED by reassuring themselves that they are "cured" of cancer. To explore this hypothesis, Penson and colleagues *(41)* compared HRQOL outcomes in 121 men without prostate cancer who had ED to 47 men with ED with a history of prostate cancer and its treat-ment. The prostate cancer group reported significantly worse sexual self-efficacy, erectile function, intercourse satisfaction, and orgasmic function than impotent men without prostate cancer. However, the impotent prostate cancer survivors reported significantly less psychological impact of erectile dysfunction on both sexual experience and emotional life than impotent men without prostate cancer. These findings appear to support the hypothesis that the psychological relief of knowing that one's prostate cancer has been successfully treated may mitigate the deleterious HRQOL effects of erectile dysfunction. All of these studies underscore the need to approach each patient individually, as each patient experiences sexual dysfunction in a profoundly personal manner, and treatment plans need to be designed around patients' psychological needs and clinical expectations.

The studies above do not specifically address the effectiveness of nerve-sparing in maintaining sexual function. To explore the effect of the nerve-sparing RP technique on quality of life outcomes, Talcott et al. *(42)* compared 28 men who underwent non-nerve-sparing RP to 66 men who underwent either unilateral or bilateral nerve-sparing surgery at a single institution. They found that men who underwent any type of nerve-sparing procedure had worse sexual function than had been previously reported. Furthermore, they noted no statistically significant differences in sexual functioning between the nerve-sparing and non-nerve-sparing groups. This study, however, reports a single center experience and may not be representative of what occurs in other centers or in the community at large. In the PCOS study mentioned above, a limited analysis was performed to assess the effectiveness of nerve-sparing *(39)*. Men who underwent bilateral nerve-sparing surgery were more likely to report erections firm enough for intercourse at 60 months (40%) than those who underwent unilateral nerve-sparing (23%) or non-nerve-sparing (23%) surgery ($p = 0.01$). The effectiveness of nerve-sparing was closely associated with age at the time of surgery ($p < 0.001$). In a report from CaPSURE, Litwin et al. *(43)* compared longitudinal HRQOL in 218 men who underwent nerve-sparing RP with 124 men who underwent the non-nerve-sparing technique. They found that the patients who underwent nerve-sparing surgery had significantly better sexual function than those who had non-nerve-sparing surgery at 6, 12, and 18 months following treatment, although the overall level of sexual function was low for both groups. These two studies confirm that nerve-sparing surgery appears to positively impact sexual outcomes.

Finally, numerous randomized clinical trials have documented the effectiveness of phosphodiesterase type-5 inhibitors (PDE5i) in aiding erectile function following bilateral and unilateral nerve-sparing radical prostatectomies *(44)*. As this is discussed elsewhere in this book, we will not go into great detail in the current chapter. However, it is interesting to contrast the findings of these randomized clinical trials to a large population-based cohort of men who elected to try sildenafil as part of routine clinical care. In randomized, blinded trials from the Cleveland Clinic, for example, 72% of patients who underwent bilateral nerve-sparing radical prostatectomy reported erections firm enough for vaginal penetration *(44)*. This population represents a group of highly motivated and selected men who had their surgery at a high-volume center that is known for superior results. In the general community, where patients' expectations may not be appropriate and where the quality of the surgery may not be as high, the results are not as encouraging. In the 520 men from the PCOS cohort who underwent radical prostatectomy and tried sildenafil and were followed for 5 years, only 45% reported that the drug helped a lot or somewhat. The amount that the drug helped was closely related to the patient's age, with 63% of men under the age of 55 years, 59% of men aged 55–60 years, 30% of men aged 60–64 years, 40% of men aged 65–70 years, and 32% of men over the age of 70 years reporting it helped a lot or somewhat *(45)*. In summary, oral PDE5i appear to be effective in aiding erectile function in men after radical prostatectomy, but probably to a lesser degree than what has been reported in clinical trials.

In summary, it is incumbent upon providers to help patients set reasonable expectations regarding erectile function after surgery. Specifically, it can take 1–2 years for functional erections to return. In addition, while oral agents are effective in restoring erectile function, they may be less effective than has been reported in randomized clinical trials, particularly in older patients. With proper counseling, it is likely that the negative effect of sexual dysfunction on HRQOL following surgery for prostate cancer can be minimizing.

4.2   External Beam Radiotherapy

Sexual dysfunction can occur following both external beam radiotherapy and interstitial brachytherapy (seeds), presumably due to radiation injury to the neurovascular bundles adjacent to the prostate, arterial inflow conduits, and erectile tissue. Because the basic techniques of external beam radiotherapy have been in use for decades, there is considerably more information regarding sexual dysfunction and HRQOL after XRT. Mantz et al. *(46)* studied 287 men with localized prostate cancer who underwent conformal EBRT. They noted actuarial potency rates of 96, 75, 59, and 53% at 1, 20, 40, and 60 months after therapy.

It is interesting to note that, similar to the situation following surgery, the effect of sexual dysfunction on quality of life is highly individualized. Reddy et al. *(47)* noted that 79% of patients who were potent prior to radiotherapy reported that the treatment qualitatively reduced their ability to obtain an erection. Despite this, 91% of patients were satisfied with their treatment, demonstrating that sexual dysfunction and satisfaction with therapy do not correlate. Helgason et al. *(48)* studied 53 men who had undergone external beam radiotherapy for localized prostate cancer and noted that 77% reported diminished sexual desire, 34% reported erections insufficient for intercourse, and 77% of men reported some loss of stiffness. However, only 50% of men reported that their overall quality of life had decreased much or very much as a direct result of their decrease in erectile function. Other researchers have also found that sexual dysfunction has less of an effect on quality of life following external beam radiotherapy. Caffo et al. *(49)* showed that, although 44% of men had significant sexual dysfunction following external beam radiotherapy, general quality of life, measured as physical, psychological, and relational well-being, all remained good.

In summary, erectile dysfunction also occurs commonly after external beam radiotherapy, although based on the currently available literature, perhaps to a somewhat lesser extent than in surgical patients. However, like surgical patients, function and bother do not always correlate and many patients who experience sexual dysfunction following external beam radiotherapy do not report concordant bother.

4.3 *Interstitial Brachytherapy (Seeds)*

Although data related to brachytherapy are relatively immature and are limited by short follow-up, it appears that this treatment may also effect erectile function and disease-specific HRQOL. Initial reports indicated that IB had minimal effect on sexual function. Arterberry et al. *(50)* reported that 87% of 35 patients who were potent pre-treatment maintained their potency 6 months following treatment. However, this study had relatively small numbers of patients and limited follow-up. In a study directly comparing outcomes between men undergoing surgery and IB and age-matched controls, Brandeis et al. *(51)* found that, at 3–17 months following treatment, sexual function in the IB group was significantly worse than in age-matched controls. There were no significant differences between the surgical and brachytherapy groups in the sexual domains. Recent reports from the CaPSURE database indicate that, while sexual function 3–4 years after seed implantation is significantly better than similar patients undergoing surgery or external beam radiotherapy, there is a still a significant decline in sexual function in the seeds group from baseline. In addition, although there are significant differences in sexual function between the three groups at 4 years after therapy, there are no differences in bother *(52)*.

5 The Psychological Effect of Post-treatment Sexual Dysfunction

In addition to the HRQOL implications discussed above, it is also important to consider the psychological impact of struggling with erectile dysfunction. In contrast to the research on coping with the diagnosis of prostate cancer, which has focused primarily on anxiety, the literature describing the psychological impact of ED concentrates on depression. Although little, if any, data exist on the association between erectile dysfunction and depression specifically in men with prostate cancer, it is clear from studies conducted in other settings that there is a relationship between these two variables. Shabsigh and colleagues *(53)* studied 120 with ED and/or benign prostatic hyperplasia (BPH). This study grouped men in three categories: 48 men with ED only, 34 men with BPH only, and 18 men with both ED and BPH. The average age of the men in the study was approximately 56 years old, and depressive symptoms were measured with the Beck Depression Inventory (BDI) *(54)*. These researchers found a remarkably high rate of depressive symptoms (56%) in the ED only group and the ED plus BPH group. This rate of 56% was significantly higher than the 21% of subjects who reported depressive symptoms in the BPH only group. These results are supported by two population-based studies that have also researched the association between depression and erectile dysfunction. Araujo et al. *(55)* presented data on 1,700 subjects from the Massachusetts Male Aging Study, a large, population-based study of the men from the greater Boston area. The men in the study ranged in age from 40 to 70 years old. In this study, the researchers measured ED with a single, self-report question and depression with the Center for Epidemiological Studies Depression Scale (CES-D) *(56)*. After controlling for variables such as age, health status, and medication use, depressive symptoms were clearly and significantly associated with ED (OR 1.8). Very similar results were reported by Nicolosi et al. *(57)* in a population-based study of 1,800 subjects from Brazil, Japan, and Malaysia. These subjects also ranged in age from 40 to 70 years old, and ED was measured with a single, self-report question while depression was assessed with the CES-D. These researchers also found a significant association between depressive symptoms and erectile dysfunction (OR 1.7).

A difficult aspect in studying this association is trying to determine which variable comes first. Does depression cause ED, or does ED cause depression? Shiri and colleagues *(58)* have suggested that it is a bidirectional relationship. These authors reported results from the large, population-based, longitudinal study conducted in Finland. The 1,680 subjects in this study ranged in age from 50 to 70 years. ED was assessed with two self-report questions and depression was measured by the 5-item Mental Health Inventory *(59)*. In this study, the incidence of depression was higher in those men who had ED as compared to men without ED $(p < 0.01)$. Likewise, the incidence of ED was higher in men who reported depression than those who did not report depression $(p < 0.05)$. The authors point to these results as evidence of a bidirectional relationship between erectile dysfunction and depression.

There are few, if any, studies that have researched this question in men with prostate cancer. Clinical experience certainly supports that the association between ED and depression exists in men treated for prostate cancer. Interestingly, there may be reason to believe men treated for prostate cancer will cope more effectively with erectile dysfunction as compared to men without prostate cancer. Penson et al. *(41)* provide preliminary evidence for this in their study discussed above. These authors suggest that men treated for prostate cancer may be able to place their ED in perspective in relation to the importance of dealing with their cancer. Additionally, many healthy men who experience ED often blame themselves; thinking that a lack of "manliness" is at fault for the loss of erections. Although many men treated for prostate cancer feel less like a "man" if they experience ED, they do not have the added psychological burden of blaming themselves for the loss of erections. The treatment clearly impacts erectile functioning and these men may possibly adjust more effectively to erectile dysfunction as a result.

6 Conclusions

Quality of life is an important concern for men with prostate cancer. The effect of this disease and the side-effects of its treatment on health-related quality of life in prostate cancer survivors cannot be understated. The literature indicates that, while the majority of men with prostate cancer do not experience significant declines in generic HRQOL directly due to the disease, a new diagnosis often causes significant psychological distress and anxiety, which can transiently have negative effects on HRQOL. While there are numerous side-effects of treatment which can affect HRQOL, sexual dysfunction, specifically erectile dysfunction, is among the most studied. While this condition is common after all therapies for prostate cancer, its HRQOL impact varies from patient to patient, based upon age, personal expectation, and the individual's psychological coping mechanisms. As healthcare providers, it is important that we be aware of the potential HRQOL impact of sexual dysfunction in prostate cancer survivors and attempt to make effective interventions to improve outcomes in these patients.

References

1. Jemal, A., Siegel, R., Ward, E., Murray, T., Xu, J., and Thun, M.J. (2007) Cancer statistics, 2007. *CA Cancer J. Clin.* **57**(1), 43–66.
2. Etzioni, R., Penson, D.F., Legler, J.M., et al. (2002) Overdiagnosis due to prostate-specific antigen screening: lessons from U.S. prostate cancer incidence trends. *J. Natl. Cancer Inst.* **94**(13), 981–990.
3. Singer, P.A., Tasch, E.S., Stocking, C., Rubin, S., Siegler, M., and Weichselbaum, R. (1991) Sex or survival: trade offs between quality and quantity of life. *J. Clin. Oncol.* **9**(2), 328–334.
4. Patrick, D.L., and Erickson, P. (1993) Assessing health-related quality of life for clinical decision-making. In: Walker, S.R., and Rosser, R.M., eds. *Quality of Life Assessment: Key Issues in the 1990's.* Dordrecht: Kluwer Academic Publishers, Chap. 19.
5. Litwin, M.S., Lubeck, D.P., Henning, J.M., and Carroll, P.R. (1998) Differences in urologist and patient assessments of health related quality of life in men with prostate cancer: results of the CaPSURE database. *J. Urol.* **159**(6), 1988–1992.
6. Litwin, M.S., and McGuigan, K.A. (1999) Accuracy of recall in health-related quality-of-life assessment among men treated for prostate cancer. *J. Clin. Oncol.* **17**(9), 2882–2888.
7. Legler, J., Potosky, A.L., Gilliland, F.D., Eley, J.W., and Stanford, J.L. (2000) Validation study of retrospective recall of disease-targeted function: results from the prostate cancer outcomes study. *Med. Care* **38**(8), 847–857.
8. Gill, T.M., and Feinstein, A.R. (1994) A Critical appraisal of the quality-of-life measurements. *JAMA*;**272**(8), 619–626.
9. Eton, D.T., and Lepore, S.J. (2002) Prostate cancer and health-related quality of life: a review of the literature. *Psycho-Oncology* **11**(4), 307–326.
10. Bacon, C.G., Giovannucci, E., Testa, M., Glass, T.A., and Kawachi, I. (2002) The association of treatment-related symptoms with quality-of-life outcomes for localized prostate carcinoma patients. *Cancer* **94**(3), 862–871.
11. Cooperberg, M.R., Lubeck, D.P., Meng, M.V., Mehta, S.S., and Carroll, P.R. (2004) The changing face of low-risk prostate cancer: trends in clinical presentation and primary management. *J. Clin. Oncol.* **22**(11), 2141–2149.
12. Litwin, M.S., Hays, R.D., Fink, A., et al. (1995) Quality-of-life outcomes in men treated for localized prostate cancer. *JAMA* **273**(2), 129–35.
13. Lubeck, D.P., Litwin, M.S., Henning, J.M., Stoddard, M.L., Flanders, S.C., and Carroll, P.R. (1999) Changes in health-related quality of life in the first year after treatment for prostate cancer: results from CaPSURE. *Urology* **53**(1), 180–186.
14. Hoffman, R.M., Gilliland, F.D., Penson, D.F., Stone, S.N., Hunt, W.C., and Potosky, A.L. (2004) Cross-sectional and longitudinal comparisons of health-related quality of life between patients with prostate carcinoma and matched controls. *Cancer* **101**(9), 2011–2019.
15. Zeliadt, S.B., Etzioni, R., Ramsey, S.D., Penson, D.F., and Potosky, A.L. (2007) Trends in treatment costs for localized prostate cancer: the healthy screenee effect. *Med. Care* **45**(2), 154–159.

16. Helgason, A.R., Adolfsson, J., Dickman, P., Fredrikson, M., Arver, S., and Steineck, G. (1996) Waning sexual function – the most important disease-specific distress for patients with prostate cancer. *Br. J. Cancer* **73**(11), 1417–1421.

17. Harlan, L.C., Potosky, A., Gilliland, F.D., et al. (2001) Factors associated with initial therapy for clinically localized prostate cancer: prostate cancer outcomes study. *J. Natl. Cancer Inst.* **93**(24), 1864–1871.

18. Penson, D.F., Feng, Z., Kuniyuki, A., et al. (2003) General quality of life 2 years following treatment for prostate cancer: what influences outcomes? Results from the prostate cancer outcomes study. *J. Clin. Oncol.* **21**(6), 1147–1154.

19. Potosky, A.L., Davis, W.W., Hoffman, R.M., et al. (2004) Five-year outcomes after prostatectomy or radiotherapy for prostate cancer: the prostate cancer outcomes study. *J .Natl. Cancer Inst.* **96**(18), 1358–1367.

20. Ware, J.E., Jr., and Sherbourne, C.D. (1992) The MOS 36-item short-form health survey (SF-36). I. Conceptual framework and item selection. *Med. Care* **30**(6), 473–483.

21. Cella, D.F., Tulsky, D.S., Gray, G., et al. (1993) The Functional Assessment of Cancer Therapy scale: development and validation of the general measure. *J. Clin. Oncol.* **11**(3), 570–579.

22. Ellman, R., Angeli, N., Christians, A., Moss, S., Chamberlain, J., and Maguire, P. (1989) Psychiatric morbidity associated with screening for breast cancer. *Br. J. Cancer* **60**(5), 781–784.

23. Ford, S., Fallowfield, L., Hall, A., and Lewis, S. (1995) The influence of audiotapes on patient participation in the cancer consultation. *Eur. J. Cancer* **31A**(13–14), 2264–2269.

24. Davison, B.J., and Goldenberg, S.L. (2003) Decisional regret and quality of life after participating in medical decision-making for early-stage prostate cancer. *BJU Int.* **91**(1), 14–17.

25. Dale, W., Bilir, P., Han, M., and Meltzer, D. (2005) The role of anxiety in prostate carcinoma: a structured review of the literature. *Cancer* **104**(3), 467–478.

26. Korfage, I.J., de Koning, H.J., Roobol, M., Schroder, F.H., and Essink-Bot, M.L. (2006) Prostate cancer diagnosis: the impact on patients' mental health. *Eur. J. Cancer* **42**(2), 165–170.

27. Korfage, I.J., Essink-Bot, M.L., Janssens, A.C., Schroder, F.H., and de Koning, H.J. (2006) Anxiety and depression after prostate cancer diagnosis and treatment: 5-year follow-up. *Br. J. Cancer* **94**(8), 1093–1098.

28. Korfage, I.J., Hak, T., de Koning, H.J., and Essink-Bot, M.L. (2006) Patients' perceptions of the side-effects of prostate cancer treatment – a qualitative interview study. *Soc. Sci. Med.* **63**(4), 911–919.

29. Roth, A.J., Kornblith, A.B., Batel-Copel, L., Peabody, E., Scher, H.I., and Holland, J.C. (1998) Rapid screening for psychologic distress in men with prostate carcinoma: a pilot study. *Cancer* **82**(10), 1904–1908.

30. Zigmond, A.S., and Snaith, R.P. (1983) The hospital anxiety and depression scale. *Acta Psychiatr. Scand.* **67**(6), 361–370.

31. Balderson, N., and Towell, T. (2003) The prevalence and predictors of psychological distress in men with prostate cancer who are seeking support. *Br. J. Health Psychol.* **8**(Pt 2), 125–134.

32. Nordin, K., Berglund, G., Glimelius, B., and Sjoden, P.O. (2001) Predicting anxiety and depression among cancer patients: a clinical model. *Eur. J. Cancer* **37**(3), 376–384.

33. Bisson, J.I., Chubb, H.L., Bennett, S., Mason, M., Jones, D., and Kynaston, H. (2002) The prevalence and predictors of psychological distress in patients with early localized prostate cancer. *BJU Int.* **90**(1), 56–61.

34. Penson, D.F., Litwin, M.S., and Aaronson, N.K. (2003) Health related quality of life in men with prostate cancer. *J. Urol.* **169**(5), 1653–1661.

35. Wei, J.T., Dunn, R.L., Marcovich, R., Montie, J.E., and Sanda, M.G. (2000) Prospective assessment of patient reported urinary continence after radical prostatectomy. *J. Urol.* **164**(3 Pt 1), 744–748.

36. Eastham, J.A., Kattan, M.W., Rogers, E., et al. (1996) Risk factors for urinary incontinence after radical prostatectomy [see comments]. *J. Urol.* **156**(5), 1707–1713.

37. Ellison, L., Heaney, J., and Birkmeyer, J. (2000) The effect of hospiral volume on mortality and resource use after radical prostatectomy. *J. Urol.* **163**(3), 867–869.

38. Potosky, A.L., Harlan, L.C., Stanford, J.L., et al. (1999) Prostate cancer practice patterns and quality of life: the Prostate Cancer Outcomes Study. *J. Natl Cancer Inst.* **91**(20), 1719–1724.
39. Penson, D.F., McLerran, D., Feng, Z., et al. (2005) Five-year urinary and sexual outcomes after tadical prostatectomy: results from the Prostate Cancer Outcomes Study. *J. Urol.* **173**(5), 1701–1705.
40. Bates, T.S., Wright, M.P., and Gillatt, D.A. (1998) Prevalence and impact of incontinence and impotence following total prostatectomy assessed anonymously by the ICS-male questionnaire. *Eur. Urol.* **33**(2), 165–169.
41. Penson, D.F., Latini, D.M., Lubeck, D.P., Wallace, K., Henning, J.M., and Lue, T. (2003) Is quality of life different for men with erectile dysfunction and prostate cancer compared to men with erectile dysfunction due to other causes? Results from the ExCEED data base. *J. Urol.* **169**(4), 1458–1461.
42. Talcott, J.A., Rieker, P., Propert, K.J., et al. (1997) Patient-reported impotence and incontinence after nerve-sparing radical prostatectomy. *J. Natl. Cancer Inst.* **89**(15), 1117–1123.
43. Litwin, M.S., Flanders, S.C., Pasta, D.J., Stoddard, M.L., Lubeck, D.P., and Henning, J.M. (1999) Sexual function and bother after radical prostatectomy or radiation for prostate cancer: multivariate quality-of-life analysis from CaPSURE. Cancer of the Prostate Strategic Urologic Research Endeavor. *Urology* **54**(3), 503–508.
44. Zippe, C.D., Kedia, A.W., Kedia, K., Nelson, D.R., and Agarwal, A. (1998) Treatment of erectile dysfunction after radical prostatectomy with sildenafil citrate (Viagra). *Urology* **52**(6), 963–966.
45. Penson, D.F., McLerran, D., Feng, Z., et al. (2005) 5-year urinary and sexual outcomes after radical prostatectomy: results from the prostate cancer outcomes study. *J. Urol.* **173**(5), 1701–1705.
46. Mantz, C.A., Song, P., Farhangi, E., et al. (1997) Potency probability following conformal megavoltage radiotherapy using conventional doses for localized prostate cancer. *Int. J. Radiat. Oncol. Biol. Phys.* **37**(3), 551–557.
47. Reddy, S.M., Ruby, J., Wallace, M., and Forman, J.D. (1997) Patient self-assessment of complications and quality of life after conformal neutron and photon irradiation for localized prostate cancer. *Radiat. Oncol. Investig.* **5**(5), 252–256.
48. Helgason, A.R., Fredrikson, M., Adolfsson, J., and Steineck, G. (1995) Decreased sexual capacity after external radiation therapy for prostate cancer impairs quality of life. *Int. J. Radiat. Oncol. Biol. Phys.* **32**(1), 33–39.
49. Caffo, O., Fellin, G., Graffer, U., and Luciani, L. (1996) Assessment of quality of life after radical radiotherapy for prostate cancer. *Br. J. Urol.* **78**(4), 557–563.
50. Arterbery, V.E., Frazier, A., Dalmia, P., Siefer, J., Lutz, M., and Porter, A. (1997) Quality of life after permanent prostate implant. *Semin. Surg. Oncol.* **13**(6), 461–464.
51. Brandeis, J.M., Litwin, M.S., Burnison, C.M., and Reiter, R.E. (2000) Quality of life outcomes after brachytherapy for early stage prostate cancer. *J. Urol.* **163**(3), 851–857.
52. Huang, G.J., Sadetsky, N., Carroll, P., and Penson, D.F. (2007) Predictors of HRQOL during long-term follow-up of men treated for prostate cancer. In: *2007 Prostate Cancer Symposium,* Orlando, FL.
53. Shabsigh, R.R., Klein, L.L.T., Seidman, S.S., Kaplan, S.S.A., Lehrhoff, B.B.J., and Ritter, J.J.S. (1998) Increased incidence of depressive symptoms in men with erectile dysfunction. *Urology* **52**(5), 848–852.
54. Schneider, B.B., and Varghese, R.R.K. (1995) Scores on the SF-36 scales and the Beck Depression Inventory in assessing mental health among patients on hemodialysis. *Psychol. Rep.* **76**(3 Pt 1), 719–722.
55. Araujo, A.A.B., Durante, R.R., Feldman, H.H.A., Goldstein, I.I., and McKinlay, J.J.B. (1998) The relationship between depressive symptoms and male erectile dysfunction: cross-sectional results from the Massachusetts Male Aging Study. *Psycho. Med.* **60**(4), 458–465.
56. van Wilgen, C.C.P., Dijkstra, P.P.U., Stewart, R.R.E., Ranchor, A.A.V., and Roodenburg, J.J.L.N. (2006) Measuring somatic symptoms with the CES-D to assess depression in cancer patients after treatment: comparison among patients with oral/oropharyngeal, gynecological, colorectal, and breast cancer. *Psychosomatics* **47**(6), 465–470.

57. Nicolosi, A.A., Moreira, E.D.E.D., Villa, M.M., and Glasser, D.B.D.B. (2004) A population study of the association between sexual function, sexual satisfaction and depressive symptoms in men. *J. Affec. Disord.* **82**(2), 235–243.

58. Shiri, R.R., Koskimäki, J.J., Tammela, T.L.T.L.J., Häkkinen, J.J., Auvinen, A.A., and Hakama, M.M. (2007) Bidirectional relationship between depression and erectile dysfunction. *J. Urol.* **177**(2), 669–673.

59. Rumpf, H.H.J., Meyer, C.C., Hapke, U.U., and John, U.U. (2001) Screening for mental health: validity of the MHI-5 using DSM-IV Axis I psychiatric disorders as gold standard. *Psychiatry Res.* **105**(3), 243–253.

Chapter 3
Pathophysiology of Erectile Dysfunction Following Radical Prostatectomy

Joshua Modder, Carol A. Podlasek, and Kevin T. McVary

Abstract Prostate cancer is the most common solid tumor in adult men, with an estimated 230,000 new cases diagnosed in the USA in 2006. There is a greater concern for quality of life after prostate cancer treatment due to the younger age of diagnosis and increased survival rate. One goal of radical prostatectomy surgery is to limit any further impairment of erectile function. We examine the current understanding of the pathophysiology of ED following radical prostatectomy.

During erection, parasympathetic tone dominates and a number of molecular pathways mediate a decrease in intracellular Ca, corporal smooth muscle relaxation, increased penile arterial inflow, and tumescence. Nitric oxide (NO) is generally agreed upon as the principle neurotransmitter involved in initiating and maintaining penile smooth muscle relaxation, and thus erection. It is clear that the extent to which the cavernous nerves are salvaged or damaged during radical prostatectomy is directly proportional to a patient's degree of postoperative ED. An emerging concept in the field of erectile dysfunction is penile homeostasis. In order for an erection to occur, the complex and unique sinusoidal morphology of the corpora cavernosa must be maintained. New light has been shed on this process with the identification and investigation of the morphogenic protein Sonic hedgehog (SHH), along

From: *Current Clinical Urology* Series, *Sexual Function in the Prostate Cancer Patient*
Edited by John P. Mulhall, DOI 10.1007/978-1-60327-555-2_3,
© Humana Press, a part of Springer Science+Business Media, LLC 2009

with its downstream targets Patched 1 (PTCH1), Hox, bone morphogenetic proteins (BMPs), vascular endothelial growth factor (VEGF), and NOS.

It is believed that chronic hypoxia and denervation of erectile tissue following radical prostatectomy result in permanent ED via apoptosis of smooth muscle cells, deposition of collagen (scar), and penile fibrosis. Hypoxia also causes an increase in release of potent vasoconstrictor molecules such as endothelin-1, a pro-fibrotic peptide, with synthesis.

Active investigation continues in the fields of penile homeostasis, the pathophysiology of ED, control of inflammation and fibrosis, prevention or limitation of smooth muscle apoptosis, and neural regenerative strategies influenced by TGF-B1.

Keywords Erectile dysfunction; prostate cancer; nitric oxide synthase; nervesparing radical prostatectomy.

1 Epidemiology of Prostate Cancer and Erectile Dysfunction

Prostate cancer is the most common solid tumor in adult men, with an estimated 230,000 new cases diagnosed in the USA in 2006 *(1)*. It is also the second leading cause of cancer death in American men, resulting in an estimated 27,000 deaths during the same calendar year *(1)*. Due to PSA screening, we have seen both an age and stage migration of prostate cancer, with a growing incidence of localized disease diagnosed in younger patients.

There is a greater concern for quality of life after prostate cancer treatment due to the younger age of diagnosis and increased survival rate. Radical prostatectomy results in erectile dysfunction (ED) in 30–87% of patients *(2–5)*, and although potency improves over time, sexual dysfunction is still common 5 years after surgery *(6,7)*. Survey studies of men electing treatment for localized prostate cancer reveal that quality of life is a primary concern in 45% of participants *(8)*, and ED caused by radical prostatectomy is associated with lowered self-esteem, self-image, and quality of life *(9)*. The Prostate Cancer Outcomes Study recorded that impaired sexual function is a "moderate" or "great" problem in 46% of patients following surgery *(6)*. Another study showed that partners are also impacted, with up to 60% of female partners having lower sexual function scores *(10)*. It is clear that ED is a significant concern in this patient population, and requires further study to determine underlying causes and potential new therapies.

Many patients with prostate cancer at baseline harbor existing ED risk factors, and preoperative potency status helps predict risk of postoperative ED *(11)*. Erectile function also correlates with a number of other parameters, including patient age, increased BMI, diabetes, hypertension, atherosclerosis, hypercholesterolemia, smoking, and cardiovascular disease *(12)*. In general, the penis can be considered an extension of the vascular tree; erections are a neurovascular phenomenon, and all of these clinical conditions impact upon neurovascular status. One example of this is age, shown to be an independent risk factor for ED. The Prostate Cancer Outcomes Study reported that 61% of men aged 39–54 had erections firm enough for intercourse following bilateral nerve-sparing prostatectomy, compared with 49% of men aged 55–59, 44% of men aged 60–64, and only 18% of men aged 65 years or greater *(6)*.

One goal of radical prostatectomy surgery is to limit any further impairment of erectile function. This chapter will examine our current understanding of the pathophysiology of ED following radical prostatectomy, and will discuss avenues of research that may lead to the development of new treatment options in the future.

2   Penile Anatomy and Physiology

Three simultaneous and integrated processes occur during normal erection:

1. Neurologically mediated increase in penile arterial inflow
2. Cavernosal smooth muscle relaxation
3. Restriction of venous outflow from the penis

ED following radical prostatectomy can be attributed to an alteration in any one or all of these processes. In order to understand how morphology and physiology of the penis is altered by prostatectomy resulting in ED, it is first necessary to have a good understanding of the normal anatomy, development, and physiology of the penis at both the histologic and molecular levels. A brief description of these processes is outlined below.

2.1   Morphology of the Penis

The paired erectile bodies of the penis, the corpora cavernosa, consist of irregularly shaped endothelium-lined vascular spaces (sinusoids) separated by trabeculae made up of smooth muscle, collagen, elastin, and loose areolar tissue containing arterioles and nerves *(13)*. The paired corpora cavernosa and the corpus spongiosum (housing the urethra) are surrounded by the tunica albuginea, a bilayered fibrous sheath composed mostly of collagenous fibers which are relaxed in the flaccid state and stretched during tumescence *(14)*. Each individual sinus is made up of a single layer of vascular endothelium surrounded by multiple layers of smooth muscle interspersed with collagen and fibroblasts (Fig. 1).

2.2   Vascular Anatomy of the Penis

The arterial supply to the penis consists of the paired dorsal penile arteries, the cavernous arteries, and the bulbourethral arteries. These are distal branches of the internal pudendal arteries, which run within Alcock's canal, anatomically positioned

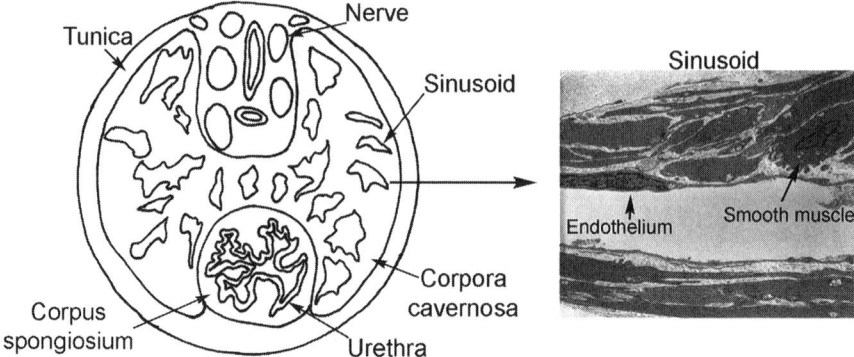

Fig. 1 (*Left*) Cross-sectional view of the penis. (*Right*) Electron microscopic scan showing a single corpora cavernosal sinus (3000× magnification)

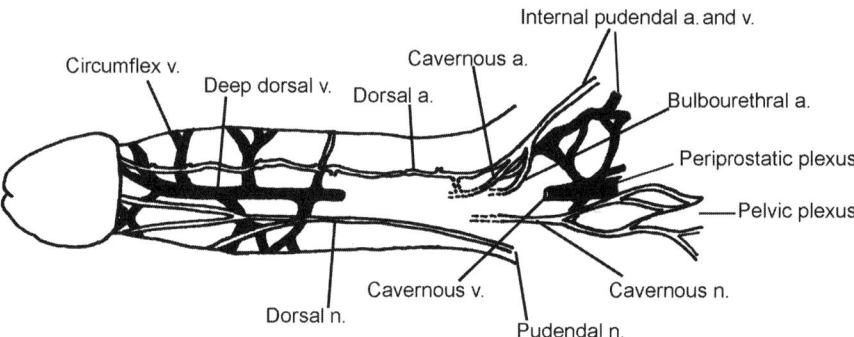

Fig. 2 Arterial, venous, and neural anatomy of the penis

such that there is little risk of injury during pelvic surgery. The cavernous arteries give off multiple tortuous branches (the helicine arteries), which empty into the sinusoidal spaces and are primarily responsible for the increase in penile blood flow during tumescence (Fig. 2).

An accessory pudendal artery may also be present. A detailed anatomic study of ten male cadavers by Breza et al. revealed an accessory pudendal artery to be present in seven of the ten dissections *(15)*. These branches originated from the obturator, inferior vesical, and superior vesical arteries, and traveled along the inferior bladder and anterolateral surface of the prostate, areas susceptible to surgical injury. Seventy percent of these accessory arteries fed the corpora cavernosa. This suggests that patients in whom these vessels are dominant or who have diseased primary pudendal arteries would experience the greatest loss of erectile function due to their damage in the course of prostatectomy *(15)*. Confirming the work of McVary et al. *(16)*, Mulhall and colleagues identified arterial insufficiency in 59% of men with ED following bilateral nerve-sparing radical prostatectomy, all of whom had excellent preoperative erectile function *(17)*. Analysis of a single surgeon database in 2004 showed that preservation of an accessory pudendal artery was associated with a significant increase in potency rates and decrease in time to recovery of spontaneous erections *(18)*. Potency rates were not increased when the vascular pedicle was not identified at the time of surgery. The authors concluded that preservation of the accessory pudendal artery, if identified, might favorably influence sexual function.

Three sets of veins drain the penis: the subcutaneous superficial veins, the intermediate system including the deep dorsal and circumflex veins, and the deep system including the cavernous and crural veins *(19)*. The corpora cavernosa drain through tiny venules leading from the peripheral sinusoids to the subtunical venular plexus. These form emissary veins which drain into the deep dorsal and circumflex veins (intermediate system) distally, and the cavernous and crural veins (deep system), proximally (Fig. 2). The venous drainage of the penis is important because histologic changes following prostatectomy can impair the ability of the penis to limit venous outflow, a necessary step in achieving and maintaining an erection.

2.3   Neural Innervation of the Penis

Erections are mediated primarily by the autonomic nervous system, with sympathetic tone predominating in the flaccid state and parasympathetic tone mediating the erect state *(20)*. The sympathetic innervation of the penis arises from the T10 to L2 spinal cord segments. Pre-ganglionic fibers pass to the paravertebral chain ganglia and synapse with post-ganglionic fibers in the pre-aortic plexus. The post-ganglionic fibers then travel to the pelvic plexus where they intermingle with pre-ganglionic parasympathetic fibers from the S2–4 spinal cord segments (termed the pelvic nerve or nervi erigentes) *(21)*. The penile sympathetic and parasympathetic fibers form a bundle called the cavernous nerve (CN), which is located posterolateral to the seminal vesicle and prostate. The CN pierces the urogenital diaphragm lateral to the membranous urethra at the 3 and 9 o'clock positions *(21)*. The CN then enters the corpus cavernosum at the hilum of the penis, piercing the tunica albuginea to innervate the helicine arteries and erectile tissue (Fig. 2). Interruption of innervation or injury to these neural pathways will result in ED.

Neural impulses mediate erections using a number of different pathways, which include sympathetic (inhibit norepinephrine release), parasympathetic (release nitric oxide and acetylcholine), and somatic (release acetylcholine) nerves. Cerebral impulses produce a "psychogenic" erection (one arising from the brain). In addition, the interplay of these neural pathways in the spinal cord results in a number of spinal reflex loops, each elicited according to the nature and intensity of genital stimulation, which can produce a "reflexogenic" erection (not mediated by the brain). These different mechanisms of erection are not mutually exclusive; instead, they serve to modulate one another. The innervation of the penis is critical to examine when discussing the development of ED following radical prostatectomy.

3 Molecular Signaling of Erections

3.1 NO/NOS

3.1.1 Normal Signaling

During erection, parasympathetic tone dominates and a number of molecular pathways mediate a decrease in intracellular Ca, corporal smooth muscle relaxation, increased penile arterial inflow, and tumescence. Nitric oxide (NO) is generally agreed upon as the principle neurotransmitter involved in initiating and maintaining penile smooth muscle relaxation, and thus erection. It is released from the nonadrenergic/noncholinergic (NANC) parasympathetic nerve terminals of the CNs, as well as from the endothelium in response to a stimulus (e.g., sexual arousal via genital stimulation or erogenous thought). NO diffuses into smooth muscle cells, activates soluble guanylyl cyclase and produces cGMP, leading to a relaxation of cavernous smooth muscle cells *(22–28)*. This results in increased penile arterial blood flow, trapping of the blood by expanding corporal sinusoids, compression of the subtunical venular plexus and the emissary veins (restricting venous outflow), increased intracavernous pressure, and erection.

Nitric oxide synthase (NOS) is the enzyme that catalyzes the production of NO from its precursor L-arginine, and exists as three separate isoforms. These are NOS-1 (neuronal or nNOS), NOS-2 (inducible or iNOS), and NOS-3 (endothelial or eNOS). nNOS and eNOS have been shown to be essential for erection to occur *(29)*. nNOS is localized and expressed primarily in NANC neuronal cells *(30)*. Its activity is Ca^{++} dependent *(31)* and is thought to be regulated by a number of proteins including protein inhibitor of NOS (PIN) and NMDA *(32,33)*. It has been shown that nNOS is responsible for the acute increase in NO production and signaling which initiates penile smooth muscle relaxation *(34–36)*. eNOS is abundant in endothelium and epithelial tissue *(37,38)*. Like nNOS, eNOS is acutely regulated in a Ca/calmodulin-dependent fashion *(31)*. However, it is constitutively activated by shear stress (i.e., increased penile arterial blood flow) via Akt-dependent phosphorylation *(35)*, and VEGF via a Ca-independent pathway to provide a sustained release of NO *(39–41)*. The integration of nNOS and eNOS presents a mechanism for both the initiation and maintenance of the NO-mediated erection.

New evidence suggests that eNOS may also be important in penile homeostasis. We know that eNOS is non-transiently phosphorylated and activated on a continual basis by vasoactive and growth factors, and the constitutive release of NO from eNOS represents a possible mechanism for protection from oxidative stress and the preservation of erectile tissue integrity *(29,35,41)*.

As opposed to nNOS and eNOS, iNOS does not appear to be involved in the physiological process of smooth muscle relaxation in the corpora cavernosa *(42)*. In fact increased iNOS which occurs with aging may lead to ED as a result of hypothalamic neuronal damage *(32)*, and to reduction of penile smooth muscle abundance through apoptosis *(32)*. However, recent studies indicate that iNOS may have anti-fibrotic (and thus cytoprotective) properties at certain sites in the penis, including the tunica albuginea *(32,42–45)* and blood vessels *(32)*. It is known that low levels of NO may stimulate collagen synthesis during normal wound healing *(46,47)*. Yet increased expression of iNOS as seen in the aging corpus cavernosum should result in higher and persistent levels of NO, eventually counteracting the excessive collagen deposition of abnormal wound healing *(43)*. This could occur by a number of different mechanisms, including direct inhibition of collagen synthesis by opposing pro-fibrotic factors (reactive oxygen species, TGF-B1), inhibition of the differentiation of fibroblasts and smooth muscle cells, or stimulation of collagen breakdown via activation of metalloproteinases *(42)*. iNOS has been localized in the lining of the corpora cavernosal sinusoidal tissue and the urethra *(37,48,49)*. More studies are needed to determine any potential function of iNOS in the development of ED.

3.1.2   NO/NOS after RRP

Non-nerve-Sparing RRP

NO signaling as a result of NOS neural stimulation is a critical component of the normal erectile process *(50)*; it is clear that the extent to which the CNs are salvaged or damaged during radical prostatectomy is directly proportional to a patient's degree of postoperative ED. Models of bilateral CN injury are associated with high rates of permanent impotence *(34)*. An analysis of the expression of the different NOS isoforms in bilateral CN injured rats revealed that the splice variant *nNOS-Ib* RNA expression was significantly decreased at 7 days following CN injury but not at 14 and 21 days post-resection. However, nNOS protein was significantly decreased between 7 and 21 days following CN injury in the penis *(34)*. Neither iNOS nor eNOS RNA or protein was altered following CN injury, indicating that these isoforms are not able to compensate for the decrease in nNOS *(34)*. Decreased smooth muscle and endothelium were observed 21 days after CN injury *(34)*, which may contribute to the observed ED following prostatectomy. These results directly link cavernous nerve injury and loss of nNOS/NO signaling with ED following radical prostatectomy. In addition, the reduced vasodilation and blood flow resulting from decreased nNOS will result in decreased eNOS activation accomplished via shear stress, and further deplete NO signaling within the penis.

Bilateral Nerve-Sparing RRP

Haffner and colleagues reported that men undergoing bilateral nerve-sparing radical prostatectomy had greater postoperative sexual function scores and were more likely to return to baseline sexual function than men who underwent unilateral or non-nerve-sparing procedures *(51)*. In one study of 129 men undergoing radical prostatectomy for prostate cancer, the 46 patients who had a nerve-sparing procedure had significantly higher postoperative erectile function scores than the 83 patients who had a non-nerve-sparing procedure *(52)*. In another series of 3,477 men with prostate cancer who were treated by radical prostatectomy, 76% of those who were potent preoperatively and underwent a bilateral nerve-sparing procedure were also potent postoperatively, compared with 53% of men who underwent a unilateral nerve-sparing procedure *(53)*.

Although erectile function (as determined by IIEF scores and sexual satisfaction surveys) is clearly the best after bilateral CN-sparing procedures, it does not approach 100%, even in men with normal preoperative erections. This has been attributed to neuropraxia or axonotmesis, as a result of thermal injury, ischemia, and mechanical stretching of the CNs during surgery. These are considered as class I or II nerve injuries according to the Sunderland classification, and are associated with a conduction block *(54)*. The nerves are capable of healing, however, and many men who are impotent immediately following surgery regain their erections over time *(6,7)*. Even if the nerve-sparing technique is meticulously employed, the CNs may be functionally inactive for a period of 6–24 months, with a mean time of 18 months to recovery of maximal erectile function *(55–57)*.

Unilateral Nerve-Sparing RRP

Whereas a bilateral CN-sparing procedure is superior for preservation of erectile function, it has been demonstrated that salvage of one neurovascular bundle is sometimes sufficient and may allow for some degree of neural regeneration *(58)*. Studies in a rodent model of unilateral CN injury revealed upregulation of both nNOS and eNOS proteins, along with the recovery of erectile function *(59)*. Another study in rats showed neural regeneration on the cut side 3 months after unilateral CN resection. This was not observed in bilateral CN injury, where ED remained permanent *(38,60)*. This is supported clinically in humans by the recovery of erectile function over time following CN-sparing procedures *(6,7)*.

3.2 Smooth Muscle/Myosin–Actin/Calcium/Rho-Kinase

The degree of tumescence or detumescence at any given time is determined by the balance between sympathetic and parasympathetic tone in the smooth muscle of the penis *(20)*. Most of the time sympathetic tone dominates, resulting in smooth muscle contraction and penile flaccidity *(61)*. Norepinephrine released from sympathetic nerve endings *(62,63)*, as well as endothelins *(64,65)* and prostaglandin F2-alpha *(66,67)* from the endothelium activate receptors on smooth muscle cells. This initiates a cascade of molecular signaling which leads to an increase in intracellular levels of calcium (Ca). Ca binds to calmodulin, activating myosin light chain (MLC) kinase which phosphorylates MLC. The phosphorylated MLC then interacts with alpha-actin leading to cycling of myosin cross-bridges (heads) and development of force (Fig. 3). It is believed that other molecules are involved in modulating

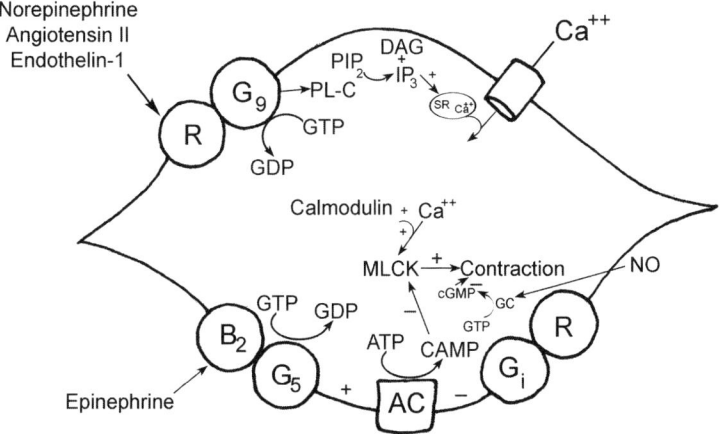

Fig. 3 Cascade of molecular signaling in smooth muscle contraction. SR = sarcoplasmic reticulum, IP3 = inositol triphosphate, DAG = diacylglycerol, PL-C = phospholipase C, NO = nitric oxide, AC = adenylate cyclase, GC = guanylyl cyclase, MLCK = myosin light chain kinase

the contractile state. For example, the protein caldesmon may create a latch state, allowing the force of contraction to be maintained at a low level of myosin phosphorylation with low energy expenditure *(68)*. Only a small amount of penile arterial blood flow occurs in the flaccid state.

The exact mechanism by which cGMP elicits smooth muscle relaxation remains uncertain but is the subject of much study. The commonly accepted pathway involves activation of potassium channels by cGMP and cGMP-specific protein kinase [as well as by NO itself *(69)*], leading to hyperpolarization and closure of voltage-dependent Ca channels *(70,71)*. This elicits a decrease in intracellular Ca, the dissociation of calmodulin from MLC kinase, its phosphorylation and inactivation, the subsequent dephosphorylation of myosin (by MLC phosphatase), and detachment from actin *(70)*.

A second potential mechanism under consideration involves inhibition of the RhoA/Rho-kinase pathway by cGMP-specific protein kinase *(72–75)*. Recent work has identified RhoA, a small G-protein, and its downstream target Rho-kinase as possible mediators of the alpha-adrenergic (norepinephrine) and endothelial (ET-1) triggered smooth muscle contraction in the penile corpora *(76–78)*. This is thought to occur by way of Rho-kinase inhibition of MLC phosphatase. MLC phosphatase de-phosphorylates MLC, stopping MLC from interacting with alpha-actin, and promoting smooth muscle relaxation and erection (Fig. 4). Inhibition of MLC phosphatase by Rho-kinase means there will be more active (phosphorylated) MLC available at the same level of MLC kinase activity (without requiring an increase in cytosolic Ca), effectively "sensitizing" the smooth muscle, and so contributes to the tonic phase of agonist-induced penile smooth muscle contraction and flaccidity *(79–81)*. In human endothelial cells, the RhoA/Rho-kinase pathway was found to inhibit the Akt-dependent phosphorylation and activation of eNOS *(82)*.

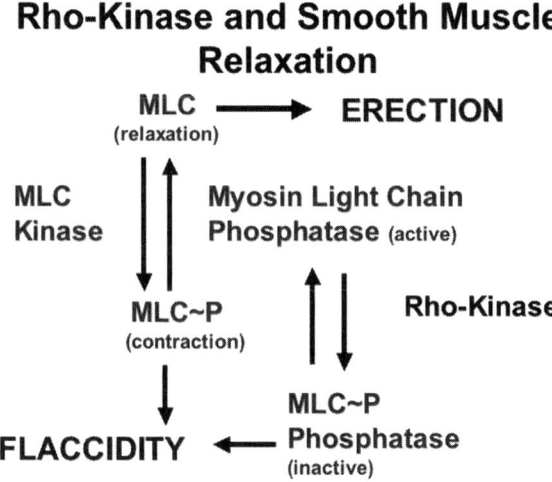

Fig. 4 The role of Rho-kinase site of action in smooth muscle relaxation

Thus an abnormally upregulated RhoA/Rho-kinase pathway could contribute to ED, and inhibition of this pathway presents a potential avenue for ED treatment development *(83)*.

cAMP is another second messenger involved in smooth muscle relaxation, and its cascade of molecular signaling is similar to that of cGMP. It involves the activation of cAMP-specific protein kinases, phosphorylation of proteins and ion channels, and an eventual drop in cytosolic free Ca. A number of studies, however, have suggested that cGMP is a more potent smooth muscle relaxant than cAMP, and a study in knockout mice revealed cGMP to be the main physiologic signal for erection, which cannot be compensated by the cAMP pathway *(84)*. Prostaglandin E-1 (PGE-1) activates adenylate cyclase in smooth muscle cells which generates cAMP. It is clear that smooth muscle physiology is a central component of erectile function, and any process that disrupts smooth muscle abundance or proper functioning can result in ED.

3.3   SHH and the Penis

An emerging concept in the field of erectile dysfunction is penile homeostasis. In order for an erection to occur, the complex and unique sinusoidal morphology of the corpora cavernosa must be maintained. New light has been shed on this process with the identification and investigation of the morphogenic protein Sonic hedgehog (SHH), along with its downstream targets Patched 1 (PTCH1), Hox, bone morphogenetic proteins (BMPs), vascular endothelial growth factor (VEGF), and NOS. SHH is a critical regulator of a conserved pathway of mesenchymal–epithelial signaling which establishes symmetry, regulates proliferation, and specifies tissue identity *(85,86)* of a number of diverse organ systems during embryogenesis. These include the CNS, eyes, axial skeleton and limbs, lungs, liver, gut, and prostate *(87–91)*. SHH also remains active after birth in some organs to regulate post-natal differentiation and homeostasis of adult tissue morphology, including the penis *(92–95)*.

SHH exists in a number of forms due to post-transcriptional modification, and is detected in both the cells that produce it as well as in target tissue *(96–99)*. Although the exact mechanism of SHH signaling in the penis remains to be elucidated, studies from other organs suggest a potential mechanism. SHH binding to PTCH1 relieves a PTCH1-mediated repression of Smoothened (Smo), a seven transmembrane protein. Smo then initiates a signaling cascade, activating targets including the Gli family of transcription factors, BMP4 (which has a negative effect on growth), and *Hox* genes (positive growth effectors) *(100)* (Fig. 5). Some long-range effects of SHH are thought to be caused by induction of secondary signals including PTCH1, Hox, BMP4, NOS, and VEGFA, a potent angiogenic growth factor *(94,101–103)*.

The essential role of *Shh* during penile embryogenesis has been shown in murine experiments, where dynamic expression of *Shh* and its targets was observed during genital tubercle outgrowth and differentiation *(104)*. The complete absence of external genitalia is observed in mice with targeted deletions of *Shh* or double knockouts of *Hoxd-13* and *Hoxa-13* *(105,106)*. The penis is unique in that it undergoes most of its differentiation in the period after birth, with postnatal differentiation of erectile tissue containing both lacunae and trabeculae occurring approximately 1 week after birth *(107)*. Androgen secretion starts to increase at 4 weeks of age, and cavernous tissue resembles the adult configuration by postnatal day 40. *Shh* is expressed in the rat penis throughout postnatal differentiation, as well as in the adult, with expression restricted to areas required for erection to occur *(95)*. SHH function is crucial for establishing and maintaining corpora cavernosal morphology. Inhibition of SHH function during postnatal development and in the adult organ results in significantly increased apoptosis in penile smooth muscle and loss of sinusoidal morphology *(95,108)*. These morphological changes are so severe that they affect the physiology of the tissue and cause ED *(95)*. Podlasek et al. have recently shown that these effects are reversible, with sinusoidal morphology being partially re-established 4

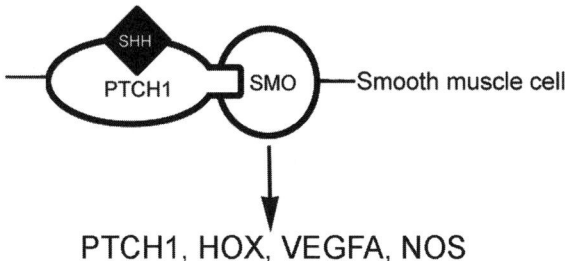

Fig. 5 The SHH signaling pathway

weeks after SHH inhibition and completely re-established by 6 weeks following inhibition *(108)*. These results suggest the potential of SHH to be developed into a therapy to treat morphology changes in the penis that accompany ED.

CN injury causes apoptosis *(108–110)* and significantly decreased SHH protein *(108)*. Significantly increased apoptosis was identified primarily in cavernosal smooth muscle of the Sprague Dawley bilateral CN cut rat model, which was assayed by TUNEL and electron microscopic analyses *(108)*. SHH inhibition in the corpora cavernosa (5E1 SHH inhibitor) caused a very similar increase in smooth muscle apoptosis in the penis *(108)*. This result is supported by previous observations of increased apoptosis and decreased SHH protein in another model of neuropathy, the BB/WOR diabetic rat *(111)*. Since SHH inhibition is a cause of smooth muscle apoptosis in the penis and SHH protein is significantly decreased in both the Sprague Dawley CN injury model and the BB/WOR diabetic model of neuropathy, this suggests that decreased SHH protein may play a role in the induction of apoptosis that occurs following neuropathy/CN injury and which leads to ED. Studies by User et al. showed the time course of apoptosis in the penis that occurs following bilateral CN resection *(109)*. Apoptosis was most abundant in the first week following CN injury, but remained elevated above baseline at 21 days post-injury *(108,109)*. If the apoptosis that occurs following CN injury/prostatectomy could be suppressed while the CN regenerates, this would lead to preservation of penile morphology, prevention of fibrosis, and resumption of normal erectile function more quickly.

A recent study examined if SHH protein treatment could prevent smooth muscle apoptosis in the penile corpora cavernosa that occurs with CN injury. This study was based on the hypothesis that decreased SHH protein is a cause of ED in neurological models of impotence by increasing apoptosis in penile smooth muscle, which leads to morphological changes within the corpora cavernosa sinusoidal tissue, and thus ED. SHH protein was soaked in Affi-Gel beads (delivery vehicle), which were injected into the corpora cavernosa at the time of CN cut surgery. TUNEL assay was then performed at 2, 4, and 8 days following CN surgery/SHH treatment *(108)*. At 2 days there was no significant change in the level of apoptosis, however, at 4 days following CN injury/SHH treatment there was a significant decrease in apoptosis in the presence of SHH protein of 1.3-fold [Fig. 6, *(108)*]. When double the concentration of SHH protein was used in the experiment the level of apoptosis was further suppressed by 2.5-fold [Fig. *6*, *(108)*]. At 8 days following CN injury/SHH treatment, apoptosis was further decreased in the presence of SHH protein by 3-fold [Fig. *6*, *(108)*]. These results are significant in that they show that SHH treatment at the time of CN injury was able to suppress/prevent CN injury-induced apoptosis, and suggests that SHH has significant potential to be developed as a treatment to prevent smooth muscle apoptosis in the penis post-prostatectomy.

3.4   Supporting Cast/Integration

Other molecules have been implicated in effecting the erectile response. Acetylcholine has been shown to contribute to penile erection by presynaptic inhibition

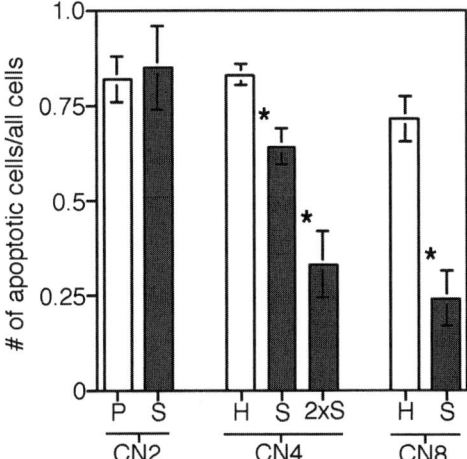

Fig. 6 The number of apoptotic cells/all cells at 2, 4, and 8 days following CN injury and SHH treatment. Apoptosis was significantly decreased by 1.3-fold at 4 days following CN injury/SHH treatment. When double the concentration of SHH protein was used in the experiment the level of apoptosis was further suppressed by 2.5-fold. At 8 days following CN injury/SHH treatment, apoptosis was further decreased in the presence of SHH protein by 3-fold. These results show that SHH treatment at the time of CN injury was able to suppress/prevent CN injury-induced apoptosis. P = PBS control, S = SHH-treated, H = heat-inactivated SHH control. *Asterisk* indicates significant differences in apoptosis/all cells

of adrenergic neurons *(112)* as well as stimulation of the release of NO from endothelial cells *(113)*. Vasoactive intestinal polypeptide (VIP) induces smooth muscle relaxation, and is thought to be mediated by NO *(114)*. Co-localization of acetylcholine, VIP, and nNOS in parasympathetic neurons suggests a role for VIP in erectile function and implies a co-operative and synergistic induction of erection *(115)*. These biochemical signals require future study to determine potential function in ED development following prostatectomy.

4 Long-Term ED

ED following radical prostatectomy appears to have two phases with separate yet related causes. The first, or immediate phase, has been attributed to a lack of NO signaling from injured or stressed CNs. It may also be due in part to compromise of the cavernosal arterial blood supply (ligation of accessory pudendal arteries). The second, or long-term phase, is due to the multiple pathophysiologic consequences resulting from nerve injury and vascular dysfunction.

4.1 Hypoxia

One end result of the derangements in these biochemical and physiologic pathways is chronic penile tissue hypoxia. During erection the oxygen tension in the penis rises by 250% (30 mm Hg flaccid and 100 mm Hg erect), and in men with intact CNs nocturnal erections provide as much as 3 h of regular oxygenation of penile tissue per day. As mentioned previously, even when a nerve-sparing procedure is performed the mean time to recovery of maximal erectile function is 18 months due to neuropraxia of the CNs. The lack of these nocturnal (as well as daytime) erections following radical prostatectomy decreases or eliminates the period of daily oxygenation and results in a persistent state of penile hypoxemia, which may contribute to penile fibrosis (116). It has been shown that there is a decrease in the oxygen tension of cavernosal blood in patients with ED due to arterial insufficiency as compared to those with psychogenic ED (117). Compounding the problem, Kim et al. showed that the NO-mediated relaxation of smooth muscle is limited under conditions of reduced oxygen tension, regardless of the integrity of the CNs and endothelium (118). Therefore penile hypoxia may contribute to ED both by inhibiting molecular signaling as well as effecting permanent morphologic changes.

4.2   Ultra-structural End Organ Changes and Long-Term ED

It is believed that chronic hypoxia and denervation of erectile tissue following radical prostatectomy result in permanent ED via apoptosis of smooth muscle cells, deposition of collagen (scar), and penile fibrosis (110,119,120). Prostaglandin E-1 and 2 (PGE-1, PGE-2) formation is oxygen dependent, and an increase in oxygen tension is associated with elevation of PGE-1 and suppression of TGF-B1 – induced collagen synthesis in rabbit and human corpus cavernosum (121–123). Recall also that PGE-1 directly promotes smooth muscle relaxation via cAMP. A recent evaluation of penile tissue in rats following bilateral CN incision revealed significant over-expression of hypoxia-related substances, including hypoxia-inducible factor-1 alpha (HIF-1A), transforming growth factor B1 (TGF-B1), and collagen 1 and 3 at 3 months post-injury (124). Hypoxia also causes an increase in release of potent vasoconstrictor molecules such as endothelin-1, a pro-fibrotic peptide, with synthesis influenced by TGF-B1 (125). Iacono et al. performed corporal biopsies in men before and after prostatectomy, documenting diminished trabecular elastic and smooth muscle fibers, as well as significantly increased collagen content at 2 months post-surgery, with further deterioration at 12 months (126). Yet another study in rats showed reduced wet weight and DNA content of the denervated penis as compared to controls (109). Clinically this manifests as penile fibrotic changes (127) and reduced penile length and circumference (128,129).

It seems reasonable that fibrotic erectile tissue will not expand as readily as normal erectile tissue, and with decreased smooth muscle abundance due to apoptosis the cavernosal sinusoids will not dilate and become engorged during arousal as well. Nehra et al. demonstrated that men with the lowest percentage of smooth muscle composition of the corpora required the highest flow to maintain erection on Doppler studies (130). Histologic analysis revealed that these men also had a relative predominance of connective tissue. Another phenomenon occurs concomitantly, which compounds the problem: venous leakage. The failure of the cavernosal bodies to expand combined with the loss of elastic fibers in the tunica albuginea results in loss of compression of the subtunical venular plexus and emissary veins; thus, venous leakage ensues. The degree of leakage worsens with time. Patients undergoing nerve-sparing radical prostatectomy were evaluated with penile Doppler ultrasound or dynamic infusion cavernosometry after surgery, and were found to have a progressive increase in venous leakage from 14% at 4 months to 50% at over 12 months *(17)*. This study also showed worse prognosis for return of functional erections in men with venous leakage (as compared to patients with ED and normal Doppler's or isolated arterial insufficiency). This does present a limited opportunity for prevention, since a significant decrease in venous leakage was observed at 6 months postoperatively in patients following a promptly instituted vasoactive recovery program *(131)*.

5 Conclusions

The causes of post-prostatectomy ED are multi-factorial since there are numerous pathways that converge to control normal erection with many complicated and interwoven layers of feedback and regulation. We are likely just scratching the surface of discovery in this field; however, each new finding presents the potential for prevention and/or treatment of ED following radical prostatectomy.

Active investigation continues in the fields of penile homeostasis, the pathophysiology of ED, control of inflammation and fibrosis, prevention or limitation of smooth muscle apoptosis, and neural regenerative strategies. In conclusion, we know that nerve-sparing radical prostatectomy is insufficient to prevent ED. The insult of surgery to the erectile mechanism occurs while in the operating room and sets off a cascade of derangements with irreversible loss of cavernosal smooth muscle. Current research by many investigators offers a wealth of possibilities for the development of new interventions to preserve normal erectile function and to treat ED as it develops in the future.

Acknowledgements   The authors would like to thank Yi Tang from Children's Memorial Hospital, Chicago for the electron microscopic analysis of normal penile tissue.

References

1. Jemal, A., et al. (2006) Cancer statistics 2006. *CA Cancer J. Clin.* **56**(2), 106–130.
2. Vale, J. (2000) Erectile dysfunction following radical therapy for prostate cancer. *Radiother. Oncol.* **57**(3), 301–305.
3. Kendirci, M., and Hellstrom, W.J. (2004) Current concepts in the management of erectile dysfunction in men with prostate cancer. *Clin. Prostate Cancer* **3**(2), 87–92.
4. Katz, A. (2005) What happened? Sexual consequences of prostate cancer and its treatment. *Can. Fam. Physician* **51**, 977–982.

5. Alivizatos, G., and Skolarikos, A. (2005) Incontinence and erectile dysfunction following radical prostatectomy: a review. *Sci. World J.* **5,** 747–758.
6. Penson, D.F., et al. (2005) 5-year urinary and sexual outcomes after radical prostatectomy: results from the prostate cancer outcomes study. *J. Urol.* **173**(5), 1701–1705.
7. Miyao, N., et al. (2001) Recovery of sexual function after nerve-sparing radical prostatectomy or cystectomy. *Int. J. Urol.* **8**(4), 158–164.
8. Crawford, E.D., et al. (1997) Comparison of perspectives on prostate cancer: analyses of survey data. *Urology* **50**(3), 366–372.
9. Litwin, M.S., et al. (1999) Sexual function and bother after radical prostatectomy or radiation for prostate cancer: multivariate quality-of-life analysis from CaPSURE. Cancer of the Prostate Strategic Urologic Research Endeavor. Urology **54**(3), 503–508.
10. Shindel, A., et al. (2005) Sexual dysfunction in female partners of men who have undergone radical prostatectomy correlates with sexual dysfunction of the male partner. *J. Sex. Med.* **2**(6), 833–841; discussion 841.
11. Rabbani, F., et al. (2000) Factors predicting recovery of erections after radical prostatectomy. *J. Urol.* **164**(6), 1929–1934.
12. Johannes, C.B., et al. (2000) Incidence of erectile dysfunction in men 40 to 69 years old: longitudinal results from the Massachusetts male aging study. *J. Urol.* **163**(2), 460–463.
13. Leeson, T.S., and Leeson, C.R. (1965) The fine structure of cavernous tissue in the adult rat penis. *Invest. Urol.* **3**(2), 144–154.
14. Goldstein, A.M.B., Meehan, J.P., and Zakhary, R. (1982) New observations on microarchitecture of corpora cavernosa in man and possible relationship to mechanism of erection. *Urology* **20,** 259.
15. Breza, J., et al. (1989) Detailed anatomy of penile neurovascular structures: surgical significance. *J. Urol.* **141**(2), 437–443.
16. Kim, E.D., Blackburn, D., and McVary, K.T. (1994) Post-radical prostatectomy penile blood flow: assessment with color flow Doppler ultrasound. *J. Urol.* **152**(6 Pt 2), 2276–2279.
17. Mulhall, J.P., et al. (2002) Erectile dysfunction after radical prostatectomy: hemodynamic profiles and their correlation with the recovery of erectile function. *J. Urol.* **167**(3), 1371–1375.
18. Rogers, C.G., Trock, B.P., and Walsh, P.C. (2004) Preservation of accessory pudendal arteries during radical retropubic prostatectomy: surgical technique and results. *Urology* **64**(1), 148–151.
19. Aboseif, S.R., et al. (1989) Penile venous drainage in erectile dysfunction. Anatomical, radiological and functional considerations. *Br. J. Urol.* **64**(2), 183–190.
20. Andersson, K.E., and Wagner, G. (1995) Physiology of penile erection. *Physiol. Rev.* **75**(1), 191–236.
21. Walsh, P.C., and Donker, P.J. (1982) Impotence following radical prostatectomy: insight into etiology and prevention. *J. Urol.* **128**(3), 492–497.
22. Ignarro, L.J., et al. (1990) Nitric oxide and cyclic GMP formation upon electrical field stimulation cause relaxation of corpus cavernosum smooth muscle. *Biochem. Biophys. Res. Commun.* **170**(2), 843–850.
23. Holmquist, F., et al. (1991) Effects of the nitric oxide synthase inhibitor NG-nitro-L-arginine on the erectile response to cavernous nerve stimulation in the rabbit. *Acta Physiol. Scand.* **143**(3), 299–304.
24. Kim, N., et al. (1991) A nitric oxide-like factor mediates nonadrenergic-noncholinergic neurogenic relaxation of penile corpus cavernosum smooth muscle. *J. Clin. Invest.* **88**(1), 112–118.
25. Pickard, R.S., Powell, P.H., and Zar, M.A. (1991) The effect of inhibitors of nitric oxide biosynthesis and cyclic GMP formation on nerve-evoked relaxation of human cavernosal smooth muscle. *Br. J. Pharmacol.* **104**(3), 755–759.
26. Burnett, A.L., et al. (1992) Nitric oxide: a physiologic mediator of penile erection. *Science* **257**(5068), 401–403.

27. Rajfer, J., et al. (1992) Nitric oxide as a mediator of relaxation of the corpus cavernosum in response to nonadrenergic, noncholinergic neurotransmission. *N. Engl. J. Med.* **326**(2), 90–94.

28. Trigo-Rocha, F., et al. (1993) The role of cyclic adenosine monophosphate, cyclic guanosine monophosphate, endothelium and nonadrenergic, noncholinergic neurotransmission in canine penile erection. *J. Urol.* **149**(4), 872–877.

29. Burnett, A.L., and Musicki, B. (2005) The nitric oxide signaling pathway in the penis. *Curr. Pharm. Des.* **11**(31), 3987–3994.

30. Rajasekaran, M., et al. (1998) Ex vivo expression of nitric oxide synthase isoforms (eNOS/iNOS) and calmodulin in human penile cavernosal cells. *J. Urol.* **160**(6 Pt 1), 2210–2215.

31. Ehren, I., Adolfsson, J., and Wiklund, N.P. (1994) Nitric oxide synthase activity in the human urogenital tract. *Urol. Res.* **22**(5), 287–290.

32. Magee, T.R., et al. (2003) Protein inhibitor of nitric oxide synthase (NOS) and the N-methyl-D-aspartate receptor are expressed in the rat and mouse penile nerves and colocalize with penile neuronal NOS. *Biol. Reprod.* **68**(2), 478–488.

33. Gonzalez-Cadavid, N.F., and Rajfer, J. (2000) Therapeutic stimulation of penile nitric oxide synthase (NOS) and related pathways. *Drugs Today (Barc)* **36**(2–3), 163–174.

34. Podlasek, C.A., et al. (2001) Analysis of NOS isoform changes in a post radical prostatectomy model of erectile dysfunction. *Int. J. Impot. Res.* **13**(Suppl 5), S1–15.

35. Hurt, K.J., et al. (2002) Akt-dependent phosphorylation of endothelial nitric-oxide synthase mediates penile erection. *Proc. Natl. Acad. Sci. USA* **99**(6), 4061–4066.

36. Burnett, A.L. (2004) Novel nitric oxide signaling mechanisms regulate the erectile response. *Int. J. Impot. Res.* **16**(Suppl 1), S15–S19.

37. Podlasek, C.A., et al. (2001) Characterization and localization of nitric oxide synthase isoforms in the BB/WOR diabetic rat. *J. Urol.* **166**(2), 746–755.

38. Jung, G.W., et al. (1999) The role of growth factor on regeneration of nitric oxide synthase (NOS) – containing nerves after cavernous neurotomy in the rats. *Int. J. Impot. Res.* **11**(4), 227–235.

39. Ujiie, K., et al. (1994) Localization and regulation of endothelial NO synthase mRNA expression in rat kidney. *Am. J. Physiol.* **267**(2 Pt 2), F296–F302.

40. Moncada, S. (1997) Nitric oxide in the vasculature: physiology and pathophysiology. *Ann. NY. Acad. Sci.* **811**, 60–67; discussion 67–69.

41. Musicki, B., et al. (2004) Phosphorylated endothelial nitric oxide synthase mediates vascular endothelial growth factor-induced penile erection. *Biol. Reprod.* **70**(2), 282–289.

42. Gonzalez-Cadavid, N.F., and Rajfer, J. (2005) The pleiotropic effects of inducible nitric oxide synthase (iNOS) on the physiology and pathology of penile erection. *Curr. Pharm. Des.* **11**(31), 4041–4046.

43. Ferrini, M.G., et al. (2002) Antifibrotic role of inducible nitric oxide synthase. *Nitric Oxide* **6**(3), 283–294.

44. Valente, E.G., et al. (2003) L-arginine and phosphodiesterase (PDE) inhibitors counteract fibrosis in the Peyronie's fibrotic plaque and related fibroblast cultures. *Nitric Oxide* **9**(4), 229–244.

45. Gholami, S.S., et al. (2003) Peyronie's disease: a review. *J. Urol.* **169**(4), 1234–1241.

46. Shi, H.P., et al. (2001) The role of iNOS in wound healing. *Surgery* **130**(2), 225–229.

47. Frank, S., et al. (2002) Nitric oxide drives skin repair: novel functions of an established mediator. *Kidney Int.* **61**(3), 882–888.

48. Seftel, A.D., et al. (1997) Advanced glycation end products in human penis: elevation in diabetic tissue, site of deposition, and possible effect through iNOS or eNOS. *Urology* **50**(6), 1016–1026.

49. Rajasekaran, M., Hellstrom, W.J., and Sikka, S.C. (2001) Nitric oxide induces oxidative stress and mediates cytotoxicity to human cavernosal cells in culture. *J. Androl.* **22**(1), 34–39.

50. Burnett, A.L., et al. (1993) Immunohistochemical localization of nitric oxide synthase in the autonomic innervation of the human penis. *J. Urol.* **150**(1), 73–76.

51. Haffner, M.C., et al. (2005) Health-related quality-of-life outcomes after anatomic retropubic radical prostatectomy in the phosphodiesterase type 5 ERA: impact of neurovascular bundle preservation. *Urology* **66**(2), 371–376.

52. Gralnek, D., et al. (2000) Differences in sexual function and quality of life after nerve sparing and nonnerve sparing radical retropubic prostatectomy. *J. Urol.* **163**(4), 1166–1169; discussion 1169–1170.

53. Kundu, S.D., et al. (2004) Potency, continence and complications in 3,477 consecutive radical retropubic prostatectomies. *J. Urol.* **172**(6 Pt 1), 2227–2231.

54. Sunderland, S. (1977) Some anatomical and pathophysiological data relevant to facial nerve injury and repair. In: Fisch, U., ed. *Facial Nerve Surgery*. Birmingham, Alabama: Aesculapius Publishers.

55. Zippe, C.D., et al. (2001) Management of erectile dysfunction following radical prostatectomy. *Curr. Urol. Rep.* **2**(6), 495–503.

56. Walsh, P.C., et al. (2000) Patient-reported urinary continence and sexual function after anatomic radical prostatectomy. *Urology* **55**(1), 58–61.

57. Walsh, P.C. (2001) Nerve grafts are rarely necessary and are unlikely to improve sexual function in men undergoing anatomic radical prostatectomy. *Urology* **57**(6), 1020–1024.

58. Carrier, S., et al. (1995) Regeneration of nitric oxide synthase-containing nerves after cavernous nerve neurotomy in the rat. *J. Urol.* **153**(5), 1722–1727.

59. El-Sakka, A.I., et al. (1998) Effect of cavernous nerve freezing on protein and gene expression of nitric oxide synthase in the rat penis and pelvic ganglia. *J. Urol.* **160**(6 Pt 1), 2245–2252.

60. Jung, G.W., Spencer, E.M., and Lue, T.F. (1998) Growth hormone enhances regeneration of nitric oxide synthase-containing penile nerves after cavernous nerve neurotomy in rats. *J. Urol.* **160**(5), 1899–1904.

61. Andersson, K.E. (2001) Pharmacology of penile erection. *Pharmacol. Rev.* **53**(3), 417–450.

62. Hedlund, H., and Andersson, K.E. (1985) Comparison of the responses to drugs acting on adrenoreceptors and muscarinic receptors in human isolated corpus cavernosum and cavernous artery. *J. Auton. Pharmacol.* **5**(1), 81–88.

63. Diederichs, W., et al. (1990) Norepinephrine involvement in penile detumescence. *J. Urol.* **143**(6), 1264–1266.

64. Holmquist, F., Andersson, K.E., and Hedlund, H. (1990) Actions of endothelin on isolated corpus cavernosum from rabbit and man. *Acta Physiol. Scand.* **139**(1), 113–122.

65. Saenz de Tejada, I., et al. (1991) Endothelin: localization, synthesis, activity, and receptor types in human penile corpus cavernosum. *Am. J. Physiol.* **261**(4 Pt 2), H1078–H1085.

66. Hedlund, H., et al. (1989) Characterization of contraction-mediating prostanoid receptors in human penile erectile tissues. *J. Urol.* **141**(1), 182–186.

67. Azadzoi, K.M., et al. (1992) Endothelium-derived nitric oxide and cyclooxygenase products modulate corpus cavernosum smooth muscle tone. *J. Urol.* **147**(1), 220–225.

68. Lue, T.F. (2002) Chapter 45: Physiology of Penile Erection and Pathophysiology of Erectile Dysfunction and Priapism. In: Walsh, P.C., Retik, A.B., Vaughan, E.D., and Wein, A.J., eds. *Campbell's Urology*, 8th edn. Philadelphia, PA: WB Saunders Co.

69. Gupta, S., et al. (1995) Possible role of Na(+)-K(+)-ATPase in the regulation of human corpus cavernosum smooth muscle contractility by nitric oxide. *Br. J. Pharmacol.* **116**(4), 2201–2206.

70. Draznin, M.B., Rapoport, R.M., and Murad, F. (1986) Myosin light chain phosphorylation in contraction and relaxation of intact rat thoracic aorta. *Int. J. Biochem.* **18**(10), 917–928.

71. Christ, G.J., et al. (1999) Ion channels and gap junctions: their role in erectile physiology, dysfunction, and future therapy. *Mol. Urol.* **3**(2), 61–73.

72. Sawada, N., et al. (2001) cGMP-dependent protein kinase phosphorylates and inactivates RhoA. *Biochem. Biophys. Res. Commun.* **280**(3), 798–805.

73. Sauzeau, V., et al. (2000) Cyclic GMP-dependent protein kinase signaling pathway inhibits RhoA-induced Ca2+ sensitization of contraction in vascular smooth muscle. *J. Biol. Chem.* **275**(28), 21722–21729.

74. Gudi, T., et al. (2002) cGMP-dependent protein kinase inhibits serum-response element-dependent transcription by inhibiting rho activation and functions. *J. Biol. Chem.* **277**(40), 37382–37393.

75. Chitaley, K., Webb, R.C., and Mills, T.M. (2003) The ups and downs of Rho-kinase and penile erection: upstream regulators and downstream substrates of rho-kinase and their potential role in the erectile response. *Int. J. Impot. Res.* **15**(2), 105–109.

76. Wang, H., et al. (2002) RhoA-mediated Ca2+ sensitization in erectile function. *J. Biol. Chem.* **277**(34), 30614–30621.

77. Rees, R.W., et al. (2002) Human and rabbit cavernosal smooth muscle cells express Rho-kinase. *Int. J. Impot. Res.* **14**(1), 1–7.

78. Mills, T.M., et al. (2001) Effect of Rho-kinase inhibition on vasoconstriction in the penile circulation. *J. Appl. Physiol.* **91**(3), 1269–1273.

79. Somlyo, A.P., and Somlyo, A.V. (2003) Ca2+ sensitivity of smooth muscle and nonmuscle myosin II: modulated by G proteins, kinases, and myosin phosphatase. *Physiol. Rev.* **83**(4), 1325–1358.

80. Somlyo, A.P., and Somlyo, A.V. (2000) Signal transduction by G-proteins, rho-kinase and protein phosphatase to smooth muscle and non-muscle myosin II. *J. Physiol.* **522**(Pt 2), 177–185.

81. Amano, M., et al. (1999) The COOH terminus of Rho-kinase negatively regulates rho-kinase activity. *J. Biol. Chem.* **274**(45), 32418–32424.

82. Ming, X.F., et al. (2002) Rho GTPase/Rho kinase negatively regulates endothelial nitric oxide synthase phosphorylation through the inhibition of protein kinase B/Akt in human endothelial cells. *Mol. Cell Biol.* **22**(24), 8467–8477.

83. Linder, A.E., et al. (2005) Rho-kinase and RGS-containing RhoGEFs as molecular targets for the treatment of erectile dysfunction. *Curr. Pharm. Des.* **11**(31), 4029–4040.

84. Hedlund, P., et al. (2000) Erectile dysfunction in cyclic GMP-dependent kinase I-deficient mice. *Proc. Natl. Acad. Sci. USA* **97**(5), 2349–2354.

85. Marti, E., and Bovolenta, P. (2002) Sonic hedgehog in CNS development: one signal, multiple outputs. *Trends Neurosci.* **25**(2), 89–96.

86. Machold, R., and Fishell, G. (2002) Hedgehog patterns midbrain architecture. *Trends Neurosci.* **25**(1), 10–11.

87. Podlasek, C.A., et al. (1999) Prostate development requires Sonic hedgehog expressed by the urogenital sinus epithelium. *Dev. Biol.* **209**(1), 28–39.

88. Niswander, L., et al. (1994) A positive feedback loop coordinates growth and patterning in the vertebrate limb. *Nature* **371**(6498), 609–612.

89. Ekker, S.C., et al. (1995) Patterning activities of vertebrate hedgehog proteins in the developing eye and brain. *Curr. Biol.* **5**(8), 944–955.

90. Bitgood, M.J., and McMahon, A.P. (1995) Hedgehog and Bmp genes are coexpressed at many diverse sites of cell-cell interaction in the mouse embryo. *Dev. Biol.* **172**(1), 126–138.

91. Bellusci, S., et al. (1997) Involvement of Sonic hedgehog (Shh) in mouse embryonic lung growth and morphogenesis. *Development* **124**(1), 53–63.

92. Traiffort, E., et al. (2001) High expression and anterograde axonal transport of aminoterminal sonic hedgehog in the adult hamster brain. *Eur. J. Neurosci.* **14**(5), 839–850.

93. Thomas, M.K., et al. (2000) Hedgehog signaling regulation of insulin production by pancreatic beta-cells. *Diabetes* **49**(12), 2039–2047.

94. Pola, R., et al. The morphogen Sonic hedgehog is an indirect angiogenic agent upregulating two families of angiogenic growth factors. *Nat. Med.* **7**(6), 706–711.

95. Podlasek, C.A., et al. (2003) Sonic hedgehog cascade is required for penile postnatal morphogenesis, differentiation, and adult homeostasis. *Biol. Reprod.* **68**(2), 423–438.

96. Zeng, X., et al. (2001) A freely diffusible form of Sonic hedgehog mediates long-range signalling. *Nature* **411**(6838), 716–720.
97. Martin, G. (1996) Pass the butter. *Science* **274**(5285), 203–204.
98. Lewis, P.M., et al. (2001) Cholesterol modification of sonic hedgehog is required for long-range signaling activity and effective modulation of signaling by Ptc1. *Cell* **105**(5), 599–612.
99. Gritli-Linde, A., et al. (2001) The whereabouts of a morphogen: direct evidence for short- and graded long-range activity of hedgehog signaling peptides. *Dev. Biol.* **236**(2), 364–386.
100. Murone, M., Rosenthal, A., and de Sauvage, F.J. (1999) Sonic hedgehog signaling by the patched-smoothened receptor complex. *Curr. Biol.* **9**(2), 76–84.
101. Lawson, N.D., Vogel, A.M., and Weinstein, B.M. (2002) Sonic hedgehog and vascular endothelial growth factor act upstream of the Notch pathway during arterial endothelial differentiation. *Dev. Cell* **3**(1), 127–136.
102. Motoyama, J., et al. (1998) Ptch2, a second mouse Patched gene is co-expressed with Sonic hedgehog. *Nat. Genet.* **18**(2), 104–106.
103. Alcedo, J., et al. (1996) The Drosophila smoothened gene encodes a seven-pass membrane protein, a putative receptor for the hedgehog signal. *Cell* **86**(2), 221–232.
104. Haraguchi, R., et al. (2001) Unique functions of Sonic hedgehog signaling during external genitalia development. *Development* **128**(21), 4241–4250.
105. Perriton, C.L., et al. (2002) Sonic hedgehog signaling from the urethral epithelium controls external genital development. *Dev. Biol.* **247**(1), 26–46.
106. Kondo, T., et al. (1997) Of fingers, toes and penises. *Nature* **390**(6655), 29.
107. Leeson, T.S., and Leeson, C.R. (1966) Penile cavernous tissue: an electron microscopic study of its development in the rat. *Acta Anat. (Basel)* **63**(3), 404–417.
108. Podlasek, C.A., et al. (2007) Regulation of cavernous nerve injury-induced apoptosis by sonic hedgehog. *Biol. Reprod.* **76**(1), 19–28.
109. User, H.M., et al. (2003) Penile weight and cell subtype specific changes in a post-radical prostatectomy model of erectile dysfunction. *J. Urol.* **169**(3), 1175–1179.
110. Klein, L.T., et al. (1997) Apoptosis in the rat penis after penile denervation. *J. Urol.* **158**(2), 626–630.
111. Podlasek, C.A., et al. (2003) Altered Sonic hedgehog signaling is associated with morphological abnormalities in the penis of the BB/WOR diabetic rat. *Biol. Reprod.* **69**(3), 816–827.
112. Saenz de Tejada, I., et al. (1989) Regulation of adrenergic activity in penile corpus cavernosum. *J. Urol.* **142**(4), 1117–1121.
113. Saenz de Tejada, I., et al. (1989) Impaired neurogenic and endothelium-mediated relaxation of penile smooth muscle from diabetic men with impotence. *N. Engl. J. Med.* **320**(16), 1025–1030.
114. Kim, Y.C., et al. (1995) Modulation of vasoactive intestinal polypeptide (VIP)-mediated relaxation by nitric oxide and prostanoids in the rabbit corpus cavernosum. *J. Urol.* **153**(3 Pt 1), 807–810.
115. Hedlund, P., Alm, P., and Andersson, K.E. (1999) NO synthase in cholinergic nerves and NO-induced relaxation in the rat isolated corpus cavernosum. *Br. J. Pharmacol.* **127**(2), 349–360.
116. Moreland, R.B. (1998) Is there a role of hypoxemia in penile fibrosis: a viewpoint presented to the Society for the Study of Impotence. *Int. J. Impot. Res.* **10**(2), 113–120.
117. Tarhan, F., et al. (1997) Cavernous oxygen tension in the patients with erectile dysfunction. *Int. J. Impot. Res.* **9**(3), 149–153.
118. Kim, N., et al. (1993) Oxygen tension regulates the nitric oxide pathway. Physiological role in penile erection. *J. Clin. Invest.* **91**(2), 437–442.
119. Yao, K.S., Clayton, M., and O'Dwyer, P.J. (1995) Apoptosis in human adenocarcinoma HT29 cells induced by exposure to hypoxia. *J. Natl. Cancer Inst.* **87**(2), 117–122.

120. Yamanaka, M., et al. (2002) Loss of anti-apoptotic genes in aging rat crura. *J. Urol.* **168**(5), 2296–2300.

121. Daley, J.T., et al. (1996) Prostanoid production in rabbit corpus cavernosum: I. regulation by oxygen tension. *J. Urol.* **155**(4), 1482–1487.

122. Nehra, A., et al. (1999) Transforming growth factor-beta1 (TGF-beta1) is sufficient to induce fibrosis of rabbit corpus cavernosum in vivo. *J. Urol.* **162**(3 Pt 1), 910–915.

123. Moreland, R.B., et al. (1995) PGE1 suppresses the induction of collagen synthesis by transforming growth factor-beta 1 in human corpus cavernosum smooth muscle. *J. Urol.* **153**(3 Pt 1), 826–834.

124. Leungwattanakij, S., et al. (2003) Cavernous neurotomy causes hypoxia and fibrosis in rat corpus cavernosum. *J. Androl.* **24**(2), 239–245.

125. Granchi, S., et al. (2002) Expression and regulation of endothelin-1 and its receptors in human penile smooth muscle cells. *Mol. Hum. Reprod.* **8**(12), 1053–1064.

126. Iacono, F., et al. (2005) Histological alterations in cavernous tissue after radical prostatectomy. *J. Urol.* **173**(5), 1673–1676.

127. Ciancio, S.J., and Kim, E.D. (2000) Penile fibrotic changes after radical retropubic prostatectomy. *BJU Int.* **85**(1), 101–106.

128. Savoie, M., Kim, S.S., and Soloway, M.S. (2003) A prospective study measuring penile length in men treated with radical prostatectomy for prostate cancer. *J. Urol.* **169**(4), 1462–1464.

129. Fraiman, M.C., Lepor, H., and McCullough, A.R. (1999) Changes in Penile morphometrics in men with erectile dysfunction after nerve-sparing radical retropubic prostatectomy. *Mol. Urol.*. **3**(2): 109–115.

130. Nehra, A., et al. (1996) Mechanisms of venous leakage: a prospective clinicopathological correlation of corporeal function and structure. *J. Urol.* **156**(4), 1320–1329.

131. Montorsi, F., et al. (1997) Recovery of spontaneous erectile function after nerve-sparing radical retropubic prostatectomy with and without early intracavernous injections of alprostadil: results of a prospective, randomized trial. *J. Urol.* **158**(4), 1408–1410.

Chapter 4
Pathophysiology of Erectile Dysfunction Following Radiation Therapy

Victoria J. Croog and Michael J. Zelefsky

Abstract   The development of erectile dysfunction (ED) after definitive prostate radiotherapy is multi-factorial in nature, and the major pathophysiologic injuries differ from those that affect patients after radical prostatectomy (RP). There is now compelling evidence that endothelial cell damage in nearby erectile tissue as a direct result of radiotherapy contributes significantly to the relatively delayed onset of post-treatment ED. Conversely, the injury to the neurovascular bundles that is central to the onset of ED after RP does not appear to be a major causative force in the setting of radiotherapy. Whether damage to the penile bulb contributes to the onset of radiation-associated impotence (RAI) is highly controversial and remains unclear. This review will examine the various functional and observational studies that have helped to highlight the injuries relevant to the development of RAI.

Keywords   Prostate radiation; brachytherapy; external beam radiotherapy; erectile dysfunction; vascular damage; penile bulb.

1   Introduction

Permanent erectile dysfunction (ED) after definitive prostate radiotherapy (RT) is a well-documented and significant source of post-treatment morbidity. The reported incidence of radiation-associated ED (RAED) after external beam irradiation or brachytherapy in previously potent patients has ranged from 15 to 60% (*4–9*).

From: *Current Clinical Urology* Series, *Sexual Function in the Prostate Cancer Patient*
Edited by John P. Mulhall, DOI 10.1007/978-1-60327-555-2_4,
© Humana Press, a part of Springer Science+Business Media, LLC 2009

Regardless of the treatment modality, the etiology of post-treatment ED is multi-factorial, making it more difficult to quantify accurately the rates of this phenomenon.

Undoubtedly, the most significant predictors of RAED are pre-treatment potency, older age, and comorbid diseases (diabetes, vasculopathy, etc.). The use of neoadjuvant androgen deprivation likely increases the chance of RAED by approximately 10% *(10)*. When these confounding factors are controlled for, impotence after prostate cancer treatment appears to result from a combination of vascular, neurogenic, and structural injuries. The relative contributions of these mechanisms are measurably different after radiotherapy compared to the post-prostatectomy setting. One noticeable manifestation of this difference is the relative delay in onset of radiation-induced ED compared to the more sudden loss of function after RP *(11)*. An outcomes study conducted by the National Cancer Institute reported continued decline in erectile function up to 5 years after prostate RT *(12)*.

2 Normal Physiology

Normal erections require vasodilatation of penile arteries (arteriogenic component) and simultaneous relaxation of the corporal sinusoidal smooth muscle (cavernosal component), with resultant venous compression and entrapment of blood. A quick review of anatomy will find the paired corpora cavernosa arising proximally as two crura before merging just below the pubic arch to lend support to the central corpus spongiosum (Fig. 1). The corpora cavernosa consist of interconnected sinusoids separated by smooth muscle trabeculae; together, the smooth muscle of the trabeculae and the arterial and arteriolar walls form the penile erectile tissue.

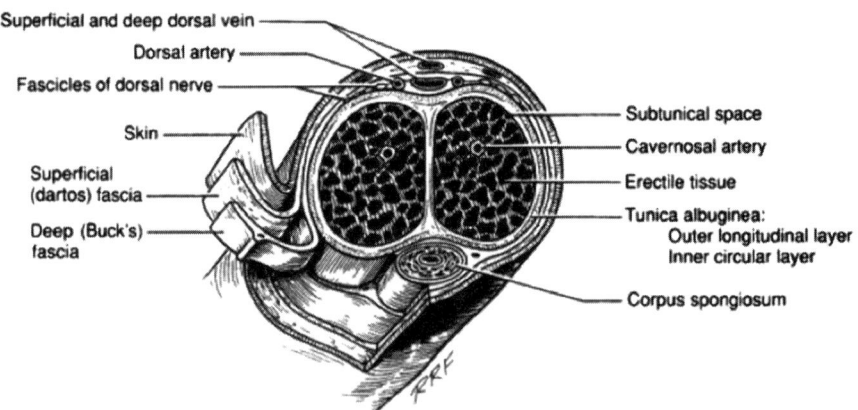

Fig. 1 Cross sectional anatomy of the penis
From Walsh: Campbell's Urology, 8th Ed., Copyright ©2002 Saunders *(1)*.

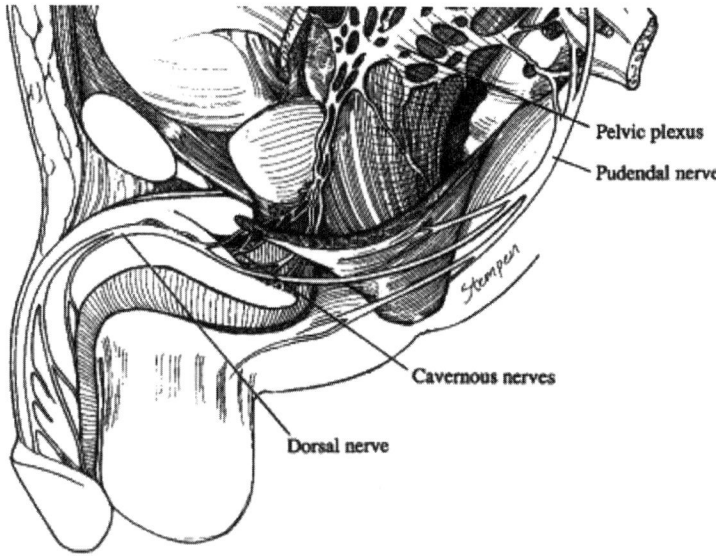

Fig. 2 Neuroanatomy of the penis
From Walsh: Campbell's Urology, 8th Ed., Copyright ©2002 Saunders *(1)*.

Cavernosal smooth muscle is moderately contracted in the flaccid state and becomes relaxed after sexual stimulation. Parasympathetic stimulation of the cavernous nerve (part of the neurovascular bundle) leads to alpha-adrenergic receptor blockade and subsequent smooth muscle relaxation (Fig. 2). Increased arterial and arteriolar inflow results in dilatation and expansion of the sinusoidal space. The venule plexuses are sandwiched between the distended sinusoids and the noncompliant tunica albuginea, resulting in entrapment of the incoming blood. The subsequent rise in intracavernous pressure and contraction of the ischiocavernosus muscles lead to the rigid erectile state.

The internal pudendal artery is the main blood supplier to the penis, with accessory arteries often existing, as well (Fig. 3). The internal pudendal artery becomes the common penile artery, which further divides into three branches: the cavernous, dorsal, and bulbourethral arteries. The cavernous artery is responsible for cavernosal engorgement. It enters proximally where the crura merge and gives off numerous helicine arteries that supply the cavernosa trabeculae and sinusoids as it courses toward the glans. The dorsal artery is responsible for glans engorgement, and the bulbourethral artery supplies the bulb of the penis and spongiosum.

In reviewing the structures responsible for normal physiologic erectile function, one can identify the areas at risk for radiation injury that may contribute to the development of erectile dysfunction. The bilateral neurovascular bundles run posterolaterally along the prostate (Fig. 4). Located therein are the cavernous nerves responsible for delivering the parasympathetic input for smooth muscle relaxation. Therefore, injury to the NVB could predictably affect erectile function. Injury to the arteries and/or trabeculae of the corpora or the proximal crura would also be

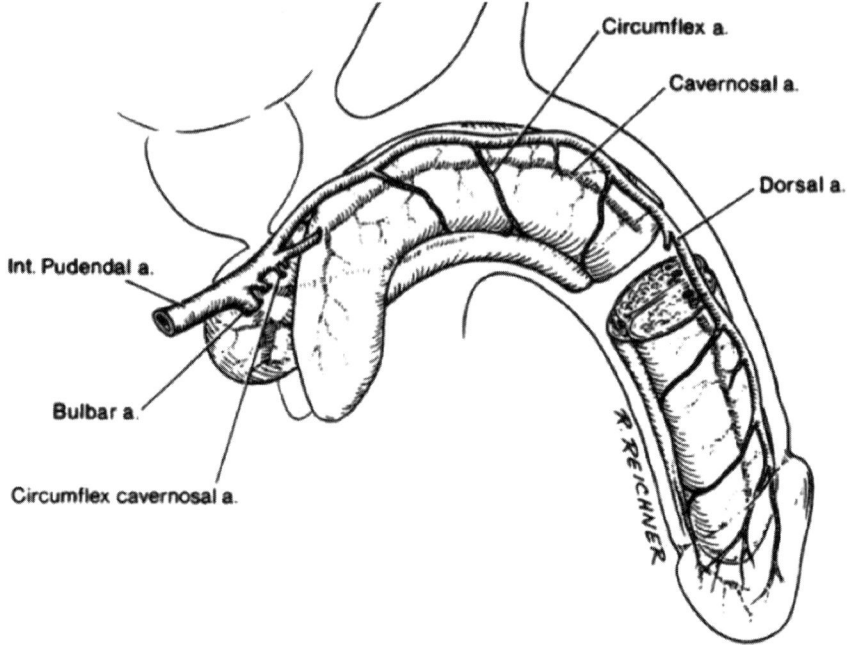

Fig. 3 Arterial supply of the penis
From Walsh: Campbell's Urology, 8th Ed., Copyright ©2002 Saunders *(1)*.

predicted to affect erectile function preservation. On the other hand, the spongio-sum and its proximal penile bulb play no role in the normal physiology of erections and one would not predict that injury to these structures would affect potency (Fig. 5).

3 Mechanisms of Injury After Prostate Irradiation

3.1 Vasculogenic Mechanisms

It is now recognized that vascular injury is a central mechanism of radiation-associated ED *(13)*. Endothelial cells are perhaps the most radiation-sensitive ele-ment of mesenchymal origin, and capillaries, sinusoids, and small arteries are the most affected vascular components in the majority of tissues *(13–16)*. Radiation-induced vasculopathy is both dose and time-dependent *(15)*. Large vessel (arterial) injury requires doses of 20 Gy and above *(17)*. In the current era of intensity-modulated radiotherapy (IMRT), most prostate cancer treatment delivers doses in excess of 75 Gy to the planned treatment volume (PTV), which by its nature includes a margin of nonprostatic tissue. Despite the rapid dose fall-off achieved with IMRT planning, the mean doses delivered to 50% of the penile bulb and proximal corpora cavernosa (D_{50}) are routinely in excess of 20 Gy.

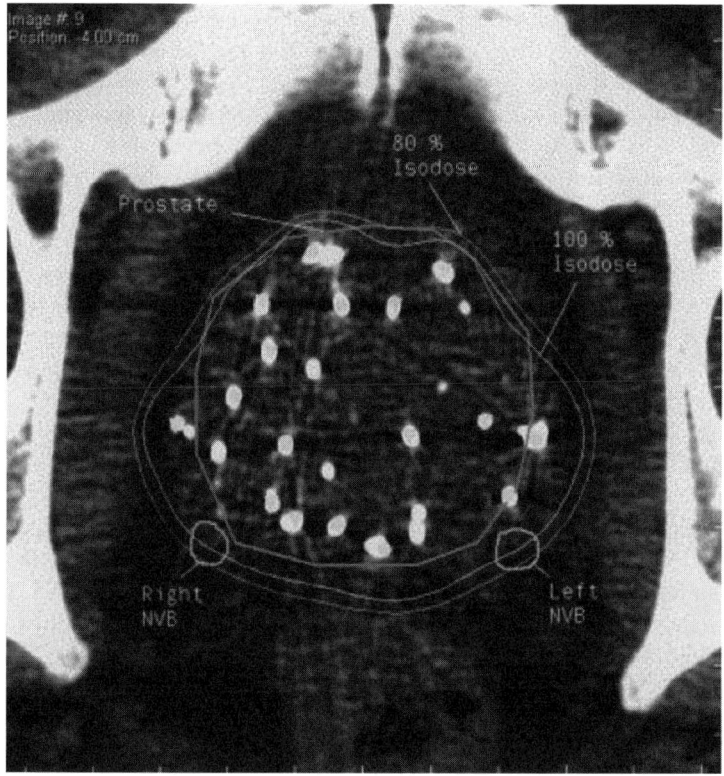

Fig. 4 Location of the neurovascular bundles
From Kiteley et al. *(2)*.

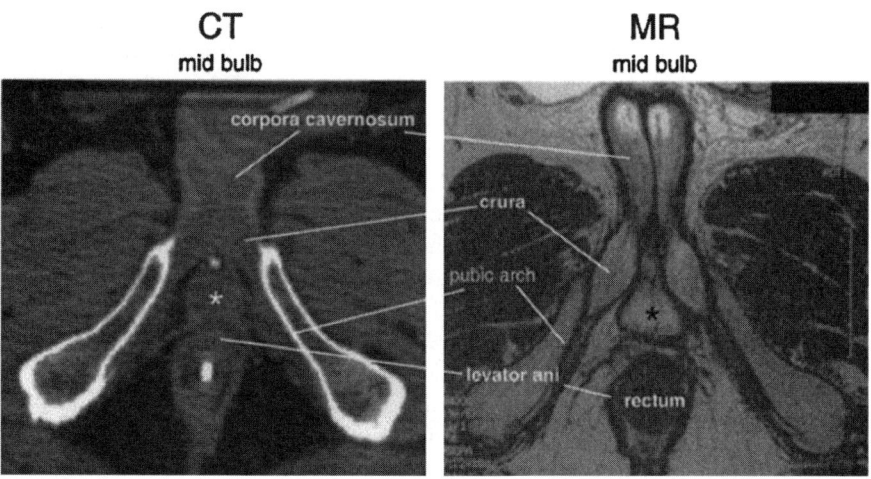

Fig. 5 Location of the penile bulb (asterisk) on CT and MR images
Wallner et al. *(3)*

Historically, doses below 12 Gy were considered less damaging since predominant vascular radiation effects at this dose occur at the microvascular level. However, Verheij et al. have demonstrated deleterious endothelial cell changes even at doses below 1 Gy that could lead to microthrombus formation and luminal occlusion *(18)*. Radiation-induced vasculopathy mediates acute and delayed radiation damages. Weeks to months following RT exposure, microvessel rupture can lead to arterial luminal occlusion *(16)*. The delayed toxicity that arises months to years after radiation exposure is attributed to the process of endarteritis obliterans *(19)*.

The pathophysiology of radiation-induced arteriopathy has been elucidated in several elegant in vitro and animal models. Up-regulation of the endothelial cell adhesion molecule ICAM-1 has been demonstrated in mouse and human tissues in response to irradiation in a dose and time-dependent manner *(20,21)*. Increased ICAM-1 expression leads to leukocyte infiltration into irradiated tissue, which eventually leads to characteristic radiation-induced functional impairment. This effect is not limited to the acute setting; enduring ICAM-1 up-regulation has been demonstrated in murine pulmonary and bladder endothelial cells *(22,23)*.

In the case of prostate irradiation, the penile vascular and erectile tissues are in close proximity to the target volume. In particular, the prostatic apex normally comes within 5–30 mm of the penile bulb, depending on the thickness of the urogenital diaphragm *(24)*. Therefore, it is expected that the penile structures will be exposed to some dose (however small). In the era of smaller radiation field sizes made possible by IMRT, damage to the erectile vasculature can be somewhat circumvented by allowing the development of collateral channels for blood flow; however, the potential for collateralization is limited by the fact that the cavernosal vasculature is an end-artery system *(25)*.

In clinical studies of penile vascular injury, arteriogenic function is assessed by peak penile blood flow measured by Doppler ultrasonography or dynamic infusion cavernosometry (DIC). Goldstein et al. published a case report on 23 patients undergoing radiation treatment for management of prostate cancer *(14)*. Of the 15 patients with intact erectile function prior to the initiation of RT, all 15 demonstrated abnormal penile Doppler ultrasonography following treatment. This finding coincided with subjective worsening of erectile function in all 15 men. Two patients were further assessed with penile arteriography, and this revealed occlusive disease within the radiation field involving the pudendal and penile arteries.

A subsequent and larger study by Zelefsky et al. confirmed these findings *(11)*. This analysis included 98 patients with new ED following definitive treatment of prostate cancer; 60 underwent prostatectomy and 38 had RT (external beam in 35 and permanent I-125 seed implantation in 3). The bilateral cavernosal arteries were assessed by observing the changes in vessel diameter and pulsed Doppler peak flows before and after intracavernous injection of Prostaglandin E_1. There was a statistically significant difference in the etiology of ED by treatment received, with 63% of RT patients displaying pure arteriogenic dysfunction compared to 32% of RP patients ($p = 0.002$). The use of neoadjuvant androgen-deprivation therapy had no significant impact on the development of permanent ED (12 patients in the RT group, 1 in the RP group).

Recently, Mulhall et al. evaluated erectile hemodynamics in 16 patients with new onset ED after external beam RT (mean dose 72 Gy) *(19)*. The time to hemodynamic testing was a mean of 11 months (95% CI 8–14 months). Arterial insufficiency was measured using cavernosal artery occlusion pressure (CAOP), namely the intracavernosal pressure at which occluded flow was demonstrated by the loss of a Doppler signal of the cavernosal artery. Among the 12 patients with assessable CAOP, all had significantly abnormal values indicative of arterial injury.

Though previously under-reported in the pelvic radiation literature, dysfunction of the veno-occlusive mechanism necessary for normal erections is another likely etiology of RAED. Cavernosal dysfunction, or venous leak, was demonstrated in 85% of the patients evaluated by Mulhall et al. *(19)*. Zelefsky et al. demonstrated abnormal corpora cavernosa distensibility under normal penile peak blood flow in 32% of patients treated with RT *(11)*. Endothelial cell dysfunction may also be central to this mechanism of ED.

The role of vasculogenic and endothelial cell injury in RAED is substantiated by the success of the phosphodiesterase type-5 (PDE-5) inhibitors in improving erectile function after prostate radiotherapy. Numerous studies have demonstrated that approximately two-thirds of men who develop ED after prostate radiotherapy will have improved erectile function that results from the use of PDE-5 inhibitors *(26–31)*. The PDE-5 inhibitors enhance the effect of nitric oxide under conditions of sexual stimulation. Nitric oxide is a vasoactive agent that is produced and released by the cavernous nerves and endothelial cells to modify the tone of adjacent smooth muscle *(1)*. Increased nitric oxide is released during sexual stimulation leading to amplified levels of cyclic guanosine monophosphate (cGMP) in the corpus cavernosum *(32,33)*. The ensuing smooth muscle relaxation increases the blood inflow to the corpus cavernosum crucial for erections.

Under normal physiologic conditions, cGMP is degraded by phosphodiesterase type-5 (PDE-5) to limit this sequence of events. The PDE-5 inhibitors block this degradation to enhance erectile function. Recently, the clinical efficacy of PDE-5 inhibitors has been correlated with objective in vivo arterial responses. As mentioned previously, Doppler ultrasound with intracavernosal injection of a vasoactive drug is considered the standard for establishing a diagnosis of vasculogenic ED. When this technique was used to assess post-occlusive changes in the diameter of cavernosal arteries with the administration of a PDE-5 inhibitor, objective improvements were mirrored by patients' experiences of drug efficacy *(34,35)*. This suggests that the effect of this class of drugs in patients with arteriogenic ED depends on the reversal of the impaired function of cavernosal endothelium.

3.2 Neurogenic Mechanisms

Though well-documented in the prostatectomy literature, neurovascular injury is thought to play only a minor role in RAED. Multiple studies have failed to demonstrate an association between dose delivered to the neurovascular bundles (NVB) and RAI *(2,11,14,36,37)*. Goldstein et al. evaluated bulbocavernous reflex latency and perineal electromyography and found post-radiotherapy neurologic assessments to be within normal limits *(14)*. Likewise, Zelefsky et al. were able to demonstrate neurogenic dysfunction in only 3% of EBRT patients (compared to 12% of post-prostatectomy patients) *(11)*.

Merrick et al. retrospectively compared the radiation dose to the NVB in 54 men with or without post-radiation ED after brachytherapy *(36)*. Average dose to the NVB was in excess of 200% of the prescription dose; 29 patients received additional EBRT. They found no significant difference in NVB dose between the 21 patients who maintained erectile function compared to the 33 who developed post-RT ED. Kiteley et al. similarly failed to show an association between NVB dose (as defined on CT) and the development of ED after brachytherapy when they compared 30 patients with RAED to 20 patients who maintained functional erections *(2)*. Wright and colleagues also failed to find a relationship between dose to the neurovascular bundles (as defined on MRI) and potency in 41 patients treated with prostate brachytherapy *(37)*.

3.3 Structural Injury

The penile bulb (PB) has been the most studied proximal penile structure in discussions of RAED, and yet its role remains highly controversial (Fig. 5). While numerous studies support a dose–volume relationship for the PB and subsequent RAED, other analyses have shed doubt on this relationship, citing the uncertain and variable anatomic and radiographic definitions of the bulb and, perhaps more importantly, the limited role the PB plays in the normal development and maintenance of erections *(2,25,36,38–44)*.

The first support for the role of the penile bulb in RAI came in 2001 from Fisch et al., who evaluated dose delivered to the penile bulb in 21 previously potent men treated with three-dimensional conformal radiotherapy (3D-CRT) for prostate cancer *(39)*. Pre- and post-treatment erectile functions were based on patients' responses on questionnaires, and not on objective measurement. The authors found that potency preservation was associated with a $D_{70} < 40$ Gy, and established the notion of dose–response for the penile bulb.

Merrick and his colleagues subsequently published data in support of these findings in patients undergoing prostate brachytherapy *(45)*. They looked at 23 previously potent men who developed ED after prostate implant and matched them to 23 similarly staged and treated men who maintained their erectile function. The penile bulb was retrospectively contoured on post-implant day 0 CT scans. They found that impotent patients received on average twice the dose to the penile bulb than their potent counterparts, and concluded that a target PB D_{50} of ≤ 50 Gy would maximize post-brachytherapy erectile function preservation. Merrick et al. next reported on dose to the bulb versus dose to the crura in 30 patients with post-brachytherapy ED and 30 potent patients matched by tumor and treatment parameters *(46)*. Pre-implant erectile function was assessed using a three-tiered system and post-implant function was based on completion of the International Index of Erectile Function (IIEF) questionnaire. Based on day 0 CT-defined dosimetry, the penile bulb D_{50} was the strongest predictor of post-implant ED, whereas the crura D_{25} merely approached statistical significance. Wernicke et al. used a questionnaire-based study to evaluate 29 patients treated with external beam RT, and concluded that higher dose–volume parameters involving the penile bulb correlated with higher risk of post-RT impotence *(44)*.

Prospective support for this hypothesis comes from the RTOG 9406 Phase I/II dose-escalation study *(42)*. For a subset of 158 patients who reported pre-treatment potency, a single, blinded observer contoured penile structures using Web-based software from a single Quality Assurance Center where all dosimetric calculations were performed. Post-radiotherapy ED was reported in 64 men, and the estimated incidence of ED at 5 years was significantly higher in men who received $\geq$52.5 Gy to the PB compared to those whose bulb received lower doses (50% vs. 25%, $p = 0.048$). A similar analysis based on patients enrolled in a Phase III dose-escalation study out of the UK supported these findings *(41)*. Of the patients initially randomized on the dose-escalation protocol, only 51 (6%) patients met the inclusion criteria for this analysis. Based on this highly selected group, the authors defended a dose–volume effect between PB radiation and subsequent development of ED at 2 years.

In contrast to the above studies, several groups have failed to substantiate an association between dose to the penile bulb and subsequent impotence. Kiteley et al. investigated this relationship in 50 men who underwent prostate brachytherapy *(2)*. They used a questionnaire to evaluate erectile function status at various intervals and calculated dose to the PB on the basis of a 1-month post-implant CT scan. At a median follow-up of 34 months, there were no differences in the PB dosimetric variables between the 20 patients who reported new ED and the 30 who maintained erectile function. A larger study out of Vancouver, Canada, also failed to demonstrate a relationship between dose to the PB after prostate brachytherapy and post-implant impotence *(40)*. Erectile status was assessed independently by both the patient and the treating physician and collected in a prospective manner for the 226 patients included in this analysis. The penile bulb was contoured on a 1-month post-implant CT scan by two independent observers, and the mean PB D_{50} and D_{95} were 52.6 Gy and 26.0 Gy, respectively. The authors concluded that deliberate dose-sparing of the proximal penile structures during brachytherapy would provide no meaningful gain in potency preservation. Rather, they found the number of needles to be an independent predictor of ED, suggesting trauma to the crura during implantation as a more plausible contributor to RAED. Lastly, a group from M.D. Anderson Cancer Center could not substantiate a dose–volume effect of penile bulb dose on ED after three-dimensional conformal RT *(43)*. Ten of the 28 potent patients who received 78 Gy and completed sexual function questionnaires reported new-onset ED at a median follow-up of 66 months. There were no differences in the dose–volume histograms calculated for the penile bulb (mean dose 42.2 Gy) between those who did and did not develop RAED.

Finally, Mulhall has argued against the involvement of the penile bulb in RAED, noting that the bulb lacks significant erectile tissue and plays no role in the physiology of normal penile erections *(2,19,25,38,40,43)*. He and others have suggested that studies supporting the role of the penile bulb could be mistakenly using PB dose as a surrogate for injury to the more important flanking erectile tissue of the crura. Indeed, studies have demonstrated that similar doses are delivered to the bulb and the crura during RT *(25–46)*.

4 Conclusion

The precise etiology of radiation-induced ED remains uncertain, and its development is likely the result of a multitude of factors. Various investigations in recent years suggest that vascular injury is a principal player, while the data supporting the roles of neurogenic damage or injury to the penile bulb have been far less persuasive (see Table 1 for a summary of the studies reviewed above). In the future,

Table 1 Summary of Important Studies

Organ at risk	Author	Patient no.	Endpoint	Effect
Arteries	Goldstein et al. *(14)*	15	Doppler ultrasound and arteriography	+
	Zelefsky and Eid *(11)*	98	Doppler ultrasound	+
	Mulhall et al. *(19)*	16	Cavernosal artery occlusion pressure	+
Cavernosa	Zelefsky and Eid *(11)*	98	Cavernosometry (venocclusive parameters)	+
	Mulhall et al. *(19)*	16	Cavernosometry (venocclusive parameters)	+
NVB	Goldstein et al. *(14)*	15	Bulbocavernous reflex, perineal electromyography	–
	Zelefsky and Eid *(11)*	98	Erectile response to prostaglandin injection	–
	Merrick et al. *(45)*	54	NVB dose	–
	Kiteley et al. *(2)*	50	NVB dose	–
	Wright et al. *(37)*	41	NVB dose	–
Penile bulb	Fisch et al. *(39)*	21	Penile bulb dose	+
	Merrick et al. *(45)*	46	Penile bulb dose	+
	Wernicke et al. *(44)*	29	Penile bulb dose	+
	Roach et al. *(42)*	158	Penile bulb dose	+
	Mangar et al. *(41)*	51	Penile bulb dose	+
	Kiteley et al. *(2)*	50	Penile bulb dose	–
	MacDonald et al. *(40)*	226	Penile bulb dose	–
	Selek et al. *(47)*	28	Penile bulb dose	–

we hope that more prospective research that includes objective measurements of erectile function-related parameters will allow us to better understand this complex phenomenon.

References

1. Walsh (2002). In: Walsh, P., ed. *Campbell's Urology*, 8th edn. Saunders.
2. Kiteley, R.A., Lee, W.R., deGuzman, A.F., et al. (2002) Radiation dose to the neurovascular bundles or penile bulb does not predict erectile dysfunction after prostate brachytherapy. *Brachytherapy* 1, 90–4.
3. Wallner, K.E., Merrick, G.S., Benson, M.L., et al. (2002) Penile bulb imaging. *Int. J. Rad. Oncol. Biol. Phys.* 53, 928–933.
4. Asbell, S.O., Krall, J.M., Pilepich, M.V., et al. (1988) Elective pelvic irradiation in stage A2, B carcinoma of the prostate: analysis of RTOG 77–06. *Int. J. Rad. Oncol. Biol. Phys.* 15, 1307–1316.
5. Roach, M., Chinn, D.M., Holland, J.J., et al. (1996) A pilot survey of sexual function and quality of life following 3D conformal radiotherapy for clinically localized prostate cancer. *Int. J. Rad. Oncol. Biol. Phys.* 35, 869–874.
6. Zelefsky, M.J., Fuks, Z., Hunt, M., et al. (2002) High-dose intensity modulated radiation therapy for prostate cancer: early toxicity and biochemical outcome in 772 patients. *Int. J. Rad. Oncol. Biol. Phys.* 53, 1111–1116.
7. Merrick, G.S., Butler, W.M., Wallner, K.E., et al. (2005) Erectile function after prostate brachytherapy. *Int. J. Rad. Oncol. Biol. Phys.* 62, 437–447.
8. Stone, N.N., and Stock, R.G. (2002) Complications following permanent prostate brachytherapy. *Eur. Urol.* 41, 427–433.
9. Banker, F.L. (1988) The preservation of potency after external beam irradiation for prostate cancer. *Int. J. Rad. Oncol. Biol. Phys.* 15, 219–220.
10. Zelefsky, M.J., Cowen, D., Fuks, Z., et al. (1999) Long term tolerance of high dose three-dimensional conformal radiotherapy in patients with localized prostate carcinoma. *Cancer* 85, 2460–2468.
11. Zelefsky, M.J., and Eid, J.F. (1998) Elucidating the etiology of erectile dysfunction after definitive therapy for prostatic cancer. *Int. J. Rad. Oncol. Biol. Phys.* 40, 129–133.
12. Potosky, A.L., Davis, W.W., Hoffman, R.M., et al. (2004) Five-year outcomes after prostatectomy or radiotherapy for prostate cancer: the prostate cancer outcomes study. *J. Natl. Cancer Inst.* 96, 1358–1367.
13. Chuang, V.P. (1994) Radiation-induced arteritis. *Semin. Roentgenol.* 29, 64–69.
14. Goldstein, I., Feldman, M.I., Deckers, P.J., et al. (1984) Radiation-associated impotence. A clinical study of its mechanism. *JAMA* 251, 903–910.
15. Fajardo, L.F. (2005) The pathology of ionizing radiation as defined by morphologic patterns. *Acta Oncologica* 44, 13–22.
16. Fajardo, L.F. (1988) Vascular lesions following radiation. *Pathol. Annu.* 23, 297–330.
17. Himmel, P.D., and Hassett, J.M. (1986) Radiation-induced chronic arterial injury. *Semin. Surg. Oncol.* 2, 225–247.
18. Verheij, M., Koomen, G.C., van Mourik, J.A., et al. (1994) Radiation reduces cyclooxygenase activity in cultured human endothelial cells at low doses. *Prostaglandins* 48, 351–366.
19. Mulhall, J., Ahmed, A., Parker, M., et al. (2005) The hemodynamics of erectile dysfunction following external beam radiation for prostate cancer. *J. Sex. Med.* 2, 432–437.
20. Hallahan, D.E., and Virudachalam, S. (1997) Ionizing radiation mediates expression of cell adhesion molecules in distinct histological patterns within the lung. *Cancer Res.* 57, 2096–2099.

21. Handschel, J., Prott, F.J., Sunderkötter, C., et al. (1999) Irradiation induces increase of adhesion molecules and accumulation of beta2-integrin-expressing cells in humans. *Int. J. Rad. Oncol. Biol. Phys.* **45**, 475–481.

22. Jaal, J., and Dörr, W. (2005) Early and long-term effects of radiation on intercellular adhesion molecule 1 (ICAM-1) expression in mouse urinary bladder endothelium. *Int. J. Rad. Biol.* **81**, 387–395.

23. Epperly, M.W., Sikora, C.A., DeFilippi, S.J., et al. (2002) Pulmonary irradiation-induced expression of VCAM-I and ICAM-I is decreased by manganese superoxide dismutase-plasmid/liposome (MnSOD-PL) gene therapy. *Biol. Blood Marrow Transplant.* **8**, 175–187.

24. Plants, B.A., Chen, D.T., Fiveash, J.B., et al. (2003) Bulb of penis as a marker for prostatic apex in external beam radiotherapy of prostate cancer. *Int. J. Rad. Oncol. Biol. Phys.* **56**, 1079–1084.

25. Mulhall, J.P., Yonover, P., Sethi, A., et al. (2002) Radiation exposure to the corporeal bodies during 3-dimensional conformal radiation therapy for prostate cancer. *J. Urol.* **167**, 539–542.

26. Ohebshalom, M., Parker, M., Guhring, P., et al. (2005) The efficacy of sildenafil citrate following radiation therapy for prostate cancer: temporal considerations. *J. Urol.* **174**, 258–262; discussion 262.

27. Kedia, S., Zippe, C.D., Agarwal, A., et al. (1999) Treatment of erectile dysfunction with sildenafil citrate (Viagra) after radiation therapy for prostate cancer. *Urology* **54**, 308–312.

28. Incrocci, L., Hop, W.C.J., and Slob, A.K. (2003) Efficacy of sildenafil in an open-label study as a continuation of a double-blind study in the treatment of erectile dysfunction after radiotherapy for prostate cancer. *Urology* **62**, 116–120.

29. Raina, R., Agarwal, A., Goyal, K.K., et al. (2003) Long-term potency after iodine-125 radiotherapy for prostate cancer and role of sildenafil citrate. *Urology* **62**, 1103–1108.

30. Merrick, G.S., Butler, W.M., Lief, J.H., et al. (1999) Efficacy of sildenafil citrate in prostate brachytherapy patients with erectile dysfunction. *Urology* **53**, 1112–1116.

31. Zelefsky, M.J., McKee, A.B., Lee, H., et al. (1999) Efficacy of oral sildenafil in patients with erectile dysfunction after radiotherapy for carcinoma of the prostate. *Urology* **53**, 775–778.

32. Rajfer, J., Aronson, W.J., Bush, P.A., et al. (1992) Nitric oxide as a mediator of relaxation of the corpus cavernosum in response to nonadrenergic, noncholinergic neurotransmission. *N. Engl. J. Med.* **326**, 90–94.

33. Boolell, M., Allen, M.J., Ballard, S.A., et al. (1996) Sildenafil: an orally active type 5 cyclic GMP-specific phosphodiesterase inhibitor for the treatment of penile erectile dysfunction. *Int. J. Impot. Res.: Official Journal of the International Society for Impotence Research* **8**, 47–52.

34. Mulhall, J., Barnas, J., Aviv, N., et al. (2005) Sildenafil citrate response correlates with the nature and the severity of penile vascular insufficiency. *J. Sex. Med.* **2**, 104–108.

35. Mazo, E.B., Gamidov, S.I., and Iremashvili, V.V. (2006) Does the clinical efficacy of vardenafil correlate with its effect on the endothelial function of cavernosal arteries? A pilot study. *BJU Int.* **98**, 1054–1058.

36. Merrick, G.S., Butler, W.M., Dorsey, A.T., et al. (2000) A comparison of radiation dose to the neurovascular bundles in men with and without prostate brachytherapy-induced erectile dysfunction. *Int. J. Rad. Oncol. Biol. Phys.* **48**, 1069–1074.

37. Wright, J.L., Newhouse, J.H., Laguna, J.L., et al. (2004) Localization of neurovascular bundles on pelvic CT and evaluation of radiation dose to structures putatively involved in erectile dysfunction after prostate brachytherapy. *Int. J. Rad. Oncol. Biol. Phys.* **59**, 426–435.

38. Mulhall, J.P., and Yonover, P.M. (2001) Correlation of radiation dose and impotence risk after three-dimensional conformal radiotherapy for prostate cancer. *Urology* **58**, 828.

39. Fisch, B.M., Pickett, B., Weinberg, V., et al. (2001) Dose of radiation received by the bulb of the penis correlates with risk of impotence after three-dimensional conformal radiotherapy for prostate cancer. *Urology* **57**, 955–959.

40. Macdonald, A.G., Keyes, M., Kruk, A., et al. (2005) Predictive factors for erectile dysfunction in men with prostate cancer after brachytherapy: is dose to the penile bulb important? *Int. J. Rad. Oncol. Biol. Phys.* **63**, 155–163.

41. Mangar, S.A., Sydes, M.R., Tucker, H.L., et al. (2006) Evaluating the relationship between erectile dysfunction and dose received by the penile bulb: using data from a randomised

controlled trial of conformal radiotherapy in prostate cancer (MRC RT01, ISRCTN47772397). Radiother. Oncol. **80**, 355–362.

42. Roach, M., Winter, K., Michalski, J.M., et al. (2004) Penile bulb dose and impotence after three-dimensional conformal radiotherapy for prostate cancer on RTOG 9406: findings from a prospective, multi-institutional, phase I/II dose-escalation study. *Int. J. Rad. Oncol. Biol. Phys.* **60**, 1351–1356.
43. Selek, U., Cheung, R., Lii, M., et al. (2004) Erectile dysfunction and radiation dose to penile base structures: a lack of correlation. *Int. J. Rad. Oncol. Biol. Phys.* **59**, 1039–1046.
44. Wernicke, A.G., Valicenti, R., Dieva, K., et al. (2004) Radiation dose delivered to the proximal penis as a predictor of the risk of erectile dysfunction after three-dimensional conformal radiotherapy for localized prostate cancer. *Int. J. Rad. Oncol. Biol. Phys.* **60**, 1357–1363.
45. Merrick, G.S., Wallner, K, Butler, W.M., et al. (2001) A comparison of radiation dose to the bulb of the penis in men with and without prostate brachytherapy-induced erectile dysfunction. *Int. J. Rad. Oncol. Biol. Phys.* **50**, 597–604.
46. Merrick, G.S., Butler, W.M., Wallner, K.E., et al. (2002) The importance of radiation doses to the penile bulb vs. crura in the development of postbrachytherapy erectile dysfunction. *Int. J. Rad. Oncol. Biol. Phys.* **54**, 1055–1062.
47. Selek, U., Cheung, R., Lii, M., et al. (2004) Erectile dysfunction and radiation dose to penile base structures: a lack of correlation. *Int. J. Rad. Oncol. Biol. Phys.* **59**, 1039–1046.

Chapter 5
Evolution of Radical Prostatectomy as It Pertains to Nerve-Sparing

Ofer Yossepowitch and James A. Eastham

Abstract Only a few decades ago, radical prostatectomy generally left patients impotent, but today, with the advent of nerve-sparing techniques, many patients can recover sexual function after surgery. We describe our contemporary technique for nerve-sparing during open radical prostatectomy. Key factors include the establishment of a bloodless surgical field prior to dissection of the neurovascular bundles, preservation of any accessory pudendal arteries, avoidance of electrocoagulation in proximity to the neurovascular bundles, and complete mobilization of the neurovascular bundles off the prostate prior to division of the urethra. Resection or partial resection of a neurovascular bundle may be warranted depending on the location of cancer. Estimates of the frequency of recovery of potency after nerve-sparing radical prostatectomy vary greatly, from 21 to 86% of patients. Recovery of potency can take up to 2 years after surgery and is more likely in patients who are younger, who were potent before surgery, and who had both neurovascular bundles preserved. Postoperative potency seems to be increased with the early use of phosphodiesterase-5 inhibitors and intracavernous injection therapy. Potential neuroprotective agents, such as immunophilin ligands, are an area of active research.

Keywords Prostate cancer; radical prostatectomy; nerve-sparing surgery; penile erection; accessory pudendal arteries; neurovascular bundles; surgical technique.

From: *Current Clinical Urology* Series, *Sexual Function in the Prostate Cancer Patient*   69
Edited by John P. Mulhall, DOI 10.1007/978-1-60327-555-2_5,
© Humana Press, a part of Springer Science+Business Media, LLC 2009

1   Introduction

After local therapy for prostate cancer, the most favorable outcome that can be achieved is complete eradication of the cancer with full recovery of urinary, bowel, and sexual function. These goals of local therapy are inextricably linked, and at times improvements in the outcome of one may occur at the expense of the others. The technical challenge of local treatment for prostate cancer is to treat sufficient periprostatic tissue to achieve cure while at the same time preserving the neuromusculature required for normal urinary and bowel function as well as the cavernosal nerves required for erectile function.

Among the most complex operations performed by urologists, radical prostatectomy challenges surgeons because the results are highly sensitive to fine details in surgical technique. The elusive goals of modern radical prostatectomy are to remove the cancer completely with minimal blood loss, no serious intra- or perioperative complications, and complete recovery of continence and potency. No surgeon achieves such results uniformly. Before the 1980s, most patients permanently lost erectile function after radical prostatectomy. Clear definition of the periprostatic anatomy has allowed the evolvement of refined surgical techniques more respectful of the intricate neurovascular structures adjacent to the prostate. Nowadays, surgical techniques based on a more precise understanding of the periprostatic anatomy and of the autonomic innervation of the corpora cavernosa, allow preservation of sexual function in many men undergoing radical prostatectomy. The purpose of this chapter is to provide surgeons with details about one approach to this operation, focusing on the preservation of erectile function. We modify our approach frequently in a continual effort to improve patient outcomes. The technique described here is not the only successful approach; various other techniques work as well. We hope that the description of our approach will clarify the important anatomical and surgical principles and allow the reader to improve his or her own technique.

2   Anatomical Considerations

Much of our current understanding of the neurovascular anatomy of the prostate derives from detailed anatomical studies conducted during the 1980 s in male fetuses and stillborn neonates, and later in adults (*1–4*). In a series of anatomical dissections, Walsh and associates determined the topographical relationship between the pelvic vasculature, pelvic nerve plexus, cavernous nerves, lateral pelvic fascia, Denonvilliers' fascia, prostate, urethra, and the urogenital diaphragm. These detailed studies formed the basis for our contemporary refined technique of nerve preservation during radical retropubic prostatectomy and cystoprostatectomy.

Penile erection is a complex phenomenon, requiring interaction between neurologic, vascular, and psychologic factors. Erection is mediated primarily through an increase in arterial blood flow to the penis, arising from the two internal pudendal arteries, the terminal branches of the hypogastric artery. Many men, however, have accessory pudendal arteries, which can originate from the external iliac, obturator, inferior vesical, or femoral arteries. These small accessory branches generally travel along the lateral aspect of the prostate and pierce the urogenital diaphragm in proximity to the urethra and the apex of the prostate *(5)*. Because these vessels may be a dominant source of arterial blood supply to the corpus cavernosum, their avulsion or intentional sacrifice may result in postoperative erectile dysfunction *(6)*. Therefore, provided that negative apical surgical margins can be assured, efforts should be made to preserve these small arterial branches when dividing the dorsal venous complex or transecting the urethra (Fig. 1). Preservation of these arteries will ensure a normal arterial inflow to the penis postoperatively. This may enable a patient to remain potent after surgery or, for a patient who is impotent, facilitate an adequate response to medical treatment *(7)*.

Innervation to the penis is both autonomic (sympathetic and parasympathetic) and somatic (sensory and motor). The somatic component is responsible for penile sensation and contraction of the bulbocavernosus and ischiocavernosus muscles during erection and ejaculation. Somatic nerve branches are delivered to the penis and pelvic muscles via the pudendal nerve, which leaves the pelvis through the greater sciatic foramen, crosses the spine of the ischium, and re-enters the pelvis through the lesser sciatic foramen to accompany the internal pudendal vessels along the ischiorectal fossa. Therefore, damage to these nerves during pelvic surgery is highly unlikely.

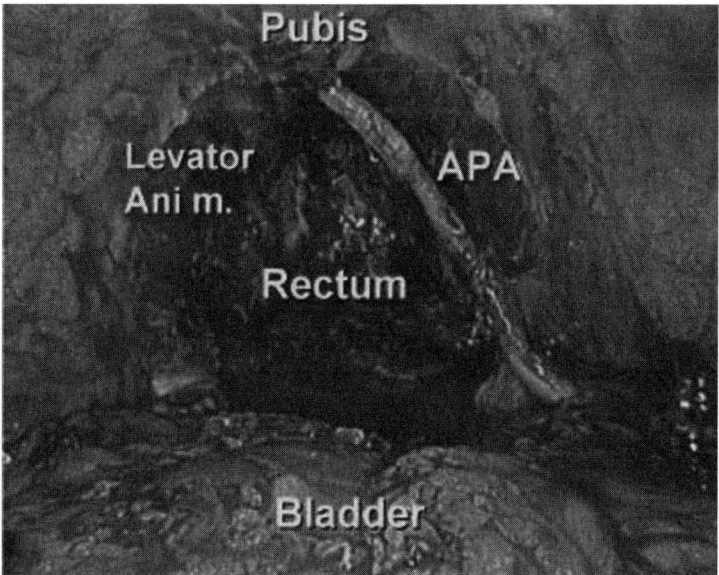

Fig. 1 Right lateral accessory pudendal artery (APA) after removing the prostate

The autonomic component of penile innervation plays a critical role in initiating and maintaining the erection. In contrast to the somatic component, the autonomic component is highly susceptible to injury during radical prostatectomy. Autonomic innervation to the corpora cavernosa arises from the pelvic plexus, which is a network of nerves forming a rectangular plate situated in a sagittal plane beside the rectum. The pelvic plexus originates from two sources: (1) sympathetic fibers from the thoracolumbar center via the hypogastric nerve; and (2) parasympathetic fibers from the sacral center via the pelvic nerve (nervus erigentes). Efferent branches from the pelvic plexus to the corpora cavernosa are bundled together to generate the cavernous nerves. These microscopic nerve fibers are encased in a dense fibro-fatty tissue and are in constant association with the capsular arteries and veins of the prostate, forming the neurovascular bundle (NVB). The NVB travels along the posterolateral aspect of prostate and provides the visual marker that is used intraoperatively to identify the efferent branches of the pelvic plexus to the corpora cavernosa. Distally, the cavernous nerves begin to approach the prostatic urethra, and at the apex of the prostate they are only a few millimeters away from the prostatic capsule at the 5 and 7 o'clock positions. Because the NVB travels outside the capsule of the prostate and outside Denonvilliers' fascia, it is possible, if one assumes that a tumor is located completely intracapsularly, to avoid injury to the cavernous nerves and to preserve sexual function without compromising surgical extirpation of the cancer.

Based upon these anatomical considerations, inadvertent injury to cavernous nerves can occur at one of three steps: (1) division of the lateral pedicle and dissection of the seminal vesicles (jeopardizing the intactness of the cavernous nerves and the main pelvic plexus); (2) dissecting the prostate off the rectum; (3) apical dissection and transection of the urethra.

While the autonomic component is highly vulnerable to damage during radical prostatectomy, the somatic component invariably remains intact. Therefore, even in the absence of an actual erection, postprostatectomy patients may still retain normal penile sensation and experience arousal and orgasms.

3   Technique

3.1   Initial Steps and Control of Bleeding

Patient positioning, exposure of the prostate, and periprostatic tissues, division of the endopelvic fascia, and control of the dorsal venous complex have been described elsewhere (8). These initial aspects of radical prostatectomy are based on a clear understanding of periprostatic anatomy and provide a bloodless field in which to work.

Bleeding from the transected dorsal venous complex is controlled by oversewing the cut edges of the lateral pelvic fascia vertically with a running suture (Fig. 2A), the last pass of which is brought through the periosteum of the pubis (Fig. 2B).

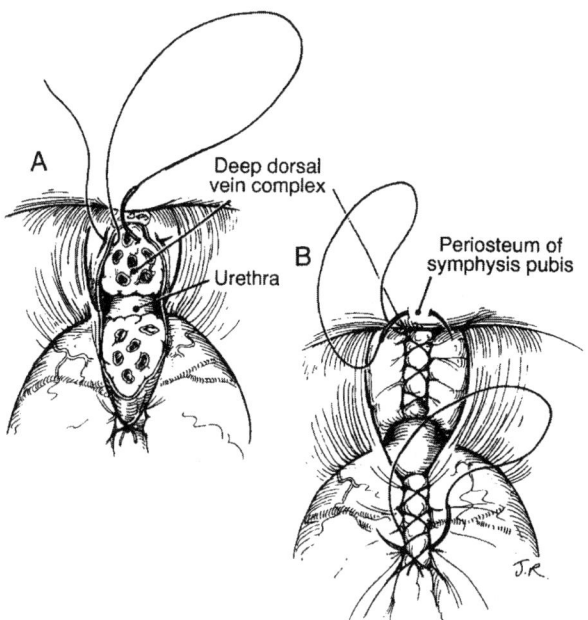

Fig. 2 Bleeding from the transected dorsal vein complex is controlled by oversewing the cut edges of the lateral pelvic fascia vertically with a continuous suture (**A**), the last pass of which is brought through the periosteum of the pubis (**B**) to compress the superficial venous complex above the lateral pelvic fascia and to fix the fascia to the periosteum, simulating the function of the puboprostatic ligaments. Back bleeding from the ventral prostate is controlled with clips or with a continuous hemostatic suture, taking care not to draw the neurovascular bundles medially (**B**)

Back-bleeding from the ventral prostate is controlled with a continuous hemostatic suture (Fig. 2B). Care should be taken to avoid suturing laterally into the dorsal aspect of the prostate, resulting in drawing the NVB medially. The latter may distort the anatomy of the NVB and hinder its subsequent release from the prostate. It is imperative to attain complete control of bleeding before initiating nerve preservation; with appropriate hemostasis, the surgeon should have a bloodless field to facilitate later steps in the procedure.

3.2 Preservation of the Neurovascular Bundle (NVB)

The surgeon can palpate and examine the course of the NVB in relation to the prostate and any palpable tumor. Additional information obtained from the diagnostic prostate biopsy and pre-operative imaging may serve to more accurately delineate cancers with extension into the capsule, for which preservation of the NVB may result in a positive margin and impaired cancer control. The prostate is rotated with a sponge stick and any remaining levator any muscle fibers are bluntly swept away.

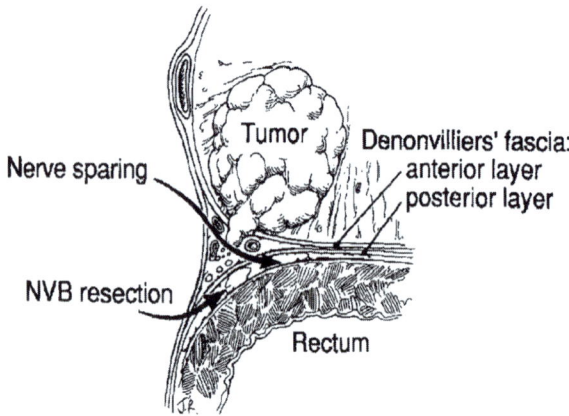

Fig. 3 The lateral plane of dissection is selected based on preoperative and intraoperative assessment of the extent of the tumor. A wider dissection, i.e., partial or complete resection of the neurovascular bundle may be required in an attempt to obtain adequate surgical margins

Frequently, a shallow groove along the lateral aspect of the prostate defines the superior margin of dissection for the preservation of the NVB. A plane of division in the lateral prostatic fascia is then chosen to assure a negative surgical margin while at the same time preserving as much of the NVB as possible (Fig. 3). Once the plane of dissection has been selected, the lateral prostatic fascia is sharply incised. The NVB is most easily dissected away from the apical third of the prostate (Fig. 4A and B). If, however, apical cancer is suspected, initating the dissection at the mid-prostate may be safer.

Small vascular branches from NVB to the prostate are carefuly defined, clipped, and divided. Avoidance of electrocoagulation, even in the presence of bleeding, is of paramount importance for maintaining the integrity of the nerves. In a recent canine study, Ong and colleagues demonstrated that use of monopolar and bipolar electrocautery as well as ultrasonic shears in proximity to the NVB is associated with significantly decreased erectile response to cavernous nerve stimulation and with a higher incidence of histologic findings (fibrosis) suggestive of nerve injury *(9)*.

The NVB is then gently dissected and displaced laterally, working from the apex toward the base. This should be done with either a Kitner (peanut) dissector and/or a right-angled clamp. Finger dissection should be avoided on the NVB. These delicate nerve fibers require gentle dissection, which will likely increase operative time. To avoid any tension on the neurovascular tissue that might result from excessive traction on the prostate, we prefer to release the entire NVB from the prostate (from the urethra to the seminal vesicle) before dividing the urethra and elevating the prostate out of the pelvis.

Denonvilliers' fascia is deliberately incised in the angle between the NVB and the prostate, completely releasing the NVB from the lateral aspect of the gland (Fig. 4C, D, and E). The risk of a positive surgical margin will be greatly reduced if this

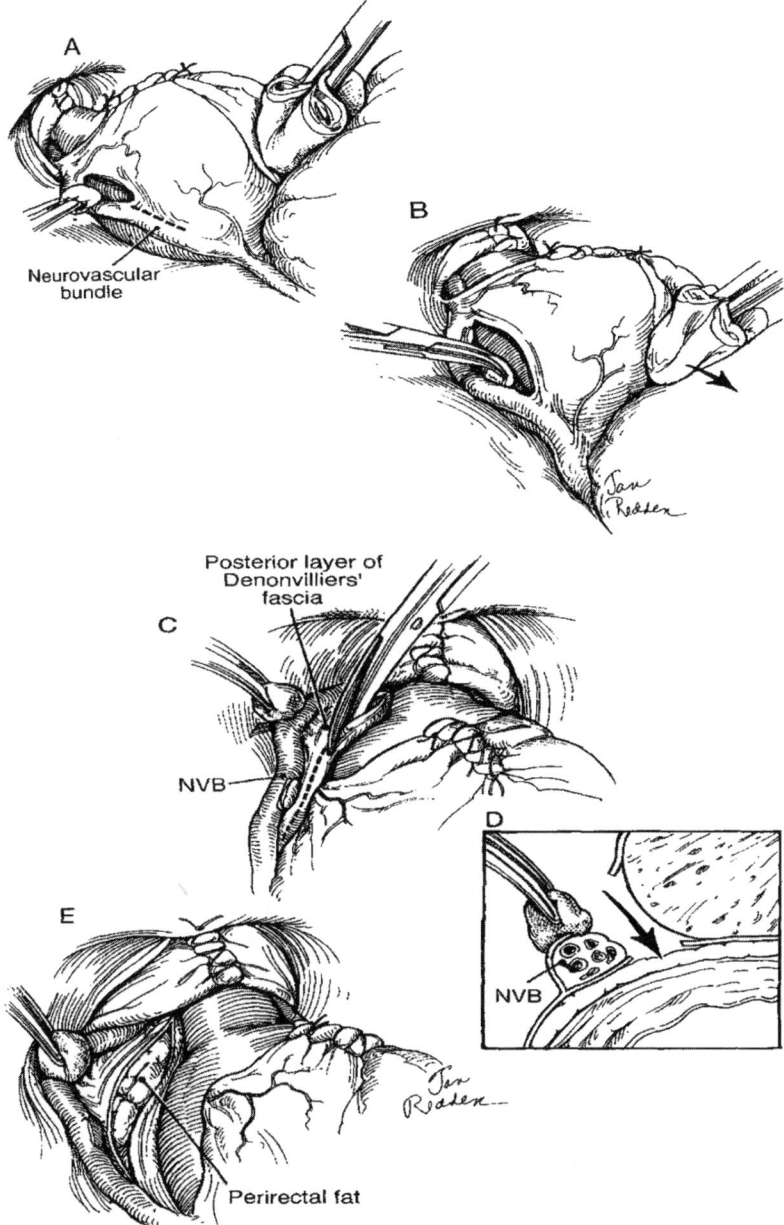

Fig. 4 Preservation of left neurovascular bundle. After the dorsal vein complex has been divided the prostate is rotated to the right and the levator muscles are bluntly dissected away. The lateral pelvic fascia is then incised in the groove between the prostate and the neurovascular bundle. The neurovascular bundle is most easily dissected away from the apical third of the prostate (**A, B**). The small branches of the vascular pedicle to the apex must be divided. The posterior layer of Denonvilliers' fascia is then incised, releasing the NVB from the prostate and urethra (**C, E**) so that the nerves will not be tethered when the urethral anastomotic sutures are tied

layer of fascia is included in the excised specimen. The appearance of perirectal fat emerging between the cut edges of this fascia will assure the surgeon that the layer has been incised completely. Special attention should be paid to avoid excessive lateral traction of the nerve while exposing and dissecting Denonvilliers' fascia. Distally, the dissection of the NVB is carried for a distance of almost 1 cm beyond the prostatourethral junction so that the nerves will not be tethered when the urethral anastomotic sutures are tied. Proximally, identification of the seminal vesicle after release of the NVB from the base of the prostate and division of the prostatic vascular pedicle will indicate complete mobilization of the NVB and prevent traction injury to the nerve during the subsequent elevation and dissection of the prostate off the rectum.

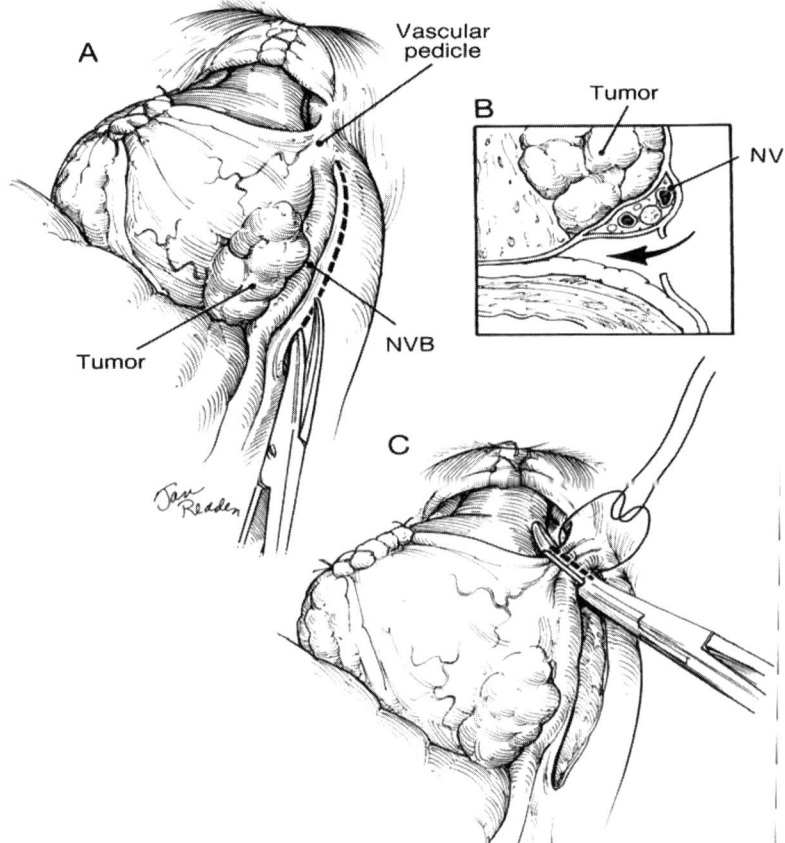

Fig. 5 Wide resection of the right neurovascular bundle (NVB). If preservation of the NVB compromises cancer control, all or part of the NVB must be resected. If the entire NVB is to be removed, dissection begins over the lateral rectal wall in the fat beneath the NVB (**A**). All tissue adjacent to the prostate is resected and left on the gland (**B**). The NVB is secured with clips or ties and divided distal to the apex of the prostate (**C**)

Should the cancer lie close to the NVB, all or part of the bundle should be resected to assure complete removal of the cancer (Figs. 3 and 5). A plane of dissection is chosen laterally. If the entire bundle is to be resected, dissection begins over the lateral rectal wall in the fat beneath the NVB (Fig. 5A and B). The incision is extended distally and the NVB is secured with clips or ties and divided distal to the apex of the prostate (Fig. 5C). Alternatively, if extension of the cancer into the capsule is suspected, the NVB may be partially resected, leaving sufficient tissue on the prostate to ensure a negative surgical margin while preserving some of the autonomic fibers to the corpora cavernosa. Partial preservation/resection of the NVB often results in bleeding from the cut edge of the NVB. This must be accepted, as excessive clip placement or cauterization will only damage the tissues of the NVB. Once the NVB has been lateralized, more precise clip placement can secure appropriate hemostasis with decreased risk of injury to the NVB.

Following complete mobilization of both NVBs off the prostate from the periurethral area to the seminal vesicle, the anterior two-thirds of the urethra is divided, exposing a previously placed catheter. The first four anastomotic sutures are placed at the 9, 11, 1, and 3 o'clock positions (Fig. 6). The catheter is withdrawn, exposing the posterior urethra, and two additional sutures are placed at the 5 and 7 o'clock positions. Attention should be given to ensure that the NVBs are not inadvertently incorporated within the latter sutures. The previously made incisions in Denonvilliers' fascia are connected across the midline beneath the divided urethra. The plane of dissection above the perirectal fat but below Denonvilliers' fascia is then developed sharply and carried cephalad and caudal paralleling the mobilized NVB (Fig. 7). This dissection should be done sharply rather than bluntly to ensure that adequate periprostatic tissue is maintained around the posterior and posterolateral aspects of the gland. A catheter may be placed through the urethra to facilitate dissection.

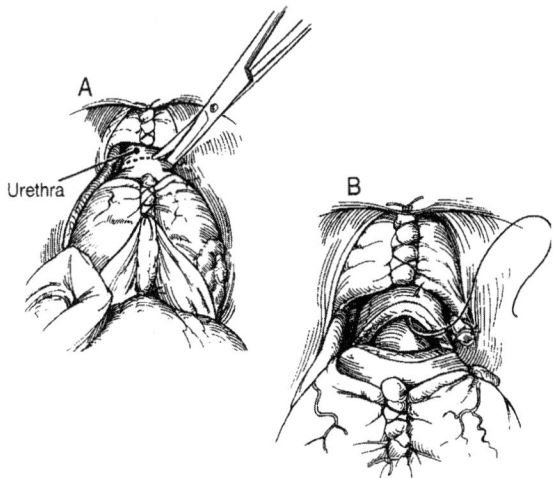

Fig. 6 Close-up views of urethra at the prostatic apex, illustrating the site of anterior division (**A**) and the placement of the anterior anastomotic sutures (**B**) beneath the mucosa of the uretha

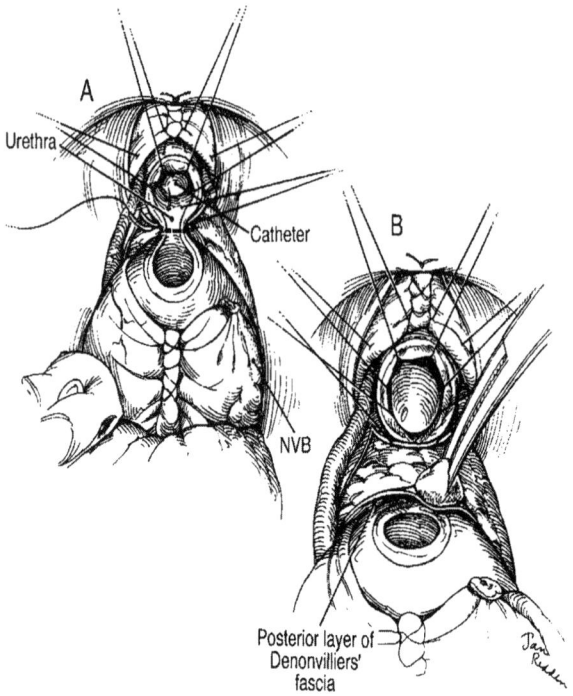

Fig. 7 After the nerves have been dissected free the remaining urethra and posterior layer of Denonvilliers' fascia beneath it are divided (**A**). The correct plane of dissection adjacent to the rectum is developed sharply after it has been identified with the aid of a Kittner dissector (**B**)

4   Erectile Function After Nerve-Sparing Radical Prostatectomy

Reported rates for the recovery of potency following radical prostatectomy vary widely. Outstanding postoperative potency rates of 62–86% have been reported *(10–12)*, but these seem to be confined to centers of excellence. The success rate drops to 44% in a large retrospective survey of non-specialists *(13)* and falls to 21% in single institutional prospective series assessing preoperative and postoperative sexual function with validated questionnaires *(14)*. Quinlan and associates found three factors associated with recovery of potency after radical prostatectomy: age, clinical and pathologic stage, and preservation of the neurovascular tissue *(15)*. Approximately 90% of men younger than 50 were potent if either one or both neurovascular bundles were preserved. For men older than 50, return of potency was more likely if both neurovascular bundles were preserved rather than only one. Catalona et al. reported potency in 68% of patients when both nerves were preserved and 47% when one nerve was spared *(11)*. They also demonstrated a strong correlation of preservation of potency with age. Rabbani and colleagues have developed a nomogram to predict the return of potency after radical prostatectomy

Table 1 Probability of Recovery of Potency by 24 and 36 Months After Radical Prostatectomy *(12)* (modified)

Preoperative potency	Probability (%) of recovery of potency by 24 (36) months		
	Age ≤ 60	*Age 60.1–65*	*Age > 65*
Bilateral nerve-sparing			
Full erection	70 (76)	49 (55)	43 (49)
Full erection, recently diminished	53 (59)	34 (39)	30 (35)
Partial erection	43 (49)	27 (31)	23 (27)
Unilateral or bilateral neurovascular bundle damage			
Full erection	60 (67)	40 (46)	35 (41)
Full erection, recently diminished	44 (50)	28 (32)	24 (28)
Partial erection	35 (40)	21 (25)	18 (21)
Unilateral neurovascular bundle resection			
Full erection	26 (30)	15 (18)	13 (15)
Full erection, recently diminished	17 (20)	10 (12)	8.5 (10)
Partial erection	13 (15)	7.5 (8.8)	6.3 (7.5)

based on a series of 314 previously potent patients treated since 1993 *(12)*. Factors significantly associated with recovery of spontaneous erections satisfactory for intercourse included the age of the patient, the quality of erections before the operation, and the degree of preservation of the neurovascular bundles. Time after surgery was also an important factor (Table 1). The median time to recovery of an International Index of Erectile Function (IIEF) score ≥ 17 was 24 months, while 42 months was required to reach an IIEF score ≥ 26.

5 Strategies to Improve Sexual Function after Radical Prostatectomy

5.1 Early Use of Intracavernosal Agents

Montorsi et al. prospectively assessed whether postoperative intracavernous injections of alprostadil could increase the rate of recovery of spontaneous erectile function after nerve-sparing radical prostatectomy *(15)*. Thirty preoperatively potent patients who underwent bilateral NVB-preserving radical prostatectomy were randomized to alprostadil injections three times per week for 12 weeks or observation without any treatment. At 6 months, 8 of 15 men (53%) receiving injections compared to 3 of 15 untreated men (20%) reported recovery of spontaneous erections sufficient for satisfactory sexual intercourse. The investigators hypothesized that alprostadil injections improve cavernosal oxygenation, thus limiting hypoxia-induced tissue damage.

5.2   Early Use of Phosphodiesterase-5 Inhibitors

Padma-Nathan et al. assessed sildenafil citrate in 76 men with normal preoperative erectile function who underwent bilateral nerve-sparing radical prostatectomy (16). Patients were randomized to sildenafil citrate (50 mg, $n = 23$; 100 mg, $n = 28$) or placebo ($n = 25$). The drug was administered nightly, double-blind, from 4 to 40 weeks after surgery. At 48 weeks after surgery, 14 of 51 (27%) men treated with sildenafil citrate but only 1 of the 25 (4%) in the placebo group had spontaneous erectile function as assessed by nocturnal penile tumescence and rigidity testing. The investigators concluded that early postoperative treatment with a phosphodiesterase-5 inhibitor improves long-term recovery of erectile function, supporting the concept of early rehabilitation of erectile function.

5.3   Perioperative Immunophilin Ligand Therapy

Immunophilin ligands have demonstrated neuroprotective activity in several animal models of nerve injury, including regeneration and/or functional recovery of sciatic, facial, and optic nerves (17,18). Histologically, axonal caliber and cross-sectional areas are significantly increased in animals with crushed nerves treated with immunophilin ligands compared to placebo. In addition, animals treated with placebo after nerve crush injury regained only 10% of their original myelination levels, while treated animals regained 30–40%.

Recently, the potential role of the immunophilin ligand FK506 and the non-immunosuppressive FK506 derivative GPI-1046 has been investigated in a model of cavernous nerve injury (19). The recovery of erections was significantly greater in treated animals compared to animals receiving placebo. Immunohistochemical studies demonstrated that the immunophilin ligand-treated animals had preserved cavernosal tissue histology. The authors suggest that the neurotropic effects of these agents may decrease the extent of cavernosal nerve degeneration and improve the recovery of erectile function after radical prostatectomy. These agents are currently being evaluated in clinical trials to determine their potential to serve as neuroprotective agents following radical prostatectomy.

References

1. Walsh, P.C., and Donker, P.J. (1982) Impotence following radical prostatectomy: insight into etiology and prevention. *J. Urol.* **128**(3), 492–497.
2. Lue, T.F., Zeineh, S.J., Schmidt, R.A., and Tanagho, E.A. (1984) Neuroanatomy of penile erection: its relevance to iatrogenic impotence. *J. Urol.* **131**(2), 273–280.
3. Lepor, H., Gregerman, M., Crosby, R., Mostofi, F.K., and Walsh, P.C. (1985) Precise localization of the autonomic nerves from the pelvic plexus to the corpora cavernosa: a detailed anatomical study of the adult male pelvis. *J. Urol.* **133**(2), 207–212.

4. Breza, J., Aboseif, S.R., Orvis, B.R., Lue, T.F., and Tanagho, E.A. (1989) Detailed anatomy of penile neurovascular structures: surgical significance. *J. Urol.* **141**(2), 437–443.
5. Secin, F.P., Karanikolas, N., Touijer, A.K., Salamanca, J.I., Vickers, A.J., and Guillonneau, B. (2005) Anatomy of accessory pudendal arteries in laparoscopic radical prostatectomy. *J. Urol.* **174**(2), 523–526; discussion 6.
6. Droupy, S., Hessel, A., Benoit, G., Blanchet, P., Jardin, A., and Giuliano, F. (1999) Assessment of the functional role of accessory pudendal arteries in erection by transrectal color Doppler ultrasound. *J. Urol.* **162**(6), 1987–1991.
7. Rogers, C.G., Trock, B.P., and Walsh, P.C. (2004) Preservation of accessory pudendal arteries during radical retropubic prostatectomy: surgical technique and results. *Urology* **64**(1), 148–151.
8. Eastham, J.A., and Scardino, P.T. (2006) Comprehensive textbook of genitourinary oncology, 3rd ed. Philadelphia: Lippincott Williams & Wilkins.
9. Ong, A.M., Su, L.M., Varkarakis, I., et al. (2004) Nerve sparing radical prostatectomy: effects of hemostatic energy sources on the recovery of cavernous nerve function in a canine model. *J. Urol.* **172**(4 Pt 1), 1318–1322.
10. Walsh, P.C., Marschke, P., Ricker, D., and Burnett, A.L. (2000) Patient-reported urinary continence and sexual function after anatomic radical prostatectomy. *Urology* **55**(1), 58–61.
11. Catalona, W.J., and Basler, J.W. (1993) Return of erections and urinary continence following nerve sparing radical retropubic prostatectomy. *J. Urol.* **150**(3), 905–907.
12. Rabbani, F., Stapleton, A.M., Kattan, M.W., Wheeler, T.M., and Scardino, P.T. (2000) Factors predicting recovery of erections after radical prostatectomy. *J. Urol.* **164**(6), 1929–1934.
13. Stanford, J.L., Feng, Z., Hamilton, A.S., et al. (2000) Urinary and sexual function after radical prostatectomy for clinically localized prostate cancer: the Prostate Cancer Outcomes Study. *JAMA* **283**(3), 354–360.
14. Talcott, J.A., Rieker P, Propert, K.J., et al. (1997) Patient-reported impotence and incontinence after nerve-sparing radical prostatectomy. *J. Natl. Cancer Inst.* **89**(15), 1117–1123.
15. Montorsi, F., Guazzoni, G., Strambi, L.F., et al. (1997) Recovery of spontaneous erectile function after nerve-sparing radical retropubic prostatectomy with and without early intracavernous injections of alprostadil: results of a prospective, randomized trial. *J. Urol.* **158**(4), 1408–1410.
16. Padma-Nathan, H., McCullough, A., and Guiliano, F. (2003) Postoperative nightly administration of sildenafil citrate significantly improves normal spontaneous erectile function after bilateral nerve-sparing radical prostatectomy. *J. Urol.* **169**(Suppl 4), 375.
17. Freeman, E.E., and Grosskreutz, C.L. (2000) The effects of FK506 on retinal ganglion cells after optic nerve crush. *Invest. Ophthalmol. Vis. Sci.* **41**(5):1111–1115.
18. Gold, B.G., Katoh, K., and Storm-Dickerson, T. (1995) The immunosuppressant FK506 increases the rate of axonal regeneration in rat sciatic nerve. *J. Neurosci.* **15**(11), 7509–7516.
19. Burnett, A.L., and Becker, R.E. (2004) Immunophilin ligands promote penile neurogenesis and erection recovery after cavernous nerve injury. *J. Urol.* **171**(1), 495–500.

Chapter 6
Laparoscopic and Robotic-Assisted Radical Prostatectomy: Sexual Function Outcome

Phillipe Paparel, Javier Romero Otero, Bertrand Guillonneau, and Karim Touijer

Abstract   The challenge of radical prostatectomy as a treatment of clinically local-ized prostate cancer lies in its goals. Achieving cancer control often competes with the preservation of sexual function. The introduction of minimally invasive tech-niques such as laparoscopic radical prostatectomy with or without robotic assistance in the last 10 years was associated with a remarkable interest in the urological com-munity. Such a rapid popularity of minimally invasive techniques is not supported by evidence demonstrating superiority over other existing surgical approaches. In fact, like the open radical prostatectomy literature, the laparoscopic and robotic-assisted laparoscopic radical prostatectomy literature reviewed in this chapter showed that a large experience with the technique has been accumulated but the subset of patients on whom the sexual function recovery is reported remain relatively small. The lit-erature also shows heterogeneity in the methodology of data acquisition, analysis, and interpretation. While prospective analyses at centers of excellence demonstrated equivalency of sexual function recovery between open and laparoscopic radical prostatectomies, the technique of radical prostatectomy regardless of the approach remains highly operator dependent.

Keywords   Laparoscopic radical prostatectomy; sexual function outcomes; erectile dysfunction; robotic-assisted LRP.

From: *Current Clinical Urology* Series, *Sexual Function in the Prostate Cancer Patient*
Edited by John P. Mulhall, DOI 10.1007/978-1-60327-555-2_6,
© Humana Press, a part of Springer Science+Business Media, LLC 2009

1 Introduction

The feasibility, reproducibility, and teachability of the laparoscopic radical prostate-ctomy are proven through its worldwide use *(1–9)*. The technique is well-established and is beyond the transition period from the initial experience of the pioneer laparo-scopic surgeons. The question remains now that the technique is reaching maturity: how is it performing? And how do we measure the quality of a laparoscopic radical prostatectomy?

The goal of modern radical prostatectomy is to excise all cancer with the least morbidity and full recovery of continence and potency. This aim is a formidable and challenging task, and resulted in a number of technical innovations contribut-ing thus far to the great strides realized in the surgical treatment of clinically localized prostate cancer *(1,10–12)*. Such an innovation is the use of the laparo-scopic approach in performing radical prostatectomy *(1,12)* with the aspiration that laparoscopic radical prostatectomy (LRP) will equal other approaches in terms of oncological efficacy and functional outcome but yet surpass them in regards to con-valescence and short-term morbidity.

In the most recent years, the DaVinci robotic system (intuitive surgical, Sunny-vale, California) has been increasingly used to perform laparoscopic radical prosta-tectomy (RALRP) in the United States particularly *(13)*. Herein, we report and analyse the results of sexual outcome after laparoscopic radical prostatectomy (LRP and RALRP) based on the published literature in the past 9 years *(14)*.

We conducted an extensive MEDLINE literature search (search terms "laparo-scopic radical prostatectomy" and "robotic assisted laparoscopic radical prostate-ctomy") from 1990 through 2007; only full length articles identified during this search were considered for the analysis. A preference was given to the articles with larger series (>100 patients). The laparoscopic results were interpreted as whole regardless of the technical differences (transperitoneal versus extraperitoneal, antegrade versus retrograde dissection, number, disposition, or size of the surgical ports, etc.).

2 Heterogeneity of Results

The lack of uniformity in defining, assessing, and reporting functional results fol-lowing radical prostatectomy in general, leads to a disparity of results between dif-ferent series. The definition used, the methodology by which the data are gathered and analyzed, and the time of assessment need to be taken into consideration while interpreting the results of potency postoperatively. This may preclude any compar-ative analyses between series.

3 Sexual Function Outcome

Preoperative potency, extent of neurovascular bundle preservation, and patient age were shown to be significant predictors of erectile function recovery after radical prostatectomy and along with the use of phosphodiesterase type 5 inhibitors (PDE5i) need to be taken into consideration when interpreting erectile function data.

Most series of LRP include potency data only on a small subset of patients, usually treated after the technique of LRP and neurovascular bundle preservation has been mastered. Stolzenburg et al. using the International Index of Erectile Dysfunction (IIEF) to measure post LRP potency, reported their experience of 700 extraperitoneal LRP. The follow-up was 6 months and nerve-sparing was performed in 185 preoperatively potent patients (26%), unilaterally in 114 patients (16%), and bilaterally in 71 (10%). At 6 months postoperatively, 8/66 men with unilateral (12%) and 16/34 with bilateral nerve preservation (47%) had erections sufficient for intercourse with or without the help of PDE5i. Baseline and postoperative IIEF scores were not reported *(15)*. Using question 3 (*How often were you able to penetrate your partner?*) and question 4 (*How often were you able to maintain your erection after you had penetrated your partner?*) of the IIEF to determine potency, Roumeguere et al. reported a 65% 1-year potency rate in 26 preoperatively potent men who underwent bilateral nerve-sparing *(16)*.

Evaluating potency with the EPIC questionnaire, Link et al. reported a decrease to 64% of baseline at 12 months for both the sexual function and bother subdomains. In the same experience, using a single question to determine potency ("During the last 4 weeks, how often did you have sexual intercourse?"), the potency rate was 79% at 12 months in a subgroup of 50 preoperatively potent men who underwent bilateral nerve-sparing. Of note, most patients used PDE5i and 11% were using vacuum erection devices, pharmacological injection therapy, or transurethral alprostadil postoperatively. The latter group of patients was asked to assess sexual function without such therapy *(17)*.

Of their initial 550 patients, the Montsouris group reported in a subset of 47 consecutive patients less than 70 years of age. Of those patients who were preoperatively potent and who had bilateral nerve-sparing LRP, 31 (66%) were able to have intercourse with or without PDE5i *(18)*. Rassweiler et al. reported in their first 180 patient LRP series, 10 patients with nerve-sparing (2 bilateral and 8 unilateral). Four patients had "*sufficient erections with sildenafil*" *(19)* (Table 1). Katz et al. reported in 143 preoperatively potent patients: 26 responded to the questionnaire at 12 months and 23% had sexual intercourse with any erectogenic therapy. The questionnaire used was a non-validated set of three questions with "yes" and "no" answers *(20)*.

Two points become obvious when reviewing the published erectile function recovery results after LRP. Firstly, neurovascular bundle preservation, rather than predominating, constitutes a minority in each reported experience. Subsequently, potency data comprise only a small number of patients in each series. Secondly, the

Table 1 Postoperative Potency Rate According to Surgical Approach

Series		No. of patients	Mean age	FU months	Intercourse after bilateral preservation (%)	Spontaneous erection (%)	Evaluation method
Laparoscopic radical prostatectomy							
Turk	(28)	58	60.2	12	38.5	—	Interview
Rozet	(29)	599	62	6	43	—	Questionnaire
Hoznek	(4)	134		12	46		Questionnaire
Stolzemburg	(30)	34	63.4	6	47	—	Questionnaire
German group	(31)	5,824	64	12	52.5	—	Questionnaire
Roumeguere	(16)	26	62.5	12	53.8		Questionnaire
Curto	(32)	137	62	12	59	—	Questionnaire
Salomon	(33)	77	63.8	12	59	—	Questionnaire
Eden	(5)	79	62.2	12	—	62	Interview
Rogers	(34)	369	57.9	12	65.7	—	Questionnaire
Guillonneau	(18)	550	—	12	66	85	Questionnaire
Rassweiler	(14)	41	64	12	67	—	Questionnaire
Su	(35)	177	—	12	76	—	Questionnaire
Link	(36)	122	58.3	12	78	—	Questionnaire
Robotic-assisted radical prostatectomy							
Bentas	(37)	37	61.3	15	—	22	Questionnaire
Ahlering	(38)	3	57.3	≤9	—	33	Questionnaire
Zorn	(13)	300	59.4	12	53 (overall)	—	Questionnaire
Menon	(21)	100	60	6	59	—	Questionnaire
Joseph	(39)	325	60	6	68	—	Questionnaire
Chien	(24)	56	58.9	12	69 (overall)	—	Questionnaire
Kaul	(40)	154	57.4	12	96	—	Questionnaire
Menon	(22)	1,113	60.2	24	100	—	Questionnaire

available results, although interesting, do not represent the current status of laparoscopic radical prostatectomy. Now that the technique is beyond the learning phase, the LRP literature is due for more substantial functional results.

Similarly in RALRP, there is a paucity of data with either limited follow-up or limited number of patients. In the published data, 20–97% of the patients were considered potent 12 months after RALRP. Menon et al. reported their erectile function outcomes after RALP with rates ranging from 59% at 6 months *(21,22)* to 100% at 24 months *(23)*. Chien et al. reported on RALP outcomes, with an overall rate of a return to baseline sexual function of 47, 54, 66 and 69% at 1, 3, 6 and 12 months postoperatively, respectively *(24)* (Table 1). These authors considered that this was a favorable outcome in comparison to open series of RRP using the same validated questionnaire, in which the percentage of patients reporting a return to baseline sexual function was 37, 41 and 50% at 3, 6 and 12 months, respectively *(24)*. Menon et al. reports that the median time to intercourse after RALP is two times shorter compared with RRP *(23)*. Interestingly, this recovery time was not found to be significantly different when a unilateral or bilateral nerve preservation was performed. In the largest RALRP published experience, 70% of the preoperatively potent patients reported intercourse at 12 months and 100% at 48 months when the neurovascular bundles were preserved bilaterally including the anterolateral aspect of the prostatic fascia *(25)*.

The laparoscopic approach to radical prostatectomy was initially met with great enthusiasm. The hope was that the magnification and the detailed anatomical visualization it provided, along with the lower intraoperative blood loss would translate into better functional outcome. The reality is that after nearly 10 years, there is no evidence to support the superiority of this approach over the open approach and the fact is that it has never been studied appropriately and it is not clear whether it will ever be.

However, the magnification and the detailed anatomical visualization allowed us to identify a higher incidence of accessory pudendal arteries, the majority of which could be preserved without compromising the oncological outcome *(26,27)*. Future studies will establish their role in the functional outcomes.

References

1. Schuessler, W.W., Schulam, P.G., Clayman, R.V., and Kavoussi, L.R. (1997) Laparoscopic radical prostatectomy: initial short-term experience. *Urology* **50,** 854.
2. Guillonneau, B., and Vallancien, G. (1999) Laparoscopic radical prostatectomy: initial experience and preliminary assessment after 65 operations. *Prostate* **39,** 71.
3. Hara, I., Kawabata, G., Miyake, H., Hara, S., Fujisawa, M., Okada, H., et al. (2002) Feasibility and usefulness of laparoscopic radical prostatectomy: Kobe University experience. *Int. J. Urol.* **9,** 635.
4. Hoznek, A., Salomon, L., Olsson, L.E., Antiphon, P., Saint, F., Cicco, A., et al. (2001) Laparoscopic radical prostatectomy. The Creteil experience. *Eur. Urol.* **40,** 38.
5. Eden, C.G., Cahill, D., Vass, J.A., Adams, T.H., and Dauleh, M.I. (2002) Laparoscopic radical prostatectomy: the initial UK series. *BJU Int.* **90,** 876.

6. Dahl, D.M., L'Esperance J,O., Trainer, A.F., Jiang, Z., Gallagher, K., Litwin, D.E., et al. (2002) Laparoscopic radical prostatectomy: initial 70 cases at a U.S. university medical center. *Urology* **60**, 859.

7. Cecchini Rosell, L., Areal Calama, J., and Saladie Roig, J.M. (2003) [Laparoscopic radical prostatectomy. Review of our first year.]. *Arch. Esp. Urol.* **56**, 287.

8. Kawabata, G., Hara, I., Hara, S., Isotani, S., Sakai, Y., Wada, Y., et al. (2001) [Laparoscopic radical prostatectomy: initial 17 case report]. *Nippon Hinyokika Gakkai Zasshi* **92**, 647.

9. Rassweiler, J., Sentker, L., Seemann, O., Hatzinger, M., Stock, C., and Frede, T. (2001) Heilbronn laparoscopic radical prostatectomy. Technique and results after 100 cases. *Eur. Urol.* **40**, 54.

10. Walsh, P.C., and Lepor, H. (1987) The role of radical prostatectomy in the management of prostatic cancer. *Cancer* **60**, 526.

11. Eastham, J.A., and Scardino, P.T. (1996) Radical prostatectomy for clinical stage T1 and T2 prostate cancer. In: Vogelzang, N.J., Scardino, P.T., Shipley W.V., et al., eds. *Comprehensive Textbook of Genitourinary Oncology*, 2nd edn. Baltimore: Williams & Wilkins, pp. 722–738.

12. Guillonneau, B., Cathelineau, X., Barret, E., Rozet, F., and Vallancien, G. (1998) [Laparoscopic radical prostatectomy. Preliminary evaluation after 28 interventions]. *Presse Med.* **27**, 1570.

13. Zorn, K.C., Gofrit, O.N., Orvieto, M.A., Mikhail, A.A., Zagaja, G.P., and Shalhav, A.L. (2006) Robotic-assisted laparoscopic prostatectomy: functional and pathologic outcomes with interfascial nerve preservation. *Eur. Urol.*

14. Rassweiler, J., Schulze, M., Teber, D., Seemann, O., and Frede, T. (2004) Laparoscopic radical prostatectomy: functional and oncological outcomes. *Curr. Opin. Urol.* **14**, 75.

15. Stolzenburg, J.U., Rabenalt, R., Do, M., Ho, K., Dorschner, W., and Waldkirch, E., et al. (2005) Endoscopic extraperitoneal radical prostatectomy: oncological and functional results after 700 procedures. *J. Urol.* **174**, 1271.

16. Roumeguere, T., Bollens, R., Vanden Bossche, M., Rochet, D., Bialek, D., Hoffman, P., et al. (2003) Radical prostatectomy: a prospective comparison of oncological and functional results between open and laparoscopic approaches. *World J. Urol.* **20**, 360.

17. Link, R.E., Su, L.M., Sullivan, W., Bhayani, S.B., and Pavlovich, C.P. (2005) Health related quality of life before and after laparoscopic radical prostatectomy. *J. Urol.* **173**, 175.

18. Guillonneau, B., Cathelineau, X., Doublet, J.D., Baumert, H., and Vallancien, G. (2002) Laparoscopic radical prostatectomy: assessment after 550 procedures. *Crit. Rev. Oncol. Hematol.* **43**, 123.

19. Rassweiler, J., Seemann, O., Hatzinger, M., Schulze, M., and Frede, T. (2003) Technical evolution of laparoscopic radical prostatectomy after 450 cases. *J. Endourol.* **17**, 143.

20. Katz, R., Salomon, L., Hoznek, A., de la Taille, A., Vordos, D., Cicco, A., et al. (2002) Patient reported sexual function following laparoscopic radical prostatectomy. *J. Urol.* **168**, 2078.

21. Menon, M., Shrivastava, A., Sarle, R., Hemal, A., and Tewari, A. (2003) Vattikuti Institute Prostatectomy: a single-team experience of 100 cases. *J. Endourol.* **17**, 785.

22. Menon, M., Shrivastava, A., Kaul, S., Badani, K.K., Fumo, M., Bhandari, M., et al. (2006) Vattikuti Institute Prostatectomy: contemporary technique and analysis of results. *Eur. Urol.*

23. Menon, M., Kaul, S., Bhandari, A., Shrivastava, A., Tewari, A., and Hemal, A. (2005) Potency following robotic radical prostatectomy: a questionnaire based analysis of outcomes after conventional nerve sparing and prostatic fascia sparing techniques. *J. Urol.* **174**, 2291.

24. Chien, G.W., Mikhail, A.A., Orvieto, M.A., Zagaja, G.P., Sokoloff, M.H., Brendler, C.B., et al. (2005) Modified clipless antegrade nerve preservation in robotic-assisted laparoscopic radical prostatectomy with validated sexual function evaluation. *Urology* **66**, 419.

25. Menon, M., Shrivastava, A., Kaul, S., Badani, K.K., Fumo, M., Bhandari, M., et al. (2007) Vattikuti institute prostatectomy: contemporary technique and analysis of results. *Eur. Urol.* **51**, 648.

26. Secin, F.P., Karanikolas, N., Touijer, A.K., Salamanca, J.I., Vickers, A.J., and Guillonneau, B. (2005) Anatomy of accessory pudendal arteries in laparoscopic radical prostatectomy. *J. Urol.* **174**, 523.

27. Secin, F.P., Karanikolas, N., Kuroiwa, K., Vickers, A., Touijer, K., and Guillonneau, B. (2005) Positive surgical margins and accessory pudendal artery preservation during laparoscopic radical prostatectomy. *Eur. Urol.* **48,** 786.

28. Turk, I., Deger, S., Winkelmann, B., Schonberger, B., and Loening, S.A. (2001) Laparoscopic radical prostatectomy. Technical aspects and experience with 125 cases. *Eur. Urol.* **40,** 46.

29. Rozet, F., Galiano, M., Cathelineau, X., Barret, E., Cathala, N., and Vallancien, G. (2005) Extraperitoneal laparoscopic radical prostatectomy: a prospective evaluation of 600 cases. *J. Urol.* **174,** 908.

30. Stolzenburg, J.U., Rabenalt, R., Do, M., Ho, K., Dorschner, W., Waldkirch, E., et al. (2005) Endoscopic extraperitoneal radical prostatectomy: oncological and functional results after 700 procedures. *J. Urol.* **174,** 1271.

31. Rassweiler, J., Stolzenburg, J., Sulser, T., Deger, S., Zumbe, J., Hofmockel, G., et al. (2006) Laparoscopic radical prostatectomy – the experience of the German Laparoscopic Working Group. *Eur. Urol.* **49,** 113.

32. Curto, F., Benijts, J., Pansadoro, A., Barmoshe, S., Hoepffner, J.L., Mugnier, C., et al. (2006) Nerve sparing laparoscopic radical prostatectomy: our technique. *Eur. Urol.* **49,** 344.

33. Salomon, L., Anastasiadis, A.G., Katz, R., De La Taille, A., Saint, F., Vordos, D., et al. (2002) Urinary continence and erectile function: a prospective evaluation of functional results after radical laparoscopic prostatectomy. *Eur. Urol.* **42,** 338.

34. Rogers, C.G., Su, L.M., Link, R.E., Sullivan, W., Wagner, A., and Pavlovich, C.P. (2006) Age stratified functional outcomes after laparoscopic radical prostatectomy. *J. Urol.* **176,** 2448.

35. Su, L.M., Link, R.E., Bhayani, S.B., Sullivan, W., and Pavlovich, C.P. (2004) Nerve-sparing laparoscopic radical prostatectomy: replicating the open surgical technique. *Urology* **64,** 123.

36. Link, R.E., Su, L.M., Sullivan, W., Bhayani, S.B., and Pavlovich, C.P. (2005) Health related quality of life before and after laparoscopic radical prostatectomy. *J. Urol.* **173,** 175.

37. Bentas, W., Wolfram, M., Jones, J., Brautigam, R., Kramer, W., and Binder, J. (2003) Robotic technology and the translation of open radical prostatectomy to laparoscopy: the early Frankfurt experience with robotic radical prostatectomy and one year follow-up. *Eur. Urol.* **44,** 175.

38. Ahlering, T.E., Woo, D., Eichel, L., Lee, D.I., Edwards, R., and Skarecky, D.W. (2004) Robot-assisted versus open radical prostatectomy: a comparison of one surgeon's outcomes. *Urology* **63,** 819.

39. Joseph, J.V., Rosenbaum, R., Madeb, R., Erturk, E., and Patel, H.R. (2006) Robotic extraperitoneal radical prostatectomy: an alternative approach. *J. Urol.* **175,** 945.

40. Kaul, S., Savera, A., Badani, K., Fumo, M., Bhandari, A., and Menon, M. (2006) Functional outcomes and oncological efficacy of Vattikuti Institute prostatectomy with Veil of Aphrodite nerve-sparing: an analysis of 154 consecutive patients. *BJU Int.* **97,** 467.

Chapter 7
Potency-Sparing Radiation: Myth or Reality?

P. William McLaughlin and Gregory Merrick

Abstract The chapter title aptly defines the fact that potency preservation following radiation therapy is not an established technique, in contrast to potency preservation through nerve-sparing prostatectomy. No prospective trials that define and prove the efficacy of potency preservation strategies have been completed, and controversies regarding the critical target and mechanism remain unsettled. The technical capability to profoundly limit dose to any defined structure through advanced planning such as intensity-modulated radiation therapy (IMRT) means that as the critical structures are defined dose limitation will be possible. Given this technical capability and the growing literature defining the critical targets, potency preservation following radiation is likely to move from myth to reality in the near future.

Keywords Erectile dysfunction post radiotherapy; potency-sparing radiotherapy; post radiation sexual function.

From: *Current Clinical Urology* Series, *Sexual Function in the Prostate Cancer Patient*
Edited by John P. Mulhall, DOI 10.1007/978-1-60327-555-2_7,
© Humana Press, a part of Springer Science+Business Media, LLC 2009

1   Introduction

Three groups of studies form the basis for strategies to preserve sexual function after radiation therapy. One group defines the *incidence of erectile dysfunction* following different forms of radiation treatments. These range in quality and follow up, but confirm that erectile dysfunction (ED) is (i) a very common outcome following radiation, (ii) progressive over years of follow up, and (iii) varies with radiation technique *(1)*. The second group of studies is *correlative*; the incidence of erectile dysfunction is related to dose to a critical structure *(2–9)*. Such studies have been limited by the poor definition of critical erectile structures by CT, and the initial correlation of erectile dysfunction with penile bulb dose was criticized on the basis that the penile bulb plays no significant role in erectile function *(8)*. The most compelling correlative evidence comes from contemporary brachytherapy series employing validated instruments. This may be due to the wide dose gradients delivered to critical structures by brachytherapy from minimal dose to prescription dose allowing for wider dose spread than external beam studies *(2,5)*. Although correlative study results are mixed, there is little doubt remaining that dose to the proximal penis region correlates with erectile dysfunction more than dose to the neurovascular bundle. This correlation has led to a variety of strategies to limit dose and preserve potency. The third group of studies is *mechanism studies*, which attempt to determine the vascular versus neurologic basis for radiation-induced ED. Such studies are limited, but suggest that vascular effects contribute more than neurological effects to radiation-induced ED *(10–13)*.

The limitations in the knowledge of mechanism and critical structure for potency preservation mean that current strategies are a "best guess" at critical targets, and current studies seek to improve potency outcomes but more importantly seek to define the critical targets and ultimate mechanism for erectile dysfunction post-therapy.

2   Critical Endpoints

An important component of improved evaluation of sexual function is in the language used to define function and dysfunction. The term *impotence*, which is analogous in emotional impact to the term *barren* in female reproductive dysfunction, is both absolute and judgmental in tone. The term erectile dysfunction (ED) removes the stigma associated with the term impotence, and also implies wide variation in degrees of dysfunction. Unfortunately, the majority of studies completed in the radiation oncology literature use the terms impotent and potent in a black and white manner, when erectile function was the actual endpoint of concern. While ED is a major advance in specificity of post-radiation evaluation, several other critical endpoints may be affected by radiation treatment. Libido, erection, ejaculation, reproductive potency, and orgasm may all be affected post-radiation, and all must be included in evaluating post-radiation changes.

Libido may be decreased if testicular exposure during radiation results in decreased androgen production *(14–17)*. There is controversy about the duration and degree of testosterone decline following external radiation, transient in most with a minority of patients experiencing long-term suppression. Androgen levels are more commonly affected by the use of systemic androgen blockade used in conjunction with radiation. The assumption that recovery of normal levels following cessation of androgen blockade is questioned by the average recovery time of 18 months and the permanent suppression in 30% reported by Padula *(18–21)*. The quality and quantity of ejaculate is a critical concern to some men, who associate potency with ejaculation as much as erection or climax. Drugs used to improve urinary function during treatment such as alpha blockers cause relaxation of the internal sphincter and loss of ejaculate in a large fraction of patients, an effect that may be incorrectly attributed to radiation treatment. Actual reproductive fertility is a concern to some men, and in spite of high likelihood of infertility by interruption of sperm production or transport, sterility is not assured, as conception has occurred after all currently available therapies *(22,23)*. Finally painful ejaculation has been reported with prostate brachytherapy in a small subset of patients, an uncommon outcome in external beam patients. Such pain may cause a limitation of sexual activity in spite of normal erectile function *(24)*.

Current scales for erectile and sexual function have limitations in elderly men diagnosed with prostate cancer. Instruments that validate erectile function on the basis of sexual function such as "sufficient firmness for penetration" may not have validity in men who masturbate but are not sexually active *(25)*. Also men who have decreased sexual performance on the basis of fear of failure may have less ED when masturbating while relaxed. Scales which address erectile function without quantifying sexual desire may not distinguish loss of libido and attendant erectile dysfunction with primary erectile dysfunction. In the author's experience decreased libido as the contributing cause for what may be reported as erectile dysfunction is common in post-radiation patients, a decrease due to widely varying causes, from low testosterone to depression to a shift in interest following a diagnosis of cancer. Standard scales may not reflect the concern of some men regarding ejaculate quantity and quality, and painful ejaculation is uncommon in untreated patients and therefore not reflected on standard, validated instruments. In spite of these limitations the employment of standard, validated instruments has improved the understanding of sexual dysfunction and improved physician understanding of the complexity of sexual function post-treatment.

Because of these limitations, validated instruments should be complemented with direct history by physicians or health care providers to address issues not included in standard instruments. Although patient-completed surveys have a research validity that physician history does not, part of the criticism of physician-derived data is that physicians have not sought out and reported negative outcomes exhaustively. If physicians do an exhaustive history and give the patient an opportunity to define problems in all domains of sexual function invaluable information and insight can be gained, even if only useful to that patient. In the author's experience, sexual dysfunction is rarely isolated to ED, and often individual patterns of dysfunction may result from two or three domains. Merely writing a prescription for a PDE5 inhibitor is not good medicine. Critical distinction of libido loss from erectile dysfunction, and sexual performance-anxiety related ED from primary ED may be accomplished in an efficient manner with limited, straightforward questions and result in more appropriately targeted interventions. One schema to assure a comprehensive history is presented in Table 1. This table suggests the complexity of sexual endpoints post-treatment and also begins to define the multiple domains of dysfunction that may result from prostate cancer or radiation treatment. The following case studies illustrate this complexity.

Carl was 2 years post-combined beam and implant therapy and had an undetectable PSA. He was thrilled with his outcome, with minimal GU or GI side effects, and offered to counsel other men struggling with the treatment decision. When asked about erections he stated they were normal. He then added, "ever since the treatment I have had severe pain with ejaculation and due to the pain we have stopped having sex. We consider it a small price to pay for saving my life."

It is ironic that this patient is pleased enough with his outcome that he would be willing to talk others into the treatment, but accepts without question an outcome (dysorgasmia and cessation of sex) many would find unacceptable. This emphasizes the difference between symptom documentation (dysorgasmia) and quality of life. This patient accepted what others would find unacceptable.

Table 1 Sexual Domains of Interest Post Therapy

Libido	Opportunity	Erectile Dysfunction in spite of normal libido and opportunity
Normal	Spouse or partner ill	
Increased	Partner with loss of libido	Decrease compared to pre-
Decreased		treatment
Fatigue from the treatment		Decreased and limiting sexuality
Depression		Responsive to Rx
Anxiety		Unresponsive to Rx
Hormonal		
Interest shift		
Ejaculation	**Orgasm**	**Potency/infertility**
Normal volume/consistency	Normal	Sperm count
Decreased volume	Change in intensity	Birth control
Post-radiation	Pain	
Alpha blockers	Intermittent	
TURP	Consistent	
No ejaculate	Worsening	
Hematospermia	Causing sex avoidance	

Jim was 2 years post-implant and had an undetectable PSA, baseline GU and GI symptoms, and moderate ED for which he tried Viagra with mixed results. When asked about libido he stated "it is not like when I was twenty," but with further questioning said it had dropped "quite a bit" in the past year, a change he attributed to aging. He was asked about other changes in lifestyle, and noted a change in "get up and go." "I think about doing things and then decide not to, and that is a change for me." He also attributed this to aging. His testosterone level was below age appropriate levels, and he opted for supplementation, with marked improvement in libido, and "get up and go." His response to Viagra remained variable but by frequency of intercourse he was more active than prior to supplementation.

This demonstrates the overlap of libido loss and ED, and emphasizes the importance of baseline testosterone levels as a reference to evaluate post-therapy changes. More importantly, it emphasizes the patient's tendency to attribute significant treatment related delayed changes to aging rather than treatment, especially when the changes occur years after treatment.

3 Post-radiation Effects on Sexual Function – Timing and Targets

3.1 Biology, Timing, and Targets

A pivotal study on the mechanism of post-radiation erectile dysfunction concluded that ED is mutifactorial, including vascular, nerve, and smooth muscle injury components *(1)*. Five months following varied doses of radiation to the prostate region of rats histological evaluation revealed a decrease in nitric oxide producing nerves. In addition smooth muscle atrophy of the corpus cavernosum resulted in decreased response to the direct smooth muscle relaxant papaverine. While this finding challenges the vascular basis of ED post-radiation, the authors concluded that damage to vessels supplying the nerves and smooth muscle may have been responsible for the loss of erectile tissues and function. Notable is the dose response variance; progressive loss of nerve density with dose, and threshold loss of smooth muscle only at extremely high dose.

In spite of the effects noted on nerve and smooth muscle the vascular basis for post-radiation toxicity is favored by an abundance of evidence, including universal vascular histologic changes post radiation in virtually every organ studied, as described by Fajardo *(26)*. In fact with the exception of rare cells vulnerable to apoptosis following radiation such as lymphocytes, the tolerance of any organ is directly related to vascular supply. The most vulnerable vascular target is the capillary endothelial cell. Tissues with large contiguous capillary and microvascular networks such as kidney and lung, or unique vascular supply such as liver, are most vulnerable to radiation damage and the tolerance is less than one half the dose of organs with ample blood supply. Tumors with extensive vascular supply such as renal cell or glioblastoma are less responsive to radiation, possibly on a vascular basis. Erectile function is a complex vascular-based mechanism based on simultaneous afferent dilation and efferent constriction and would be predicted to be extremely vulnerable to radiation damage. On this basis one would predict the terminal internal pudendal artery junction with the corpus cavernosum to be the most vulnerable to disruption.

The manifestation of endothelial cell damage is delayed for several reasons. The universal initial response to radiation is arrest of cell division. Cells may remain in a dormant state for months and are "doomed but not dead." The mitotic rate of endothelial cells is extremely slow and the arrest phase is extremely prolonged. For example, when canine brains receive a necrosis-causing dose of radiation there may be no clinical manifestation of the damage for months (27) and the brain appears normal on scan until 3–6 weeks prior to death. As the cells resume division the lethal damage is expressed, resulting in microvascular disruption including separation of the endothelial cell from the basal lamina, thrombosis, and rupture. The most critical outcome is ischemia and the triggering of a non-vascular response resulting in compensatory new vessel formation termed telangiectasia. Telangiectasias are compensatory for ischemia but not for function, as they form in locations apart from the normal vascular supply. One would not predict that telangiectasias could restore disruption of the erectile vessels by radiation.

While the endothelial cell's vulnerability is well-established, vascular damage following radiation included damage to every layer of the artery wall, including subendothelial and adventitial fibrosis and hyalinization of the media in small vessels. Medium and larger arteries display extensive intimal fibrosis. The timing of such lesions and the clinical manifestations are delayed relative to the endothelial response. Loss of elasticity limits the capacity for full dilation and rapid filling critical to normal erection function.

Nerve damage from radiation is not universally present in radiated tissues as vascular damage is, but at large doses per fraction nerve damage is encountered in the clinical radiation literature. This was first noted as a problem in intra-op studies of single large dose fraction for sarcomas (28). Although such high doses in a single fraction are unusual with external beam, such fractions are routinely applied with high dose rate radiation (HDR) for prostate boost. Also permanent implants may develop extreme high-dose regions with potential for direct nerve damage and disruption of erectile function on this basis. At lower dose per fraction reversible demyelination is seen in nerve tissue, manifest as Lhermitte or subacute CNS neurologic dysfunction. Demyelination has not been commonly reported outside the CNS, but the subacute timing of the process with slow onset and slow recovery is consistent with reversible ED seen in some radiated patients.

3.2 Radiation Reactions

Acute radiation reactions are due to irritation from inflammation. Prostate cancer treatment is associated with irritation of bowel and bladder. Such reactions are self-limited and generally resolve to a significant degree by 1 month following therapy. Acute erectile dysfunction is rare with external beam therapy, but is seen following brachytherapy in approximately 15% of patients *(24)*. The mechanism of the acute sexual dysfunction is uncertain but may be due to trauma to the erectile tissues by needles passed through the perineum. A subset of men with acute ED post-implant do not recover erectile function.

Subacute radiation reactions beginning weeks to months following radiation are reversible and resolve slowly over months. The mechanism is nerve demyelination. Although such injuries are documented extensively in treatment of central nervous system malignancies, the injury can be induced by radiation in peripheral nerves experimentally or after intra-op abdominal radiation. It may be speculated that such neural injury could explain reversible erectile dysfunction seen in brachytherapy patients in a time frame consistent with demyelination injury and recovery, but mechanism studies will be necessary to confirm this. The target nerves could be the neurovascular bundle or the terminal cavernosal nerves. The clinical pattern of ED that would correlate with this is ED progressing during the first 12 months post-brachy with dependence on Viagra or equivalent, followed at 18–24 months by improvement and decreased requirement for Viagra. We have noted this pattern in an ongoing prospective study of brachytherapy patients.

Late reactions include vascular changes and fibrosis. Late reactions which are vascular may be divided into microvascular and macrovascular. Radiation results in diminution of the capillary and adjacent microvascular network, rendering tissue hypoxic, which initiates a neovascular response. Typically radiated tissues have telangiectasia as evidence of this compensatory response. Such telangiectasias appear 9–18 months following radiation. Possible microvascular targets include the terminal internal pudendal arteries supplying the corpus cavernosum, the vasa nervosa supplying the cavernosal nerves, or where present accessory pudendal arteries. The timing of microvessel damage correlates with the timing of progressive erectile dysfunction following radiation and in theory may be due to disruption of the terminal vessels supplying the corpus cavernosum.

The timing of fibrosis following radiation parallels the microvascular effects in onset (months to years) but may progress continuously over decades. Fibrosis may contribute to ED by compounding the direct injury to vessel and nerves, and by restricting expansion of the CC.

Macrovascular changes are delayed and are manifested as increased arteriosclerosis of radiated tissues. Such changes are typically seen more than 5 years post-radiation and are well-established in a variety of malignancies. Such delayed reactions may cause obstruction of the internal pudendal arteries and accelerate the process responsible for the majority of erectile dysfunction in the untreated population.

Correlation of clinical dysfunction with the above injuries is challenging due to variation in timing of the above injuries and the variable timing of the response. A schema of potential correlations is presented in Table 2 and summarized below.

Table 2 Radiation Response of Normal Tissues with Time

Timing	Onset	Resolution	Mechanism	Target	XRT type
Acute Reversible	Immediate	Weeks	Trauma	CN, IPA CC	B
Acute Irreversible	Immediate		Trauma	CN, IPA CC	B
Subacute Reversible	Weeks	Months	Demyelination	CN, NVB	B>E
Chronic Progressive	9 months	Progressive	Microvascular fibrosis	IPA, CC	E, B
Delayed Progressive	5 years	Progressive	macrovascular	IPA	E>B

E = external beam radiation, B = brachytherapy. CN = cavernosal nerve, NVB = neurovascular bundle, CC = corpus cavernosum, IPA = internal pudendal artery

3.3   Clinical Syndromes

Acute, reversible erectile dysfunction may occur after implant therapy and is likely due to reversible traumatic vascular or nerve injury. It is not typically seen during external beam therapy

Acute, irreversible ED may occur immediately following brachytherapy and may be permanent. The mechanism is not defined but likely involves traumatic disruption of vascular or neural pathways in the course of the needles. This includes the terminal internal pudendal artery (IPA), proximal corpus cavernosum (CC), and cavernosal nerves (CN).

Subacute, reversible ED is seen post-brachytherapy in approximately 1/4 patients. The onset is within weeks and duration may be 12–24 months. The hallmark of the dysfunction is its reversibility. Although the timing is consistent with demyelination and repair, no direct evidence for a demyelination mechanism is available. Potential targets include the neurovascular bundle (NVB) and CN.

Chronic, progressive erectile dysfunction has its onset 9 months to years following radiation and is likely a function of microvascular injury and fibrosis. It is typically responsive to phosphodiesterase inhibitors, but the response may diminish with time. Chronic, progressive ED is well-established post-external beam and brachytherapy.

Delayed progressive *erectile dysfunction* due to macrovascular change is not well-established due to the overlap of microvascular and macrovascular injury. In studies of internal pudendal artery-sparing radiation therapy, a subset of patients have approximation of the IPA and the prostate and separation of the terminal IPA and CC. Such patient may have late onset ED on the basis of the macrovascular change from radiation but the distinction between vascular occlusive disease and non-radiation etiologies is impossible, unless the IPA obstruction occurs in the high-dose region of the vessel. Such patterns of occlusion and dose have been established in head and neck cancers but no evidence is available for discrete high-dose radiation and occlusive disease for pelvic vessels responsible for erectile function.

4 Potential Target Definition

4.1 Prostate Apex Definition

The prostate apex is poorly defined on CT and genitourinary diaphragm (GUD) elements contiguous with the prostate are often included in the prostate contour. MRI is superior in definition of this region relative to CT (Figs. 1 and 2 and Color Plate 1, following p. 264). Because most of the critical erectile structures (CES) are variable distances below the apex, accurate definition of the apex position is more critical to potency sparing than defining the CES, and the degree to which CES can be spared is directly proportional to the distance between the apex and CES. Accurate apex definition and conformal planning or IMRT will result in sparing of the CES, even without formal definition of CES. Multiple strategies have evolved to define the apex, including marker seeds, apex relationship to identifiable structures such as penile bulb or urethrogram apex, MRI imaging in axial, coronal, and sagittal views *(29)*, and genitourinary diaphragm (GUD) recognition on CT following MRI training *(30)* (Table 3).

   MRI studies suggest wide variation in thickness of the GUD (Fig. 3), nullifying rules commonly employed based on apex distance to the penile bulb (PB) or urethrogram apex. The actual distance from the prostate apex to penile bulb on MRI ranges from 0.6 to 2.3 cm. The average distance rules (apex is 1.5 cm above the PB and 1 cm above the urethrogram apex) may lead to overestimating and underestimating the actual distance, a twofold hazard for marginal miss or unneces-

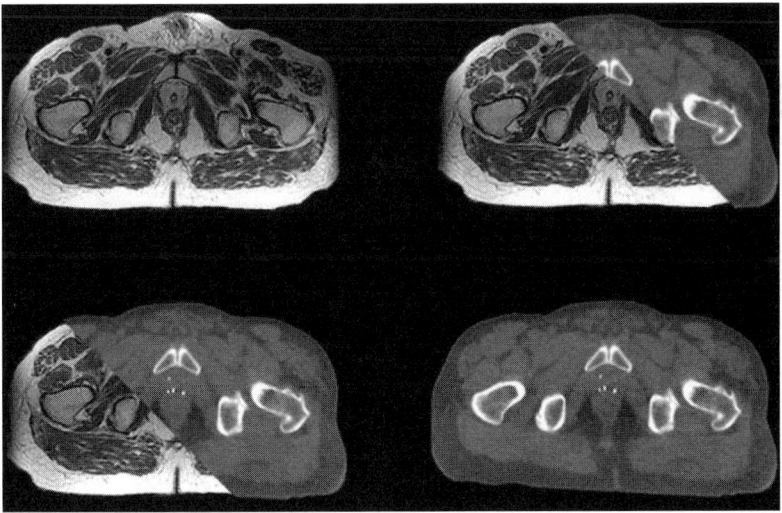

Fig. 1 Fused CT and MRI demonstrating the clarity of detail on MRI versus CT at the same level in the prostate

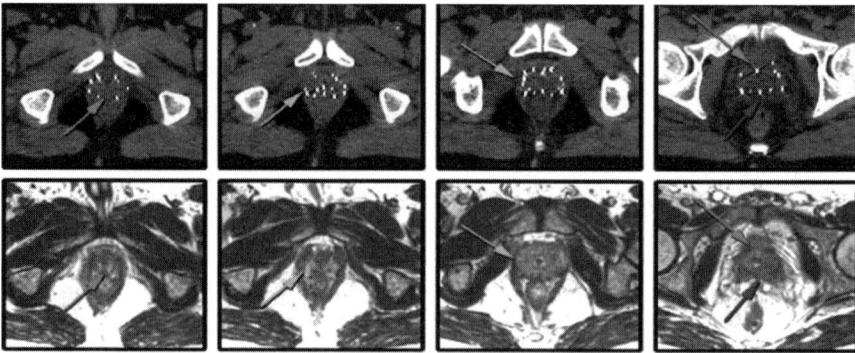

Fig. 2 Comparison of prostate interface clarity at different levels within the prostate. *Arrow* represents an interface with the prostate clarified by MRI, unclear on CT. *Left to right panels*: Genitourinary diaphragm, apex, mid-prostate, and base (*See* Color Plate 1, following p. 264)

sary high dose to the CES. Such average distance rules should not be employed. Coronal MRI accurately defines the separation of the prostate apex and penile bulb and the direct measurement can be applied to CT. Another method to define the apex is GUD recognition. In this method the CT is reviewed from the PB level and moving superior the triangular, circular, and slit forms typical of the GUD levels can be recognized and the apex is defined as the next slice above the last recognizable GUD element. GUD recognition was formally tested in ten patients with three observers and it was possible to define the apex within 0.5 cm *(30)*.

4.2   Definition of Critical Erectile Structures (CES)

CES include the neurovascular bundle (NVB), cavernosal nerves (CN), corpus cavernosum (CC), and internal pudendal artery (IPA). These structures are depicted in Fig. 4 and Color Plate 2, following p. 264, a 3D reconstruction following fusion of MRI, time-of-flight angiogram, and CT of a patient on a potency preservation proto-

Table 3 Preferred Imaging Method for Prostate Apex and CES

Structure	Preferred imaging method
Prostate apex	MRI coronal >
	MRI axial >
	GUD recognition
NVB	MRI = CT
Cavernosal nerves	MRI (relationship to external sphincter)
Corpus cavernosum	MRI > CT
Internal pudendal artery	Time-of-flight MRI >
	T2 MRI > CT

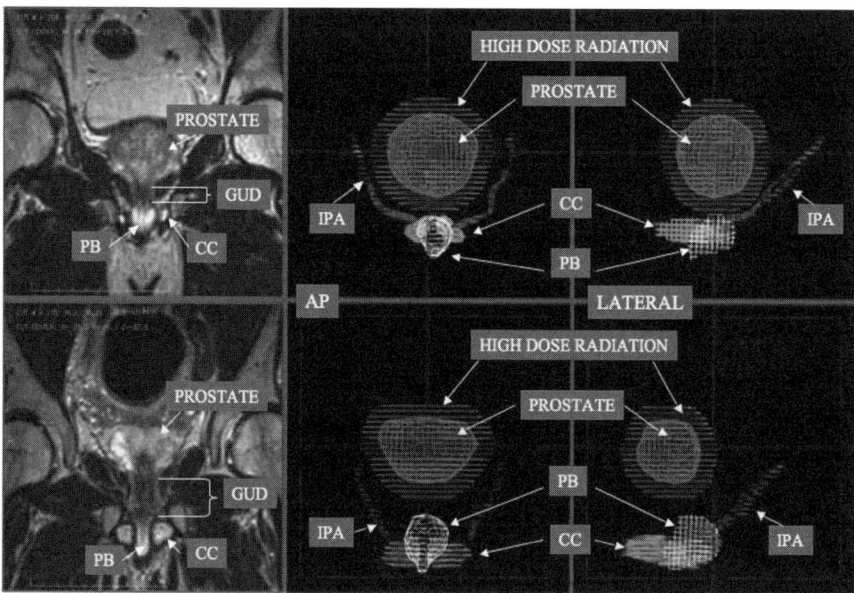

Fig. 3 Variation in genitourinary diaphragm (GUD) thickness. Patient in *upper panel* has minimal distance from prostate apex and penile bulb on coronal MRI. Patient in *lower panel* has a thicker GUD and greater separation of prostate and CES. Figures to the *left* represent prostate, critical structures, and high-dose radiation volume. Note the high-dose region is separable from the CES in the patient in the *lower panels*

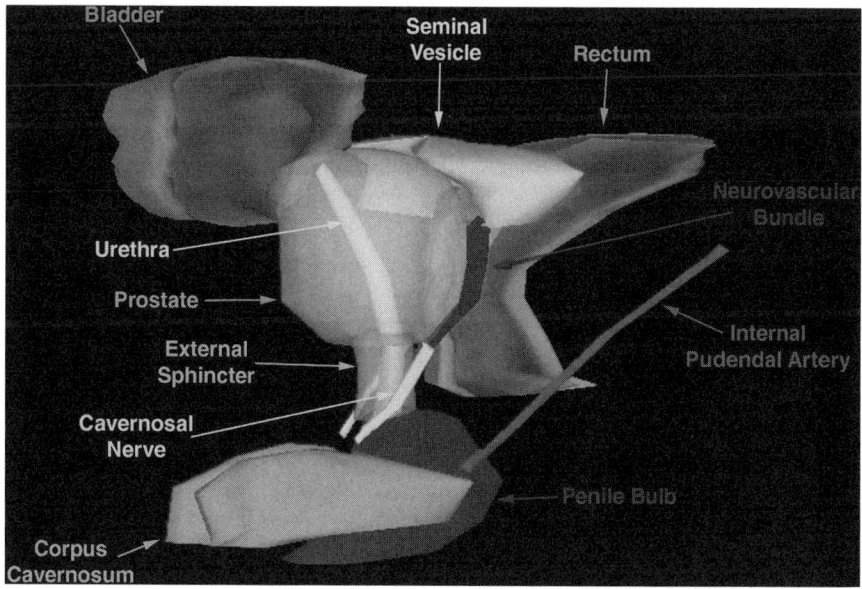

Fig. 4 Prostate and CES defined by fusion of CT and MRI (*See* Color Plate 2, following p. 264)

col. The penile bulb has no role in erectile function but has been used as a surrogate for the proximal penis. All CES except the cavernosal nerves may be defined on CT after MRI training but are usually more clearly defined on MRI.

The NVB is visible at the posterior lateral prostate border in approximately 50% of patients. In those in which the bundle is poorly defined a location has been specified by empirical contouring of the posterior lateral region. The problem with this approach is that in pathologic examination of surgical specimens only 50% of patients had an NVB which could be defined. In the remaining 50% the neurovascular bundle was a neurovascular plexus, which was spread over the lateral surface of the prostate *(31–33)*. Such a configuration limits not only the efficacy of nerve-sparing prostatectomy but also complicates correlative studies after radiation. Practically speaking it is impossible with current technology to limit dose to the neurovascular bundle or plexus except in permanent implants with a distinct NVB visible under color Doppler. In the subset of patients with a clearly defined NVB it is possible to vary seed position and limit actual implant of seeds into the bundle, but the NVB still receives prescription dose.

The cavernosal nerves which are the extension of the NVB through the GUD, are not visible on any current imaging modality, but are defined by their relationship to the external sphincter, which is clearly visible on T2 MRI. The cavernosal nerves proceed from the 5 and 7 o'clock positions relative to the external sphincter at the prostate apex to the 11 and 1 o'clock positions at the inferior GUD level just above the penile bulb.

In the anatomy literature, the cavernosal nerves are split into lesser cavernosal nerves and greater cavernosal nerves *(34,35)*. The cavernosal nerves referred to in the surgical literature are the lesser cavernosal nerves *(36)*. The greater cavernosal nerves proceed anterior and pierce the GUD anterior to the lesser cavernosal nerves and proceed under the pubic arch. The wide variation in NVB anatomy, from bundle to plexus, may also terminate in a highly varied cavernosal nerve complex, which may vary from two distinct trunks (greater and lesser cavernosal nerves) to a plexus without distinct and definable trunks. For correlation studies and expansion of the external sphincter, or the GUD, can be used as a surrogate for the lesser cavernosal nerve dose. Both the GUD and external sphincter are clearly defined on T2 MRI and allow definition of the lesser cavernosal nerve pathway by its fixed relationship to the external sphincter as specified by Walsh.

The IPA can be defined by a time-of-flight sequence, which allows definition of location and potency (Fig. 5). With training it is possible to trace the course of the IPA through the pudendal canal on T2 MRI, and if calcified it is visible on CT. Although the IPA is the main blood supply to the corpus cavernosum, and IPA obstruction is a common etiology for ED in the non-radiated population, wide variations in blood supply to the CC have been documented. In some patients vessels supplying the CC are in closer proximity to the prostate (accessory pudendal arteries) and may not be sparable without compromising treatment. In a majority of patients the IPA contributes to the CC blood supply, and sparing of the IPA may prevent acclerated arteriosclerosis.

The corpus cavernosum is visible on CT but more clearly visible on T2 MRI. In addition the T2 MRI allows the clear distinction of the muscle and parenchyma

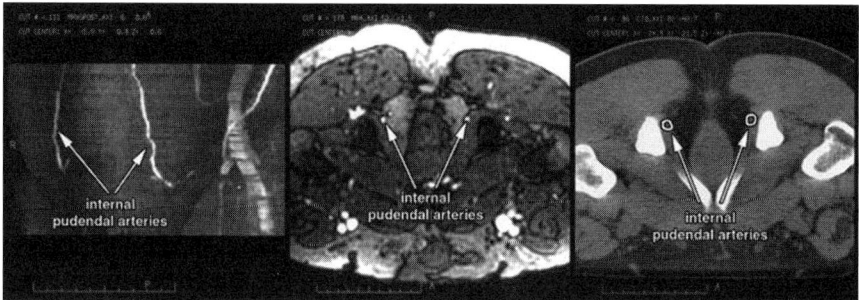

Fig. 5 Internal pudendal artery. *Left and mid-panels* are time-of-flight sequences (non contrast). *Right panel* is location on CT after fusion of time-of-flight and CT

components of the CC. The CC are easily distinguished from the penile bulb, also visible on CT but more clearly defined on MRI. Correlative studies of ED and PB dose have been criticized on the basis that the PB does not have a role in erections *(8)*. Yet, terminal branches of the cavernosal nerves pass over the superior and lateral surface of the PB to reach the CC. It is possible that exposure of this region could disrupt the terminal cavernosal nerve branches before they reach the CC.

4.3 Radiation Treatment Planning

The separation of the structures relative to the prostate directly impacts the sparing potential of the radiation delivery plan. IMRT and tomotherapy are superior to 3D conformal, and IMRT planning allows a specific dose restriction to be assigned to CES. However, 3D conformal with MRI-defined targets has been shown to be superior in CES sparing compared to CT-planned IMRT *(29)*. The CT planning with IMRT was based on the use of rules to define the apex, and failed to define the population of men with extreme separation of the prostate and CES, a group easily spared with 3D conformal radiation. Thus accurate MRI-based imaging plus IMRT combine to take full advantage of available technology. This in turn allows correlative studies of dose and ED to ultimately define a mechanism of failure and critical targets to avoid. The influence of CES on treatment planning is that fields not commonly employed in standard treatment planning become advantageous when CES are considered. Standard treatment planning based on limiting dose to the rectum favors lateral field approaches, while the inclusion of CES in planning often results in use of anterior fields.

5 Potency-Sparing Radiotherapy – Preliminary Results

As stated in the introduction potency-sparing radiotherapy is far less defined than nerve-sparing surgical procedures. Although exhaustive prospective data with long follow up are not available, compelling preliminary data using validated instruments are now available. Merrick has a large series in progress in which initial correlations of ED to proximal penis dose were established, followed by studies in which PB and CC dose were consciously restricted in an effort to preserve potency. The strength of these studies is that they are prospective, with validated baseline potency scales used in both early and later potency-sparing approaches. These studies move beyond studies which define the feasibility of defining and restricting dose *(7,29)* to actual correlation of outcomes after dose restriction.

Using the International Index of Erectile Function (IIEF) Merrick et al. reported a 39% 6-year rate of potency preservation following brachytherapy *(37)*. When implant technique was modified to spare the PB in a later series, potency post-brachytherapy improved *(38)* (Fig. 6). The addition of supplemental XRT resulted in a deleterious effect on potency preservation (26% vs. 52%). By carefully restricting dose to the proximal penis, overall potency preservation rates using the IIEF questionnaire increased from 39 to 51% without a deleterious effect on erectile function in patients receiving supplemental beam *(38)* (Fig. 7). Using day 0 CT-based dosimetry, maximal potency preservation was dependent on limiting the penile bulb D_{50} to $\leq 30\%$ of prescription dose and the proximal crural D_{50} to $\leq 50\%$ of prescription *(38)* (Fig. 8A,B). With adherence to these cut-points, greater than 70% of patients maintained potency compared to only approximately 30% in patients who received higher doses. Although the site-specific structure in the proximal penis remains unclear, radiation doses to the corpora cavernosa may be more important than those to the penile bulb because the corpora cavernosa represents the true erectile tissue, whereas the corpora spongiosum is believed to play little role in the development or maintenance of erectile rigidity *(6,7)*.

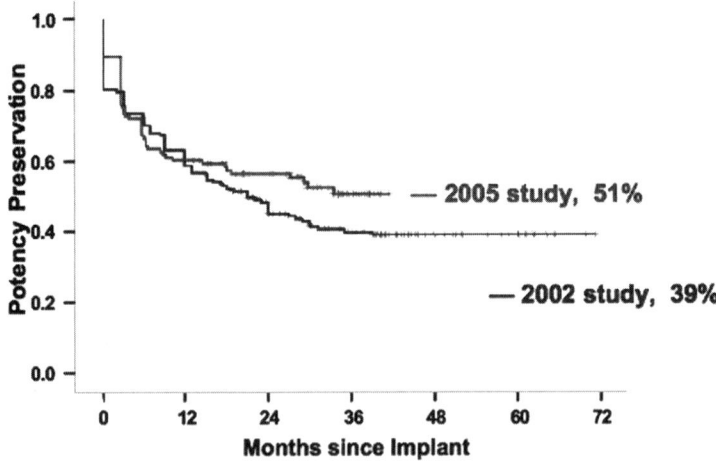

Fig. 6 Comparison of ED in two eras differing by dose limitation to the PB and CC

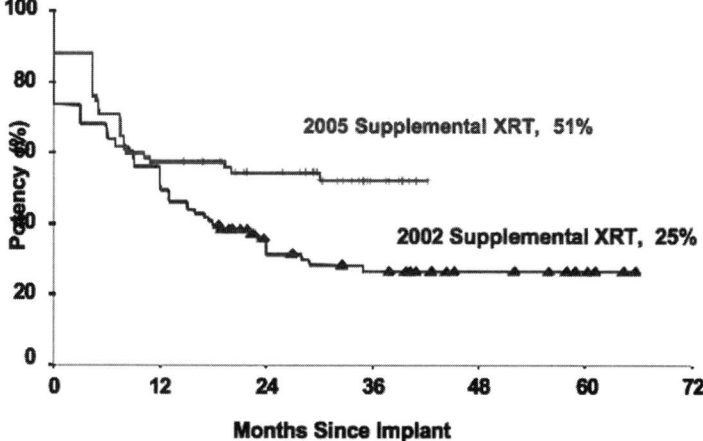

Fig. 7 Effect of external beam in combination with implant in two eras differing by limitation in dose to the PB and CC

The above studies confirm the importance of the proximal penile region in contributing to post-radiation erectile dysfunction and begin to define a dose tolerance for the CES. They are limited by the use of CT to define CES and prostate apex, and further dose restriction may be possible using MRI-based planning with IMRT *(29)*.

Besides dose to CES, a key predictor of potency preservation for all forms of radiation is the baseline function *(38)*. Patients with a pre-treatment IIEF of 29–30, 24–30, 18–23 and 13–17 have potency preservation rates of 79, 58, 48 and 22%, respectively, following brachytherapy *(38)* (Fig. 9). However, the post-implant IIEF scores are routinely less than the pre-implant value. For example, patients with a pre-implant IIEF of 29 or 30 had a median post-implant IIEF of 24 *(38)*. In addition patient age and presence or absence of nocturnal erections predicted post-radiation potency preservation *(38)*.

6 Summary

Potency following radiation therapy is a complex function of baseline function, age, radiation dose to CES, radiation technique, and the use of hormone therapy. There is no evidence from prospective studies that brachytherapy is more sparing of erectile function than other modalities, provided dose to the proximal penile structures is limited appropriately. Improvements in imaging employing MRI-based imaging can improve the definition of prostate apex and CES and allow further reduction of dose over CT-based approaches, especially when combined with IMRT planning. Androgen blockade remains a critical factor in affecting potency post-radiation, especially long-term blockade. Currently, there are wide differences in the hormone therapy

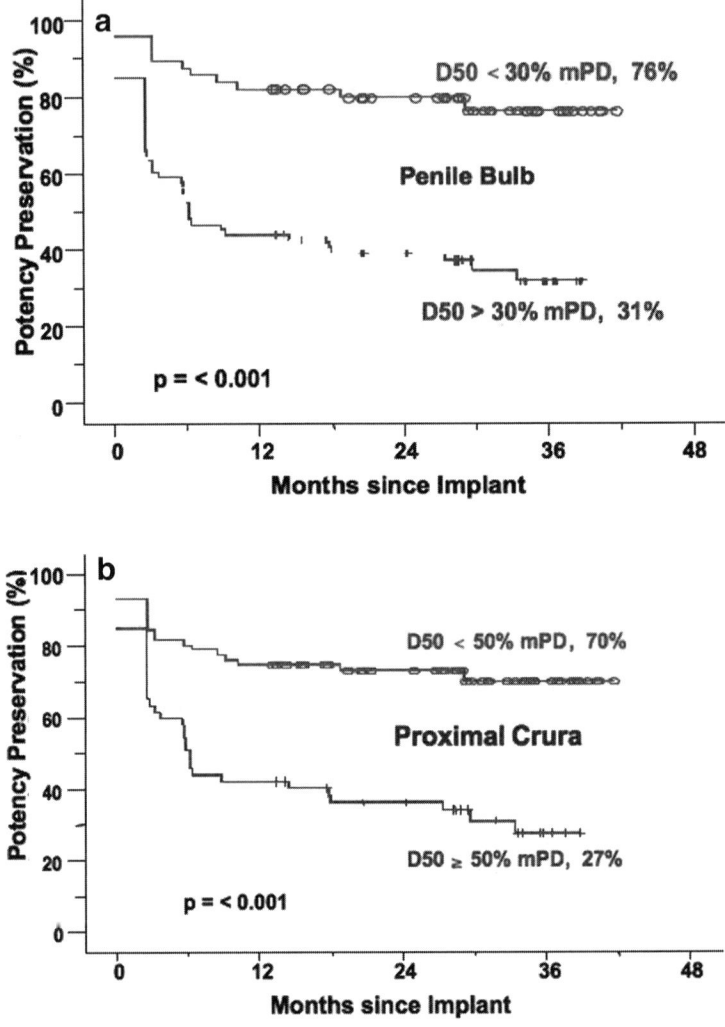

Fig. 8 Dose response correlating ED and dose to PB (**A**) and proximal CC (**B**)

recommendations that are dependent on the radiation modality chosen. In general
when brachytherapy with confirmed excellent post-implant coverage is included in
the therapy, either in primary or combined, the role of hormone therapy is diminished *(39,40)*. In contrast prospective randomized trials suggest that 6 months of
androgen blockade improve outcome compared to external radiation alone *(41)*.
Few studies of combined hormone therapy and implant suggest a benefit in this
group, especially when implant quality is confirmed *(39,40)*. For high-risk patients
treated with external beam therapy current evidence suggests a 2–3-year course
of hormone therapy *(42)*. High-risk patients treated with combined implant plus

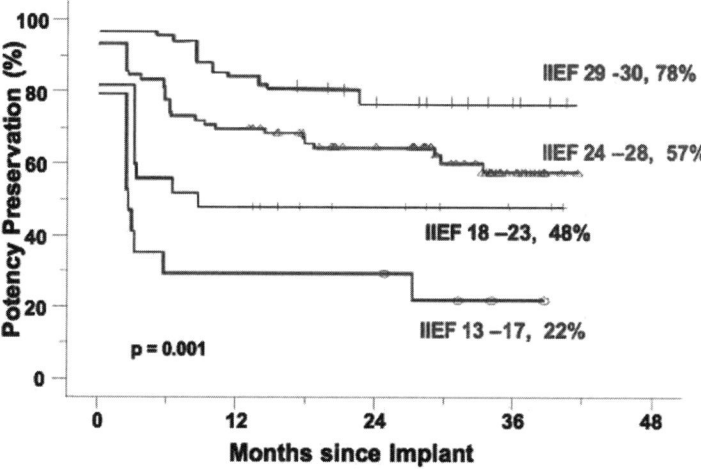

Fig. 9 Relationship of ED post-radiation to baseline function

beam may require 6–9 months of hormone therapy *(39,40)*. These data suggest that potency preservation radiation techniques must factor in the current requirement for hormone therapy, and the decision for potency preservation may compel some patient to consider combined modality or primary brachytherapy. While prospective trials will have to confirm this excellent long-term biochemical control and survival can be achieved in the vast majority of patients with radiation modalities, which do not require hormonal therapy.

References

1. Incrocci, L., Slob, A.K., and Levendag, P.C. (2002) Sexual (dys) function after radiotherapy for prostate cancer: a review. *Int. J. Radiat. Oncol. Biol. Phys.* **52**, 681–693.
2. Merrick, G.S., Butler, W.M., Dorsey, A.T., et al. (2000) A comparison of the radiation dose to the neurovascular bundles in men with and without prostate brachytherapy induced erectile dysfunction. *Int. J. Radiat. Oncol. Biol. Phys.* **46**, 1069–1074.
3. Fisch, B.M., Pickett, B., Weinberg, V., et al. (2001) Dose of radiation received by the bulb of the penis correlates with risk of impotence after three-dimensional conformal radiotherapy for prostate cancer. *Urology* **57**, 955–959.
4. Pickett, B., Fisch, B.M., Weinberg, V., et al. (1999) Dose to the bulb of the penis is associated with the risk of impotence following radiotherapy for prostate cancer. *Int. J. Radiat. Oncol. Biol. Phys.* **45**, 263.
5. Merrick, G.S., Wallner, K., Butler, W.M., et al. (2001) A comparison of radiation dose to the bulb of the penis in men with and without prostate brachytherapy induced erectile dysfunction. *Int. J. Radiat. Oncol. Biol. Phys.* **50**, 597–604.
6. Mulhall, J.P. (2001) Minimizing radiation-induced erectile dysfunction. *J. Brachytherapy Int.* **17**, 221–227.
7. Mulhall, J.P., Yonover, P., Sethi, A., et al. (2002) Radiation exposure to the corporeal bodies during 3-dimensional conformal radiotherapy for prostate cancer. *J. Urol.* **167**, 539–542.

8. Mulhall, J.P., and Yonover, P. (2002) Correlation of radiation dose and impotence risk after three-dimensional conformal radiotherapy for prostate cancer (Letter). *Urology* **58**, 828.

9. Merrick, G.S., Butler, W.M., Wallner, K.E., Leif, J.H., Anderson, R.L., Smeiles, B.S., Galbreath, R.W., and Benson, M.L. (2002) The importance of radiation doses to the penile bulb vs. crura in the development of post brachytherapy erectile dysfunction. *Int. J. Radiat. Oncol. Biol. Phys.* **54**(4), 1055–1062.

10. Goldstein, I., Feldman, M.I., Deckers, P.J., et al. (1994) Radiation-associated impotence. *JAMA* **251**, 903–910.

11. Zelefsky, M.J., and Eid, J.F. (1998) Elucidating the etiology of erectile dysfunction after definitive therapy for prostatic cancer. *Int. J. Radiat. Oncol. Biol. Phys.* **40**, 129–133.

12. Mittal, B. (1985) A study of penile circulation before and after radiation in patients with prostate cancer and its effect on impotence. *Int. J. Radiat. Oncol. Biol. Phys.* **11**, 11

13. Carrier, S., Hricak, H., Lee, S., et al. (1995) Radiation induced decrease in nitric oxide synthase – containing nerves in the rat penis. *Radiology* **195**, 95–99.

14. Pickles, T., and Graham, P. (2002 Jun) Members of the British Columbia Cancer Agency Prostate Cohort Outcomes Initiative. What happens to testosterone after prostate radiation monotherapy and does it matter?. [Journal Article. Research Support, Non-U.S. Gov't] *J. Urol.* **167**(6), 2448–2452.

15. Grigsby, P.W., and Perez, C.A. (1986) The effects of external beam radiotherapy on endocrine function in patients with carcinoma of the prostate. *J. Urol.* **135**, 726.

16. Zagars, G.K., and Pollack, A. (1997) Serum testosterone levels after external beam radiation for clinically localized prostate cancer. *Int. J. Radiat. Oncol. Biol. Phys.* **39**, 85.

17. Daniell, H.W., Clark, I.C., Pereira, S.E., et al. (2001) Hypogonadism following prostate-bed radiation therapy for prostate carcinoma. *Cancer* **91**, 1889.

18. Padula, G.D., Zelefsky, M.J., Venkatraman, E.S., Fuks, Z., Lee, H.J., Natale, L., and Liebel, S.A. (2002) Normalization of serum testosterone levels in patients treated with neoadjuvant hormonal therapy and three-dimensional conformal radiotherapy for prostate cancer. *Int. J. Radiat. Oncol. Biol. Phys.* **52**(2), 439–443.

19. Oefelein, M.G. (1998) Time to normalization of serum testosterone after 3-month luteinizing hormone-releasing hormone agonist administered in the neoadjuvant setting: implications for dosing schedule and neoadjuvant study consideration. *J. Urol.* **160**, 1685.

20. Nejat, R.J., Rashid, H.H., Bagiella, E., Katz, A.E., and Benson, M.C. (2000 Dec) A prospective analysis of time to normalization of serum testosterone after withdrawal of androgen deprivation therapy. [Journal Article] *J. Urol.* **164**(6), 1891–1894.

21. Wilke, D.R., Parker, C., Andonowski, A., et al. (2006) Testosterone and erectile function recovery after radiotherapy and long-term androgen deprivation with luteinizing hormone-releasing hormone agonists. *BJU Int.* **97**, 962–968.

22. Mydlo, J.H., and Lebed, B. (2004) Does brachytherapy of the prostate affect sperm quality and/or fertility in younger men? *Scand. J. Urol. Nephrol.* **38**, 221–224.

23. Grocela, J.,Mauceri, T., and Zeitman, A. (2005) New life after prostate brachytherapy? Considering the fertile female partner of the brachytherapy patient. *BJU Int.* **96**, 781–782.

24. Merrick, G.S., Wallner, K.E., Butler, W.M., et al. (2001) Short-term sexual function after prostate brachytherapy. *Int. J. Cancer* **96**, 313–319.

25. Rosen, R.C., Riley, A., Wagner, G., et al. (1997) The International Index of Erectile Function (IIEF): a multidimensional scale for assessment of erectile dysfunction. *Urology* **49**, 822–830.

26. Fajardo, L.F. (1997) Morphology of radiation effects on normal tissues. In: Perez, C.A., and Brady, L.W., eds. *Principles and Practice of Radiation Oncology*, 3rd edn. Philadelphia: J.B. Lippincott Company, pp. 143–154.

27. Brennan, K.M., Poos, M.S., Budinger, T.F., et al. (1993) A study of radiation necrosis and edema in the canine brain using positron emission tomography and magnetic resonance imaging. *Rad. Res.* **134**, 43–53.

28. Hu, K.S., and Harrison, L.B. (2000) Results and complications of surgery combined with intra-operative radiation therapy for the treatment of locally advanced or recurrent cancers in the pelvis. Semin. *Surg. Oncol.* **18**, 269–278.

29. McLaughlin, P.W., Narayana, V., Meriowitz, A., Troyer, W., Roberson, P.L., Gonda, Jr., R., Sandler, H., Marsh, L., Lawrence, T., and Kessler, M. (2005 Jan 2) Vessel-sparing prostate radiotherapy: dose limitation to critical erectile vascular structures (internal pudendal artery and corpus cavernosum) defined by MRI. *Int. J. Radiat. Oncol. Biol. Phys.* **61**, 1, 20–31.

30. McLaughlin, P.W., Feng, M., Berri, S., and Narayana, V. (2006) Improved CT prostate apex definition by genitourinary diaphragm recognition. Abstract *ASTRO*.

31. Kiyoshima, K., Yokomizo, A., Yoshida, T., Tomita, K., Yonemasu, H., Nakamura, M., Oda, Y., Naito, S., and Hasegawa, Y. (2004 Aug) Anatomical features of periprostatic tissue and its surroundings: a histological analysis of 79 radical retropubic prostatectomy specimens. *Jpn. J. Clin. Oncol.* **34**(8),463–468.

32. Takenaka, A., Murakami, G., Matsubara, A., Han, SH., and Fujisawa, M. (2005 Jan) Variation in course of cavernous nerve with special reference to details of topographic relationships near prostatic apex: histologic study using male cadavers. *Urology* **65**(1), 136–142.

33. Costello, A.J., Brooks, M., and Cole, O.J. (2004 Nov) Anatomical studies of the neurovascular bundle and cavernosal nerves. *BJU Int.* **94**(7), 1071–1076.

34. Standing, S., ed. (2005) *Gray's Anatomy*, 39th edn. Edinburgh: Elsevier.

35. Netter, F. (1989) *Atlas of Human Anatomy*. Summit, NJ: Ciba Geigy Corp.

36. Schlegel, P.N., and Walsh, P.C. (1987 Dec) Neuroanatomical approach to radical cystoprosta-tectomy with preservation of sexual function. *J. Urol.* **138**(6), 1402–1406.

37. Merrick, G.S., Wallner, K.E., Butler, W.M., and Galbreath, R.W. (2002) Erectile function after permanent prostate brachytherapy. *Int. J. Radiat. Oncol. Biol. Phys.* **52**, 893–902.

38. Merrick, G.S., Butler, W.M., and Wallner, K.E. (2005) Erectile function after prostate brachytherapy. *Int. J. Radiat. Oncol. Biol. Phys.* **62,** 437–447.

39. Merrick, G.S., Butler, W.M., Wallner, K.E., et al. (2006) Androgen deprivation therapy does not impact cause specific or overall specific survival after permanent prostate brachytherapy. *Int. J. Radiat. Oncol. Biol. Phys.* **65,** 669–677.

40. Merrick, G.S., Butler, W.M., Wallner, K.E., et al. (2005) Impact of supplemental external beam radiotherapy and/or androgen deprivation therapy on biochemical outcome after permanent prostate brachytherapy. *Int. J. Radiat. Oncol. Biol. Phys.* **61**(1), 32–43.

41. D'Amico, A.V., Chen, M., Renshaw, A., Loffredo, M., and Kantoff, P. (2008) Androgen sup-pression and radiation vs radiation alone for prostate cancer. *JAMA* **299**(3), 289–295.

42. Damico, A.V. (2007 Jan 1) Toward the optimal use of androgen suppression therapy in the radiotherapeutic management of prostate cancer. *J. Clin. Oncol.* **25**(1), 8–9.

Chapter 8
Neuromodulatory Drugs for the Radical Prostatectomy Patient

Arthur L. Burnett II

Abstract Neurogenic erectile dysfunction remains a common complication of radical prostatectomy despite current modifications of the surgery, which include preservation of the cavernous nerves essential for autonomically nerve-regulated penile erection. An imperative exists to address this problem with the primary objective of rapidly restoring natural, medically unassisted erections. Neuromodulation is an exciting, innovative field of endeavor developed to meet this objective. With the acknowledgement that penile neuropathy is a major pathogenic basis for the complication, this field promotes neuroprotective and nerve regenerative strategies for facilitating cavernous nerve functional recovery. Several possibilities have been investigated at the preclinical level and in early clinical trials, directly relevant to this context, suggesting likely therapeutic directions to be developed further in the near future. Other possibilities are conjectured at this time to have likely utility in this clinical context, borrowing from concepts advanced in basic science and clinical medicine disciplines distinct from the neuro-urologic field. For moving this particular field forward, emphasis is given to elucidating the molecular basis of the pathologic injury associated with radical prostatectomy and characterizing the role of molecular effectors responsible for cavernous nerve injury and recovery. Such focused molecular neurobiologic investigation can be expected to reveal highly effective pharmacologic approaches to address the problem and maximize erectile function restoration following surgery.

From: *Current Clinical Urology* Series, *Sexual Function in the Prostate Cancer Patient*
Edited by John P. Mulhall, DOI 10.1007/978-1-60327-555-2_8,

Keywords Erectile dysfunction; penis; penile erection; cavernous nerve; peripheral neuropathy; neurogenesis; neuroprotection; regeneration; neurotrophic; neurotropic.

1 Introduction

The description of the anatomic radical prostatectomy just over 20 years ago by Walsh impacted greatly on the field of urology *(1)*. This original modification of the procedure of radical prostatectomy was based on an improved understanding of the course of the cavernous nerves adjacent to the prostate, which supplied the penis and allowed for their structural preservation when performing this pelvic surgery. The significance of the discovery is that it advanced concepts of functional outcome preservation, which in the context of autonomic "nerve-sparing" specifically pertains to erectile function, while adhering to sound surgical oncologic principles. Although the exact degree of erection recovery achieved with this pioneering advance has remained hotly debated at present, there is no question that erection recovery rates following modern procedures for radical prostatectomy have improved dramatically from that of the prior surgical era *(2,3)*.

The advance can be thought of too as inaugurating a new field of study in neuro-urology, focused on the development and implementation of strategies for preserving the functional integrity of the cavernous nerves in the context of pelvic surgery. Several strategies have been proposed in recent years with the goal of even better preserving the neurogenic basis of penile erection following radical prostatectomy and thereby maximizing postoperative erectile function outcomes. Such strategies have included intraoperative cavernous nerve neurostimulation *(4,5)*, cavernous nerve interposition grafting *(6,7)*, and further refinements in cavernous nerve preservation techniques during the performance of the surgery *(8,9)*. Neuromodulatory therapy, in reference to therapeutic approaches for protecting and recovering the function of cavernous nerves injured during radical prostatectomy, has also received intense interest in recent years.

The interest in this strategy largely stems from the knowledge that many men experience a delay or failure in the full recovery of natural penile erection postoperatively today despite current surgical improvements *(10)*. The concern is that even the very best surgical proficiency for cavernous nerve preservation will foreseeably remain imperfect in consistently obtaining prompt, functional erectile responses postoperatively and some additional means of facilitating the recovery of cavernous nerve function required for this outcome remain most purposeful in this setting. The reality of erectile dysfunction as a lingering potential complication of radical prostatectomy at this time is further underscored by the frequent use of erectile aids in the interim for many men while awaiting natural erection recovery *(11,12)* and by the enthusiasm for vasoactive pharmacological erection rehabilitative strategies to promote this recovery *(13,14)*.

This chapter conveys the rapidly growing scientific interest in addressing the penile neuropathy associated with the performance of radical prostatectomy, which is inherent in the temporary or permanent occurrence of erectile dysfunction following this iatrogenic event. It highlights an assortment of initiatives considered to be neuromodulatory in nature, which could be offered adjunctively with the surgery to produce possible therapeutic benefit. To be discussed are several exciting scientific directions, from preclinical studies to early clinical trials, aimed toward promoting cavernous nerve functional preservation, and thereby maximizing erection ability, after surgery-related cavernous nerve injury. However, in recognition that progress in this specific field of endeavor is relatively immature to date, discussion is also provided with respect to the potential utility of neuromodulatory prospects that might be introduced to this clinical arena based on advances in other clinical disciplines in which nerve injury occurs. For the latter concern, literature relating to both nerve injury and functional nerve recovery in non-urological contexts including such areas as peripheral nerve injury, spinal cord injury as well as neurodegenerative diseases of the central nervous system has been reviewed. Further, advances in the molecular basis of neuroprotection and neuroregeneration after nerve injury, including the roles of molecular factors and signal transduction pathways, were deemed to be informative for this undertaking. Molecular concepts may broadly apply to settings of nerve injury and wholly translate to innovative mechanism-based interventions.

2   Pathogenesis of Acute, Traumatic Penile Neuropathy

In many respects, the proceedings of radical prostatectomy resulting in cavernous nerve injury parallel the description of nerve injury in other contexts of traumatic nerve injury. Accordingly, there is an initial traumatic insult, which then triggers a secondary pathological cascade of biochemical and metabolic derangements leading to functional loss (Table 1). The neuropathy and nerve recovery process associated with cavernous nerve injury are presumed to involve events resembling that of peripheral neuropathy and peripheral nerve regeneration, respectively.

2.1   Peripheral Nerve Degeneration and Regeneration

Broadly speaking, peripheral neuropathy implies derangement in structure and function of peripheral motor, sensory, and autonomic neurons in their entirety or involving select parts of the neuron. The diverse nature of neurons invokes a range of potential target sites and mechanisms that may be associated with nerve injury and neuronal dysfunction. However, a fairly well-understood consistent manner of neuronal loss follows peripheral nerve injury. After axonal injury of a peripheral nerve, such as by axotomy or crush, cellular and molecular mechanisms are

Table 1 Pathobiology of Traumatic Cavernous Nerve Injury

Primary mechanisms
    Contusion
    Compression
    Traction
    Avulsion
    Transection
Secondary mechanisms
    Extracellular factors
        Microcirculatory vascular damage
        Ischemia
        Hemorrhage
        Edema
        Cytokine-mediated inflammation
    Intracellular factors
        Ischemia-reperfusion
        Electrolyte imbalance
        Edema
        Neurotransmitter excess
        Amino acid excitotoxicity
        Lipid peroxidation
        Reactive oxygen species generation
        Neurotrophic factor deprivation
        Apoptosis

put in play signifying neuronal cell death and recovery *(15,16)*. Nerve fibers distal to the site of injury undergo a process referred to as Wallerian degeneration. The retrograde transport of neurotrophins (neurotrophic factors) released from the target tissue to the nerve cell body to support its survival and facilitate axonal regeneration is additionally disrupted, further signifying neuronal cell death and impaired regeneration.

A microenvironmental change accompanies neuronal cell death and likewise links with the events involved in neuronal cell survival. Intracellular calcium levels rise, while free radicals and reactive oxygen species are generated and activated. These events signal the reactivity of neighboring Schwann cells, glial cells of peripheral nerves, which respond by producing extracellular matrix components, remyelinating regenerating axons, and secreting neurotrophins. Neurotrophins interact with specific plasma membrane receptors, e.g., TrkA, TrkB, p75, in neurons thereby activating Akt (protein kinase B) and/or mitogen-activated protein kinases, i.e., extracellular signal-regulated kinase (ERK), c-Jun NH_2-terminal kinase (JNK) and p38, which regulate downstream effectors in neuronal proliferation and survival pathways *(17)*. The range of effects includes neuronal proliferation, differentiation, and changes in cell motility, structure, and phenotype. Neurite outgrowth from the proximal nerve segment, as governed by neurotrophins, proceeds either in a trophic manner, i.e., related to protein synthesis and regulation, or in a tropic manner, i.e., related to directionality. Cell adhesion molecules (CAM), i.e., N-CAM, N-cadherin, and the L1 glycoprotein, also play important roles in governing the directional growth of axons *(18)*. Negative extracellular signals have recently been described as inhibiting neurite outgrowth. Neuronal growth inhibitory proteins include Nogo, myelin-associated glycoprotein, and the growth collapsing semaphorins/neuropilins, and their actions may involve Rho-kinase-mediated signaling *(18,19)*. Upon the regeneration of neurons and their reconnection with target locations, the axonal growth and recovery process is terminated.

2.2   *Cavernous Nerve Injury*

During radical prostatectomy, the surgical dissection as dictated by oncologic principles may require intentional wide excision of periprostatic tissues including all or a portion of the cavernous nerves when performing a non-nerve-sparing procedure. Alternatively, such principles may still permit preservation of periprostatic tissues including the cavernous nerves when performing a nerve-sparing procedure. In the former instance, nerve injury is easily contended to consist of direct nerve transection, which generally produces a permanent interruption of autonomic nerve connections with the penis. In the latter instance, which implies the intention to maintain the anatomic integrity of the cavernous nerves, several conceivable mechanisms of nerve injury may nonetheless occur in the course of prostate removal including contusion, compression, traction, and avulsion as well as transection (Table 1). These mechanisms, depending upon their extent and severity, correspond to the commonplace variable loss of neurogenic erectile function which arises in this setting. For the nerve-sparing modification of the surgery, erection loss frequently results from nerve injury albeit it was unintentional. At the same time, the observation that erectile function to some degree recovers in time with the nerve-sparing modification and sometimes even with the non-nerve-sparing approach establishes the neuroregenerative potential of this clinical setting.

Following denervation injury to the penis, it is likely that a process of penile neuropathy ensues. Erectile tissue health and the erectile response are conceivably affected adversely by the disruption of the cavernous nerve supply. Experimental animal studies and clinical observations support functional, morphological, and metabolic consequences following penile denervation. The functional loss of erections following cavernous nerve injury is attributable to defective neurotransmission required for penile erection. Grossly apparent atrophic and fibrotic changes of the penis have been reported after cavernous nerve injury *(20,21)*, which on the microscopic level correlate with degeneration of nerve terminations in the erectile tissue, corporal smooth muscle deterioration, and infiltration of the erectile tissue with collagen *(22,23)*. An active process of corporal smooth muscle apoptosis has been shown to occur in rats following penile denervation *(24,25)*. In sum, these changes result in an altered biophysical compliance of the penis that predisposes to cavernous (veno-occlusive) dysfunction *(26)*.

3 Therapeutic Penile Neurogenesis

Neurogenesis is a developmental biology concept that refers to the growth and regeneration of neurons in organ systems. The concept also relates to the basic science of neurotrophic growth factors, neural development, neuroprotection, neural regeneration, and the prevention of neuronal cell death. The association of neurogenesis with the penis corresponds to the premise that nerve development and reconstitution are required for preserving neurobiological functions of this organ particularly in the face of cavernous nerve injury. This area of study has evolved at the level of preclinical investigation as well as in the form of early clinical trials in men undergoing radical prostatectomy.

The clinical pertinence of this research effort is that it may introduce therapies to counteract the neuropathic effects of cavernous nerve injury associated with radical prostatectomy. With this purpose in mind, a body of research discoveries in penile neurogenesis and neurobiology has formed suggesting several possible neuromodulatory directions to pursue for this clinical application. These advances readily fit categories within a schema of neuroprotective and nerve regenerative strategies, similarly considered for a variety of nerve injury contexts *(27–33)* (Tables 2 and 3). This schema is consistent with principles discussed in the aforementioned section on the pathology of nerve injury and the neurobiology of nerve recovery. Possibilities range then from specific strategies which would minimize injury from all aspects of inflammation, ischemia, excitotoxicity, lipid peroxidation, free radical production, and apoptosis to strategies which would promote functional nerve recovery via actions of neurotrophic factors, neuronal repair mechanisms, and nerve reconstructive techniques.

3.1 Preclinical Investigation

Basic science research in this field has largely relied on experimental animal models, both to evaluate the consequences of cavernous nerve injury and to advance neuromodulatory therapeutic objectives. Animal models have provided useful paradigms for investigative work, and they have permitted integrative studies of both anatomical (i.e., quantitative morphological, histological, histochemical) and functional (i.e., behavioral, electrophysiologic) components of penile neuropathy and cavernous nerve regeneration. Further, animal models have offered insight into molecular mechanisms involved in cavernous nerve neuronal degeneration and regeneration.

Studies in the rat have confirmed collagen infiltration of cavernosal tissue and corporal smooth muscle apoptosis resulting from cavernous nerve injury *(22,24,25)*. The rat has been used additionally to evaluate the existence and function of neurotrophic factors in the penis. As demonstrated by molecular expression studies, several growth factors are localized to the rat penis including nerve growth factor, basic fibroblast growth factor, transforming growth factors α and β1-3, and

Table 2 Strategies for Mechanism-Based Neuroprotection

Anti-inflammatory agents
    Steroids (glucocorticoids, 21-aminosteroids)
    Sex steroids (estrogen, testosterone)
    Cyclo-oxygenase-2 inhibitors
    Minocycline
    Poly (adenosine diphosphate-ribose) polymerase inhibitor

Anti-oxidants
    Melatonin
    Nicotine
    Acetylcholine
    α-Tocopherol
    Flavonoids (quercetin)
    Thioredoxin

Immune modulators
    Immunophilin ligands
    Monoclonal antibodies

Ischemia counteractive agents
    Nimodipine
    Dopamine
    Atropine
    Angiotensin receptor antagonists

Anti-excitotoxicity agents
    Gangliosides
    Opiate blockers
    Thyrotropin-releasing hormone
    Glutamate receptor-selective drugs

Ionic/membrane stabilizers
    Calcium channel blockers
    Sodium channel blockers
    Beta-blockers
    Mitochondrial ATP-sensitive potassium channel activators

Anti-apoptotic agents
    Calpain antagonists
    Caspase inactivators
    Erythropoietin

N.B. This list is not meant to be exhaustive or complete. Some agents may act through more than one mechanism.

insulin-like growth factor *(34,35)*. The rat has also served to define the roles of neurotrophic factors such as nerve growth factor, acidic fibroblast growth factor, brain-derived neurotrophic factor, and insulin-like growth factor in promoting penile nerve fiber regeneration and erectile function recovery after cavernous nerve injury *(36–39)*. Atypical neurotrophic factors either shown or proposed to play roles in cavernous nerve regeneration after injury include growth hormone *(40)*, the glial cell line-derived neurotrophic factor neurturin *(41)*, the morphogenic factor Sonic

Table 3 Strategies for Mechanism-Based Nerve Regeneration

Neurotrophic factors
    Classic neurotrophins
        Nerve growth factor
        Brain-derived neurotrophic factor
        Neurotrophin-3, neurotrophin-4
        Acidic fibroblast growth factor
    Neuropeptide growth factors
        Bombesin
        Neurotensin
    Atypical neurotrophic factors
        Growth hormone
        Neurturin
        Sonic hedgehog protein
        Erythropoietin
        Vascular endothelial growth factor

Axonal outgrowth inhibitory neutralizers
        Inhibitory myelin protein antagonists
        Myelin-reactive T-lymphocyte vaccines
        Activated autologous macrophages
        Rho-kinase pathway antagonists
        Phosphodiesterase inhibitors
        Nitric oxide donors
        Chondroitinase

Axonal reconstructive substances
        Fusogens (polyethylene glycol)
        Nerve guides

Tissue engineering/stem cell therapy
        Non-glial cells (neurons, fibroblasts)
        Glial cells (Schwann cells, macrophages)
        Stem/progenitor cells
        Genetically modified cells
        Tissues (peripheral nerves, omentum)

Electrical stimulation

N.B. This list is not meant to be exhaustive or complete. Some agents may act through more than one mechanism.

hedgehog protein *(42)*, and the cytokine-hormone/anti-apoptotic agent erythropoietin *(43)*.

The rat model of cavernous nerve injury has also served to demonstrate the cavernous nerve neuroprotective and/or nerve regenerative effects of the immunophilin ligand FK506 (tacrolimus) and its derivatives *(44–46)* as well as the anti-inflammatory agent poly (adenosine diphosphate-ribose) polymerase (PARP) inhibitor *(47)*. Additionally, studies in the rat model of cavernous nerve injury have demonstrated the utility of an assortment of nerve guides, which offer directional guidance for regenerating nerves and otherwise act as nerve conduits for reconstituting innervation to the penis. Autologous genitofemoral nerve *(48)*, amniotic membrane *(36)*, silicone nerve tubes *(37)*, Schwann cell seeded nerve guidance tubes *(49)*, and biodegradable L-lactic acid and E-caprolactone copolymer conduit, and collagen sponge *(50)* all have served effectively as nerve guides. As an extension of the latter principle for cavernous nerve reconstruction, tissue engineering and stem cell approaches have had preliminary success in enhancing penile nerve fiber growth and recovering erection responses in cavernous nerve injured rats *(51,52)*. Lastly, the potential use of gene therapy for recovering erectile function in the face of cavernous nerve injury was demonstrated in rats using gene constructs for delivering neuronal nitric oxide synthase (the gene synthesizing the erection mediator nitric oxide) and brain-derived neurotrophic growth factor *(38,53)*.

The progress in this area is most exciting, suggesting multiple neuromodulatory directions which could be pursued for clinical advancement. While these strategies show promise, further investigation is needed in most instances before assigning their likely roles to the clinical arena.

3.2   Clinical Trials

Several clinical treatments have been proposed as offering potential therapeutic benefit as neuromodulatory drugs in the setting of radical prostatectomy. The rationale for their use has variably followed exciting results from preceding preclinical studies in this scientific area or suggestions of potential benefit based on reports of therapeutic efficacy in clinical settings distinct from pelvic surgery or pelvic disease conditions. The adherence to controlled clinical trial methodology to investigate prospective therapies is most appropriate before claiming their true benefit clinically.

A few clinical trials have been done in this area specifically. Corticosteroids have been briefly investigated, based on proposals that they would counteract inflammatory conditions associated with the surgery. In one study, the corticosteroid methylprednisolone was administered for a short course immediately following surgery *(54)* and in another betamethasone cream 0.1% was locally applied to the cavernous nerves at the time of surgery *(55)*. Neither study demonstrated appreciable improvement compared with the absence of treatment up to 12 months postoperatively. While there were no complications associated with either of these treatments, support for the use of corticosteroids with radical prostatectomy is lacking at this time.

Immunophilin ligands, e.g., FK506 (tacrolimus) and its derivatives, have received a great deal of attention for this clinical purpose. Their potential use has been supported by successful findings resulting from the application of such agents in animal models of cavernous nerve injury *(44–46)*. The mechanism of action of these drugs has remained elusive. Initial considerations were given to possible immune modulatory effects, based on the knowledge that the prototype FK506 has been used clinically as an immunosuppressant drug. However, evidence in support of the fact that these drugs do not require calcineurin inhibition to exert neuroprotection has dampened the fervor of this contention *(56,57)*. A further consideration is that non-immunosuppressant immunophilin ligands have shown neuroprotective effects *(56,57)*. In this light, current thought is that the drugs operate through specialized receptor proteins called immunophilins expressed in injured nerve tissue whereupon downstream intracellular events conceivably result in their beneficial effects *(56–59)*. Recent studies have supported their anti-oxidative effects, as evinced by their ability to produce glutathione upregulation *(60,61)*.

At the clinical trial level, a phase 2, multicenter, randomized, double-blind, placebo-controlled trial using the non-immunosuppressant immunophilin ligand GPI-1485 in approximately 200 preoperatively potent men undergoing nerve-sparing radical prostatectomy has been initiated to explore whether the treatment improves erectile function recovery beyond currently untreated conditions *(62)*. Features of the study include both preoperative and postoperative dosing and the allowance of phosphodiesterase 5 inhibitor use on demand at 1 month following surgery. The study is designed to assess erectile function along with safety and pharmacokinetic profiles of the therapy for a duration of 12 months postoperatively. While final results of this major trial await analysis and reporting, it is anticipated that they will support immunophilin ligands as a promising neuromodulatory approach for radical prostatectomy. As well, it is certain that the trial will impart important, new insights regarding the conduct of clinical trials for the promotion of erectile function recovery following this pelvic surgery.

4 New Frontiers in Molecular Neurobiology

In the excitement of bringing promising neuromodulators to clinical practice not just for radical prostatectomy but additionally for other clinical conditions, a great deal of attention has been given to identifying molecular mechanisms underlying the neuroprotective and/or nerve regenerative effects of prospective neuromodulators. These mechanisms refer to such elements as nerve plasma membrane receptors, nerve membrane channels, subcellular molecules/transcription factors, and intracellular signaling pathways. A purpose in carrying out this line of research is that it may reveal exact target sites of convergence for developing effective neuromodulatory intervention. Such targets would ideally be exploited by currently available drugs and compounds, and their identification may further direct the synthesis of neuromodulatory drugs that are predicted to be most advantageous for future study. It is acknowledged that much of this work has been done using in vitro neuronal cell culture systems, in which specific pharmacologic activation and inhibition methodologies were applied. Another tool, having particular relevance for the study of central neurodegenerative disorders, is the engineering and application of genetically manipulated mice targeting specific neuromodulatory cytokines or neurotrophic factors.

4.1 Signal Transduction Mechanisms

In recent investigations exploring the molecular basis for neuromodulation, significant focus has been given to the actions of survival kinase pathways and their associated transcription factors (Table 4). Nuclear factor-κB (NFκB) *(63,64)* and Ca^{2+}/cAMP-response element binding protein (CREB) *(65,66)* are prominent intracellular signaling factors, which operate in the setting of apoptosis and in association with stimulated actions of neurotrophins. The NFκB transcription factor is purported to exert anti-apoptotic effects in neurons by increasing Akt-1 activity, which affects Bcl-2-associated death protein (Bad) phosphorylation and Bcl-x_L upregulation. Meanwhile, Akt-1 is also activated by phosphatidylinositol-3-kinase [PI(3)K], while Ras-mitogen-activated protein-kinases (MAPKs) and *S*ignal *T*ransducers and *A*ctivators of *T*ranscription 5 (STAT-5) control Bcl-x_L upregulation. Akt-1 activation is proposed to contribute to neuronal survival by stabilizing mitochondrial membrane potential and preventing the release of cytochrome *c* *(67)*. Cytochrome *c* release from mitochondria supposedly signals the activation of a family of executioner cysteine proteases (caspases) in concert with the occurrence of cellular death *(68,69)*. CREB, which is activated by intracellular Ca^{2+} increases via Ca^{2+} channels, serves to modulate the activities of NFκB, PI(3)K/Akt, MAPK, and STAT-5. Separately, with reference to the cell adhesion molecule pathway, the fibroblast

Table 4 Molecular Effectors and Putative Mechanistic Targets

Positive effectors (to be activated)	*Pathogenic mechanism*
Janus-tyrosine-kinase-2	Apoptosis
Nuclear factor-κB	Apoptosis
Ras-mitogen-activated kinases	Apoptosis
Signal transducers and activators of transcription 5	Apoptosis
Akt-1 (protein kinase B)	Mitochondrial depolarization
	Apoptosis
Ca^{2+}/cAMP-response element binding protein	Apoptosis
	Excitotoxicity
	Neurotrophic factor deprivation
Transforming growth factor-β	Ischemia
	Excitotoxicity
	Oxidative stress
Tyrosine kinase	Neurite outgrowth
Negative effectors (to be inhibited)	
Tumor necrosis factor-α	Inflammation
Interleukin-6	Inflammation
Bcl	Apoptosis
Cytochrome *c*	Mitochondrial depolarization
Caspases	Mitochondrial depolarization
Rho-kinase	Neurite outgrowth

N.B. This list is not meant to be exhaustive or complete.

growth factor receptor tyrosine kinase is identified as the primary signal transduction molecule *(18)*.

A salient matter is that intracellular signaling pathways appear to be intricately linked as a basis for mediating the effects of neuromodulators. For instance, the neuroprotective effects of transforming growth factor-β (TGF β)1, which activates NFκB, result from cross-talk between the PI(3)K/Akt and MAPK/ERK 1/2 pathways *(70)*. Also, the novel neuroprotective cytokine erythropoietin acts by binding to its specific erythropoietin receptor, which dimerizes and becomes activated to autophosphorylate Janus-tyrosine-kinase-2 (JAK-2), a critical step toward phosphorylation of several downstream signaling pathways *(71–73)*. These signaling pathways include MAPKs, PI(3)K/Akt, and STAT-5. JAK-2 further interacts with the NFkB signal transduction system in mediating the protection of cortical neurons by erythropoietin from excitotoxic- and nitric oxide-induced apoptosis *(74)*. Further exemplified, androgens exert neuroprotective actions by activating MAPK/ERK while also increasing p90 kDa ribosomal S6 kinase (Rsk) phosphorylation and phosphorylation-dependent inactivation of Bad *(75)*.

Of further interest, neuromodulatory drugs may exert their actions employing alternative molecular routes resulting in neuroprotection. For instance, although erythropoietin perceptibly operates through its receptor pathway and then engages a likely signal transduction pathway in this fashion, it also induces both mRNA expression and the production of biologically active brain-derived neurotrophic factor (BDNF) *(76,77)*. BDNF expression in neuronal cells is induced by the activation of voltage Ca^{2+} channels and recruitment of CREB. Consequently, erythropoietin actions may directly oppose excitotoxic neuronal injury mechanisms *(78)* or deprived neurotrophic factor expression *(79)*.

For central neurodegenerative disorders specifically such as stroke and Alzheimer's disease, recent studies have established the importance of several factors and their signal transduction pathways. Such examples include TGF β, which operates via serine/threonine kinase cascades; tumor necrosis factor-alpha (TNF α), which acts via a p55 receptor linked to a sphingomyelin-ceramide-NFκB pathway; and secreted forms of beta-amyloid precursor protein (beta APP), which employs receptor guanylate cyclase-cGMP-cGMP-dependent kinase K+ channel activation *(80)*. Protein kinase C delta and epsilon are identified to exert roles in the apoptosis following central ischemic events *(81)*. Additional recently described novel signaling pathways with possible roles in central neurodegenerative disorders include the Wnt signaling pathway *(82)* and the nuclear transcription factor 2-antioxidant response element (Nrf2-ARE) pathway *(83)*.

5   Special Considerations

Clinical progress advancing the concept of neuromodulatory drugs in other areas should help in bringing forward this intervention for radical prostatectomy. A historical review of clinical trial efforts in other disciplines is instructive. Clinical experience with the use of neurotrophins, for instance, suggests that significant progress is still required before introducing this form of therapy to the setting of radical prostatectomy or elsewhere. Nerve growth factor has been investigated in phase II and III clinical trials for diabetic polyneuropathy and HIV-related neuropathy *(84)*. Results have shown questionable efficacy for ameliorating symptoms, and the treatment could not be tolerated because of painful side effects. Ciliary neurotrophic factor, BDNF, and insulin growth factor-1 have also been studied for treating amyotrophic lateral sclerosis, but they have demonstrated limited efficacy *(85)*. Thus, prior work in the field for a seemingly promising form of intervention would be questionably offered for radical prostatectomy. In addition to worries that neurotrophic compounds may produce adverse effects elsewhere in the nervous system, issues persist as to whether such therapy may exert growth stimulatory effects on malignant cells. This latter issue arises because evidence exists to suggest that classic neurotrophins and neuropeptide growth factors in preclinical models increased tumor invasiveness and enhanced growth of prostate cancer *(86–88)*. Clearly, prior lessons learned in combination with seeming scientific limitations associated with the use of classic neurotrophins question the likely future use of these agents at a clinical therapeutic level for radical prostatectomy.

Radical prostatectomy represents a special scenario for evaluating and advancing neuromodulatory therapy. As just stated, forthcoming therapies for this application must be assessed for their potential mitogenic risk with respect to prostate cancer cells that may have escaped the organ at local resection or were pre-existent as micrometastases before surgery. On the other hand, radical prostatectomy may offer advantages for the application of neuromodulatory therapy. One apparent advantage is that the occurrence of the injury is predetermined, affording a truly preventive opportunity for neuromodulatory intervention. Another conceivable advantage is associated with the peripheral circumstances of the injury. Accordingly, systemic therapy would not be required to cross the blood–brain/spinal cord barrier, as would be required with such administrations invoked in the treatment of brain and spinal cord injuries. In fact, a proposal for therapy is that it may be advantageously administered locally in the pelvic region at the time of surgery. Further, radical prostatectomy offers a unique experimental paradigm for furthering advances in neuromodulatory therapy. The paradigm is ideal in this respect, given the frequency with which this surgery is performed, its reproducibility, the predictability of nerve injury associated with it, its temporal characteristics in terms of the precise onset of the injury and a fairly well-defined time line for nerve function recovery, and the availability of a measurable endpoint to evaluate the success of the therapy, in this case erectile function restoration.

6 Conclusion

Neuromodulatory therapy for radical prostatectomy encompasses interventions which are either neuroprotective or nerve regenerative for the cavernous nerves injured at the time of the surgery. The therapy is meant to counteract the penile neuropathy that ensues postoperatively, thereby maximizing the potential for rapid, complete erectile function restoration. The science of penile neurogenesis as well as concepts in molecular neurobiology applied to the penis are fruitful areas for scientific investigation and can be expected to guide the development of promising pharmacotherapeutic prospects in this field. However, forthcoming therapy in this clinical context may also derive from exciting non-pharmacologic options as well including stem cell therapy and electrical stimulation. Conceivably, these multiple dimensions of the field suggest their application not just independently but possibly in combination for a maximal therapeutic benefit. In all, it appear that enormous opportunities exist ahead to yield improved sexual function outcomes for patients undergoing radical prostatectomy.

References

1. Walsh, P.C. (1998) Anatomic radical prostatectomy: evolution of the surgical technique. *J. Urol.* **160**, 2418–2424.
2. Han, M., Partin, A.W., Pound, C.R., Epstein, J.I., and Walsh, P.C. (2001) Long-term biochemical disease-free and cancer-specific survival following anatomic radical retropubic prostatectomy. The 15-year Johns Hopkins experience. *Urol. Clin. North Am.* **28**, 555–565.
3. Begg, C.B., Riedel, E.R., Bach, P.B., et al. (2002) Variations in morbidity after radical prostatectomy. *N. Engl. J. Med.* **346**, 1138–1144.
4. Klotz, L., and Herschorn, S. (1998) Early experience with intraoperative cavernous nerve stimulation with penile tumescence monitoring to improve nerve sparing during radical prostatectomy. *Urology* **52**, 537–542.
5. Walsh, P.C., Marschke, P., Catalona, W.J., et al. (2001) Efficacy of first-generation cavermap to verify location and function of cavernous nerves during radical prostatectomy: a multi-institutional evaluation by experienced surgeons. *Urology* **57**, 491–494.
6. Scardino, P.T., and Kim, E.D. (2001) Rationale for and results of nerve grafting during radical prostatectomy. *Urology* **57**, 1016–1019.
7. Walsh, P.C. (2001) Nerve grafts are rarely necessary and are unlikely to improve sexual function in men undergoing anatomic radical prostatectomy. *Urology* **57**, 1020–1024.
8. Menon, M., Kaul, S., Bhandari, A., Shrivastava, A., Tewari, A., and Hemal, A. (2005) Potency following robotic radical prostatectomy: a questionnaire based analysis of outcomes after conventional nerve sparing and prostatic fascia sparing techniques. *J.Urol.* **174**, 2291–2296.
9. Montorsi, F., Salonia, A., Suardi, N., et al. (2005) Improving the preservation of the urethral sphincter and neurovascular bundles during open radical retropubic prostatectomy. *Eur. Urol.* **48**, 938–945.
10. Burnett, A.L. (2005) Erectile dysfunction following radical prostatectomy. *JAMA* **293**, 2648–2653.
11. Gralnek, D., Wessells, H., Cui, H., and Dalkin, B.L. (2000) Differences in sexual function and quality of life after nerve sparing and nonnerve sparing radical retropubic prostatectomy. *J. Urol.* **163**, 1166–1169.
12. Stephenson, R.A., Mori, M., Hsieh, Y.C., et al. (2005) Treatment of erectile dysfunction following therapy for clinically localized prostate cancer: patient reported use and outcomes from the Surveillance, Epidemiology, and End Results Prostate Cancer Outcomes Study. *J. Urol.* **174**, 646–650.
13. Montorsi, F., Guazzoni, G., Strambi, L.F., et al. (1997) Recovery of spontaneous erectile function after nerve-sparing radical retropubic prostatectomy with and without early intracavernous injections of alprostadil: results of a prospective, randomized trial. *J. Urol.* **158**, 1408–1410.

14. Mulhall, J., Land, S., Parker, M., Waters, W.B., and Flanigan, R.C. (2005) The use of an erectogenic pharmacotherapy regimen following radical prostatectomy improves recovery of spontaneous erectile function. *J. Sex. Med.* **2**, 532–540.
15. Frostick, S.P., Yin, Q., and Kemp, G.J. (1998) Schwann cells, neurotrophic factors, and peripheral nerve regeneration. *Microsurgery* **18**, 397–405.
16. Semkova, I., and Krieglstein, J. (1999) Neuroprotection mediated via neurotrophic factors and induction of neurotrophic factors. *Brain Res. Brain Res. Rev.* **30**, 176–188.
17. Xu, Z., Maroney, A.C., Dobrzanski, P., Kukekov, N.V., and Greene, L.A. (2001) The MLK family mediated c-Jun N-terminal kinase activation in neuronal apoptosis. *Mol. Cell Biol.* 21, 4713–4724.
18. Skaper, S.D. (2005) Neuronal growth-promoting and inhibitory cues in neuroprotection and neuroregeneration. *Ann. NY Acad. Sci.* **1053**, 376–385.
19. Kim, J., Schafer, J., and Ming, G.L. (2006) New directions in neuroregeneration. *Expert Opin. Biol. Ther.* **6**, 735–738.
20. Fraiman, M.C., Lepor, H., and McCullough, A.R. (1999) Changes in penile morphometrics in men with erectile dysfunction after nerve-sparing radical retropubic prostatectomy. *Mol. Urol.* **3**, 109–115.
21. Savoie, M., Kim, S.S., and Soloway, M.S. (2003) A prospective study measuring penile length in men treated with radical prostatectomy for prostate cancer. *J. Urol.* **169**, 1462–1464.
22. Podlasek, C.A., Gonzalez, C.M., Zelner, D.J., Jiang, H.B., McKenna, K.E., and McVary, K.T. (2001) Analysis of NOS isoforms changes in a post radical prostatectomy model of erectile dysfunction. *Int. J. Impot. Res.* **13**(Suppl 5), S1–S15.
23. Iacono, F., Giannella, R., Somma, P., Manno, G., Fusco, F., and Mirone, V. (2005) Histological alterations in cavernous tissue after radical prostatectomy. *J. Urol.* **173**, 1673–1676.
24. Klein, L.T., Miller, M.I., Buttyan, R., et al. (1997) Apoptosis in the rat penis after penile denervation. *J. Urol.* **158**, 626–630.
25. User, H.M., Hairston, J.H., Zelner, D.J., McKenna, K.E., and McVary, K.T. (2003) Penile weight and cell subtype specific changes in a post-radical prostatectomy model of erectile dysfunction. *J. Urol.* **169**, 1175–1179.
26. Nehra, A., Goldstein, I., Pabby, A., et al. (1996) Mechanisms of venous leakage: a prospective clinicopathological correlation of corporeal function and structure. *J. Urol.* **156**, 1320–1329.
27. Schwartz, M. (2001) Harnessing the immune system for neuroprotection: therapeutic vaccines for acute and chronic neurodegenerative disorders. *Cell Mol. Neurobiol.* **21**, 617–627.
28. Levi, M.S., and Brimble, M.A. (2004) A review of neuroprotective agents. *Curr. Med. Chem.* **11**, 2383–2397.
29. Bialek, M., Zaremba, P., Borowicz, K.K., and Czuczwar, S.J. (2004) Neuroprotective role of testosterone in the nervous system. *Pol. J. Pharmacol.* **56**, 509–518.
30. Sosa, I., Reyes, O., and Kuffler, D.P. (2005) Immunosuppressants: neuroprotection and promoting neurological recovery following peripheral nerve and spinal cord lesions. *Exp. Neurol.* **195**, 7–15.
31. Tsai, E.C., and Tator, C.H. (2005) Neuroprotection and regeneration strategies for spinal cord repair. *Curr. Pharm. Des.* **11**, 1211–1222.
32. Schwab, J.M., Brechtel, K., Mueller, C.A., et al. (2006) Experimental strategies to promote spinal cord regeneration-an integrative perspective. *Prog. Neurobiol.* **78**, 91–116.
33. Chiang, Y.H., Borlongan, C.V., Zhou, F.C., Hoffer, B.J., and Wang Y. (2005) Transplantation of fetal kidney cells: neuroprotection and neuroregeneration. *Cell Transplant.* **14**, 1–9.
34. Te, A.E., Santarosa, R.P., Koo, H.P., et al. (1994) Neurotrophic factors in the rat penis. *J. Urol.* **152**, 2167–2172.
35. Dahiya, R., Chui, R., Perinchery, G., Nakajima, K., Oh, B.R., and Lue, T.F. (1999) Differential gene expression of growth factors in young and old rat penile tissues is associated with erectile dysfunction. *Int. J. Impot. Res.* **11**, 201–206.
36. Burgers, J.K., Nelson, R.J., Quinlan, D.M., and Walsh, P.C. (1991) Nerve growth factor, nerve grafts and amniotic membrane grafts restore erectile function in rats. *J. Urol.* **146**, 463–468.

37. Ball, R.A., Lipton, S.A., Dreyer, E.B., Richie, J.P., and Vickers, M.A. (1992) Entubulization repair of severed cavernous nerves in the rat resulting in return of erectile function. *J. Urol.* **148,** 211–215.
38. Bakircioglu, M.E., Lin, C.S., Fan, P., Sievert, K.D., Kan, Y.W., and Lue, T.F. (2001) The effect of adeno-associated virus mediated brain derived neurotrophic factor in an animal model of neurogenic impotence. *J. Urol.* **165,** 2103–2109.
39. Bochinski, D., Hsieh, P.S., Nunes, L., et al. (2004) Effect of insulin-like growth factor-1 and insulin-like growth factor binding protein-3 complex in cavernous nerve cryoablation. *Int. J. Impot. Res.* **16,** 418–423.
40. Jung, G.W., Spencer, E.M., and Lue, T.F. (1998) Growth hormone enhances regeneration of nitric oxide synthase-containing penile nerves after cavernous nerve neurotomy in rats. *J. Urol.* **160,** 1899–1904.
41. Laurikainen, A., Hiltunen, J.O., Thomas-Crusells, J., et al. (2000) Neurturin is a neurotrophic factor for penile parasympathetic neurons in adult rat. *J. Neurobiol.* **43,** 198–205.
42. Podlasek, C.A., Meroz, C.L., Korolis, H., Tang, Y., McKenna, K.E., and McVary, K.T. (2005) Sonic hedgehog, the penis and erectile dysfunction: a review of sonic hedgehog signaling in the penis. *Curr. Pharm. Des.* **11,** 4011–4027.
43. Allaf, M.E., Hoke, A., and Burnett, A.L. (2005) Erythropoietin promotes the recovery of erectile function following cavernous nerve injury. *J. Urol.* **174,** 2060–2064.
44. Sezen, S.F., Hoke, A., Burnett, A.L., and Snyder, S.H. (2001) Immunophilin ligand FK506 is neuroprotective for penile innervation. *Nat. Med.* 7, 1073–1074.
45. Burnett, A.L., and Becker, R.E. (2004) Immunophilin ligands promote penile neurogenesis and erection recovery after cavernous nerve injury. *J. Urol.* **171,** 495–500.
46. Hayashi, N., Minor, T.X., Carrion, R., Price, R., Nunes, L., and Lue, T.F. (2006) The effect of FK1706 on erectile function following bilateral cavernous nerve crush injury in a rat model. *J. Urol.* **176,** 824–829.
47. Kendirci, M., Zsengeller, Z., Bivalacqua, T.J., et al. (2005) Poly (Adenosine diphosphate-ribose) polymerase inhibition preserves erectile function in rats after cavernous nerve injury. *J. Urol.* **174,** 2054–2059.
48. Quinlan, D.M., Nelson, R.J., and Walsh, P.C. (1991) Cavernous nerve grafts restore erectile function in denervated rats. *J. Urol.* **145,** 380–383.
49. May, F., Weidner, N., Matiasek, K., et al. (2004) Schwann cell seeded guidance tubes restore erectile function after ablation of cavernous nerves in rats. *J. Urol.* **172,** 374–377.
50. Hisasue, S., Kato, R., Sato, Y., Suetomi, T., Tabata, Y., and Tsukamoto, T. (2005) Cavernous nerve reconstruction with a biodegradable conduit graft and collagen sponge in the rat. *J. Urol.* **173,** 286–291.
51. Graziottin, T.M., Resplande, J., Nunes, L., Rogers, R., Gholami, S., and Lue, T. (2002) Long-term survival of autotransplanted major pelvic ganglion in the corpus cavernosum of adult rats. *J. Urol.* **168,** 362–366.
52. Bochinski, D., Lin, G.T., Nunes, L., et al. (2004) The effect of neural embryonic stem cell therapy in a rat model of cavernosal nerve injury. *BJU Int.* **94,** 904–909.
53. Magee, T.R., Ferrini, M., Garban, H.J., et al. (2002) Gene therapy of erectile dysfunction in the rat with penile neuronal nitric oxide synthase. *Biol. Reprod.* **67,** 1033–1041.
54. Parsons, J.K., Marschke, P., Maples, P., and Walsh, P.C. (2004) Effect of methylprednisolone on return of sexual function after nerve-sparing radical retropubic prostatectomy. *Urology* **64,** 987–990.
55. Deliveliotis, C., Delis, A., Papatsoris, A., Antoniou, N., and Varkarakis, I.M. (2005) Local steroid application during nerve-sparing radical retropubic prostatectomy. *BJU Int.* **96,** 533–535.
56. Gold, B.G., and Villafranca, J.E. (2003) Neuroimmunophilin ligands: the development of novel neuroregenerative/neuroprotective compounds. *Curr. Top. Med. Chem.* **3,** 1368–1375.
57. Klettner, A., and Herdegen T. (2003) FK506 and its analogs – therapeutic potential for neurological disorders. *Curr. Drug Targets CNS Neurol. Disord.* **2,** 153–162.

58. Avramut, M., and Achim, C.L. (2003) Immunophilins in nervous system degeneration and regeneration. *Curr. Top. Med. Chem.* **3**, 1376–1382.
59. Zawadzka, M., and Kaminska, B. (2005) A novel mechanism of FK506-mediated neuroprotection: downregulation of cytokine expression in glial cells. *Glia* **49**, 36–51.
60. Tanaka, K., Yoshioka, M., Miyazaki, I., Fujita, N., and Ogawa, N. (2002) GPI1046 prevents dopaminergic dysfunction by activating glutathione system in the mouse striatum. *Neurosci. Lett.* **321**, 45–48.
61. Tanaka, K., Fujita, N., Yoshioka, M., and Ogawa, N. (2001) Immunosuppressive and non-immunosuppressive immunophilin ligands improve H(2)O (2)-induced cell damage by increasing glutathione levels in NG108-15 cells. *Brain Res.* **889**, 225–228.
62. Burnett, A.L., and Lue, T.F. (2006) Neuromodulatory therapy to improve erectile function recovery outcomes after pelvic surgery. *J. Urol.* **176**, 882–887.
63. Kaltschmidt, B., Widera, D., and Kaltschmidt, C. (2005) Signaling via, N.F.-kappaB in the nervous system. *Biochim. Biophys. Acta* **1745**, 287–299.
64. Mattson, M.P., and Meffert, M.K. (2006) Roles for, N.F.-KappaB in nerve cell survival, plasticity, and disease. *Cell Death Differ.* **13**, 852–860.
65. Masutani, H., Bai, J., Kim, Y.C., and Yodoi, J. (2004) Thioredoxin as a neurotrophic cofactor and an important regulator of neuroprotection. *Mol. Neurobiol.* **29**, 229–242.
66. Papadia, S., Stevenson, P., Hardingham, N.R., Bading, H., and Hardingham, G.E. (2005) Nuclear Ca2+ and the cAMP response element-binding protein family mediate a late phase of activity-dependent neuroprotection. *J. Neurosci.* 25, 4279–4287.
67. Kennedy, S.G., Kandel, E.S., Cross, T.K., and Hay, N. (1999) Akt/Protein kinase B inhibits cell death by preventing the release of cytochrome c from mitochondria. *Mol. Cell Biol.* **19**, 5800–5810.
68. Mitra, D., Kim, J., MacLow, C., Karsan, A., and Laurence, J. (1998) Role of caspases 1 and 3 and Bcl-2-related molecules in endothelial cell apoptosis associated with thrombotic microangiopathies. *Am. J. Hematol.* **59**, 279–287.
69. Chong, Z.Z., Lin, S.H., and Maiese, K. (2002) Nicotinamide modulates mitochondrial membrane potential and cysteine protease activity during cerebral vascular endothelial cell injury. *J. Vasc. Res.* **39**, 131–147.
70. Zhu, Y., Culmsee, C., Klumpp, S., and Krieglstein, J. (2004) Neuroprotection by transforming growth factor-beta 1 involves activation of nuclear factor-kappaB through phosphatidylinositol-3-OH kinase/Akt and mitogen-activated protein kinase-extracellular-signal regulated kinase 1,2 signaling pathways. *Neuroscience* **123**, 897–906.
71. Chong, Z.Z., Lin, S.H., Kang, J.Q., and Maiese, K. (2003) Erythropoietin prevents early and late neuronal demise through modulation of Akt1 and induction of caspase 1, 3, and 8. *J. Neurosci. Res.* **71**, 659–669.
72. Chong, Z.Z., Kang, J.Q., and Maiese, K. (2003) Erythropoietin fosters both intrinsic and extrinsic neuronal protection through modulation of microglia, Akt1, Bad, and caspase-mediated pathways. *Br. J. Pharmacol.* **138**, 1107–1118.
73. Ghezzi, P., and Brines, M. (2004) Erythropoietin as an antiapoptotic, tissue-protective cytokine. *Cell Death Differ.* **11**(Suppl 1), S37–S44.
74. Digicaylioglu, M., and Lipton, S.A. (2001) Erythropoietin-mediated neuroprotection involves cross-talk between Jak2 and NF-kappaB signaling cascades. *Nature* **412**, 641–647.
75. Nguyen, T.V., Yao, M., and Pike, C.J. (2005) Androgens activate mitogen-activated protein kinase signaling: role in neuroprotection. *J. Neurochem.* **94**, 1639–1651.
76. Wang, L., Zhang, Z., Wang, Y., Zhang, R., and Chopp, M. (2004) Treatment of stroke with erythropoietin enhances neurogenesis and angiogenesis and improves neurological function in rats. *Stroke* **35**, 1732–1737.
77. Viviani, B., Bartesaghi, S., Corsini, E., et al. (2005) Erythropoietin protects primary hippocampal neurons increasing the expression of brain-derived neurotrophic factor. *J. Neurochem.* **93**, 412–421.

78. Morishita, E., Masuda, S., Nagao, M., Yasuda, Y., and Sasaki, R. (1997) Erythropoietin receptor is expressed in rat hippocampal and cerebral cortical neurons, and erythropoietin prevents in vitro glutamate-induced neuronal death. *Neuroscience* **76,** 105–116.

79. Koshimura, K., Murakami, Y., Sohmiya, M., Tanaka, J., and Kato, Y. (1999) Effects of erythropoietin on neuronal activity. *J. Neurochem.* **72,** 2565–2572.

80. Mattson, M.P., Barger, S.W., Furukawa, K., et al. (1997) Cellular signaling roles of TGF beta, TNF alpha and beta APP in brain injury responses and Alzheimer's disease. *Brain Res. Brain Res. Rev.* **23,** 47–61.

81. Perez-Pinzon, M.A., Dave, K.R., and Raval, A.P. (2005) Role of reactive oxygen species and protein kinase C in ischemic tolerance in the brain. *Antioxid. Redox. Signal.* **7,** 1150–1157.

82. Inestrosa, N.C., Urra, S., and Colombres, M. (2004) Acetylcholinesterase (AChE)—amyloid-beta-peptide complexes in Alzheimer's disease, the Wnt signaling pathway. *Curr. Alzheimer. Res.* **1,** 249–254.

83. van Muiswinkel, F.L., and Kuiperij, H.B. (2005) The Nrf2-ARE Signaling pathway: promising drug target to combat oxidative stress in neurodegenerative disorders. *Curr. Drug Targets CNS Neurol. Disord.* **4,** 267–281.

84. Apfel, S.C. (2002) Nerve growth factor for the treatment of diabetic neuropathy: what went wrong, what went right, and what does the future hold? *Int. Rev. Neurobiol.* **50,** 393–413.

85. Apfel, S.C. (2001) Neurotrophic factor therapy—prospects and problems. *Clin. Chem. Lab. Med.* **39,** 351–355.

86. Djakiew, D., Pflug, B.R., Delsite, R., et al. (1993) Chemotaxis and chemokinesis of human prostate tumor cell lines in response to human prostate stromal cell secretory proteins containing a nerve growth factor-like protein. *Cancer Res.* **53,** 1416–1420.

87. Miknyoczki, S.J., Wan, W., Chang, H., et al. (2003) The neurotrophin-trk receptor axes are critical for the growth and progression of human prostatic carcinoma and pancreatic ductal adenocarcinoma xenografts in nude mice. *Clin. Cancer Res.* **8,** 1924–1931.

88. Lee, L.F., Guan, J., Qiu, Y., and Kung, H.J. (2001) Neuropeptide-induced androgen independence in prostate cancer cells: roles of nonreceptor tyrosine kinases Etk/Bmx, Src, and focal adhesion kinase. *Mol. Cell Biol.* **21,** 8385–8398.

Chapter 9
Nerve Grafting at Radical Retropubic Prostatectomy: Rationale, Technique, and Results

Joseph A. Pettus and Farhang Rabbani

Abstract While cavernous nerve preservation is ideal for optimal recovery of erectile function after radical prostatectomy, unilateral or bilateral nerve resection may be necessary in a given individual at increased risk for extracapsular extension in order to achieve a negative surgical margin. In such patients cavernous nerve grafting with autogenous sural or genitofemoral nerve may improve recovery of erectile function. While pilot studies demonstrated efficacy in over 40% of men undergoing bilateral nerve grafting, more recent data have been more sobering with only 11% of men undergoing bilateral nerve grafting able to consistently obtain adequate erections. A randomized trial of unilateral nerve grafting has demonstrated no significant improvement in potency with unilateral sural nerve grafting. Ultimately, a randomized trial of bilateral nerve grafting will be necessary to determine its role in the management of men needing bilateral nerve resection at the time of radical prostatectomy.

Keywords Nerve grafting; retropubic prostatectomy; erectile function recovery; penile rehabilitation.

1 Introduction

Cavernous nerve preservation is the cornerstone to regaining potency following RP *(1–4)*. The cavernous nerve fibers arise from the spinal cord at S2–S4 and travel within the pelvic plexus, then coalescing within the neurovascular bundle located

From: *Current Clinical Urology* Series, *Sexual Function in the Prostate Cancer Patient*
Edited by John P. Mulhall, DOI 10.1007/978-1-60327-555-2_9,
© Humana Press, a part of Springer Science+Business Media, LLC 2009

posterolateral to the prostate in the groove between the rectum and prostate, reaching the corpora cavernosa distal to the prostatic apex. In patients at high risk of having extracapsular extension (ECE), resection of the neurovascular bundle is often necessary to optimize cancer control and achieve negative surgical margins. Postoperative potency is quantitatively related to the number of cavernous nerve fibers preserved at surgery *(4)*. Recovery of potency has been reported at 55–76% with bilateral nerve-sparing versus 21–56% with unilateral nerve resection *(4–6)*. Recovery of erectile function after bilateral wide resection is minimal *(7,8)*.

Quinlan and colleagues were first to perform genitofemoral nerve grafting in a rat model with bilaterally ablated cavernous nerves *(9)*. At 4 months, the nerve-grafted rats had better erectile function than sham-treated controls. In 1999, Kim et al. reported the first pilot study in humans, reporting that 2/9 patients undergoing bilateral cavernous nerve grafts had erectile function sufficient for intercourse *(10)*. In an update with at least 1-year follow-up, they reported that 10/23 (43%) patients had erections adequate for penetration using sildenafil with functional return delayed until at least 5 months, reaching a plateau at 18 months *(7)*. These early reports of success have provided the foundation for subsequent studies of cavernous nerve grafting.

2 Fundamentals

Nerve regeneration is a complex, highly orchestrated process *(11)*. Within hours of peripheral nerve injury, the distal end undergoes Wallerian degeneration, characterized by demyelination, and cell membrane degeneration and leakage of various neurotropic factors with subsequent phagocytosis by macrophages. The proximal nerve stump retracts to the level of the most proximal node of Ranvier and starts to sprout axons *(12)*. Within 3 days of axotomy, the distal axonal membrane and surrounding Schwann cells are phagocytosed by macrophages. The macrophages and other surrounding cells elaborate cytokines and neurotropic factors that stimulate Schwann cells to proliferate. The new Schwann cells form conduits for the regenerating axons and provide neurotrophic stimuli allowing for appropriate dendritic connections to be made with ultimate reinnervation of the end organ *(13–15)*. Without Schwann cell stimuli, regenerating axons may grow inappropriately, failing to reinnervate the end organ. Axonal regeneration is slow, occurring at only 1–2 mm/day, and end organ reinnervation is inversely proportional to the distance of regeneration. A nerve graft also experiences the same phagocytosis and Schwann cell proliferation which act as a guide for axonal regeneration by providing physical structural support and a favorable microenvironment.

In animal models, researchers have explored a number of techniques which facilitate nerve regrowth. Quinlan *(9)* was the first to apply genitofemoral nerve grafts to the cavernous nerves in a rat model, performing 3 mm cavernous nerve ablations bilaterally, and comparing nerve-grafted rats to those without nerve grafts. The grafted rats had significantly better erectile function at 4 months than controls, with functional recovery in 50% versus 11%, respectively. Burger and colleagues *(16)* compared erectile function in rats with 3 mm bilateral cavernous nerve grafts which had local application of nerve growth factor (NGF) to bilaterally grafted rats without NGF, demonstrating 64% versus 33% of rats having erectile function. Cavernous nerve regeneration has also been demonstrated using silastic tube grafts; *(17)* May et al. *(18)* reported that silastic conduits lined with cultured Schwann cells restored erectile function comparable to sham controls.

The rodent model has several short-comings. Rats are known to have excellent nerve regenerative capacity, the cavernous nerve is a more distinct entity than in humans, and the ability to create a large gap is limited. The canine cavernous nerve anatomy is more similar to that of humans. In dogs, the cavernous nerve is a plexus, rather than a distinct structure, containing both myelinated and unmyelinated fibers. Lowe and colleagues *(19)* performed 3 cm bilateral cavernous nerve ablation in dogs and on comparison of bilaterally grafted to non-grafted dogs, reported that grafted dogs had return of preoperative erectile function by 4 months while ablated animals still had significant deficits by 8 months. Further, histologic examination of the grafts at 8 months demonstrated evidence of regeneration in the mid and distal segments of the graft with minimal Wallerian degeneration in the distal cavernous nerve stump. Return of parasympathetic function has been demonstrated in humans with phrenic nerve grafts for vocal cords *(20)* and in cardiac transplantation *(21)*. Even though the sural and genitofemoral grafts are myelinated, they undergo the same degeneration as described above, leaving proliferating Schwann cells whose basement membranes seem to be most important for regenerating nerves *(14)*.

3 Indications

Assessment of the risk of ECE prior to RP is paramount to determination of the need for wide excision and hence nerve grafting. Using the information from the expanded sextant prostate biopsy regarding the number of positive cores and the length and percentage of tumor in each core as well as the Gleason score, along with preoperative PSA and DRE findings, we can estimate the probability of ECE using a nomogram *(22,23)*. In addition, we frequently perform preoperative endorectal coil MRI of the prostate to evaluate tumor location and volume which may indicate the presence of ECE and preoperative planning for dissection of the neurovascular bundle *(24)*. Based on these data, we can advise patients at high risk for ECE or tumor close to the neurovascular bundle that nerve resection may be necessary to obtain complete tumor extirpation and clear surgical margins. Such patients who are potent may be offered a nerve grafting procedure in order to optimize recovery of potency and possibly continence. Patients are then consented for unilateral or bilateral nerve grafting using either the sural or the genitofemoral nerves. If the caliber of the genitofemoral nerves is inadequate, the sural nerve may be harvested. The final decision to widely resect the neurovascular bundles is made intraoperatively based on the adherence of the neurovascular bundles to the prostate and the palpation of the tumor within the prostate.

4 Surgical Technique

The patient is placed supine on the operating table, and the right leg is prepped into the surgical field. Our radical prostatectomy technique has been described in detail elsewhere *(25)*. In general, if the genitofemoral nerve is easily accessible and of sufficient caliber, generally 2–3 mm in diameter or larger, it is considered adequate for nerve grafting, otherwise the sural nerve should be used because its caliber is reliably large enough for the neural anastomosis. The advantage of use of a larger caliber nerve is that if the distal cavernous nerve stump is indistinct, the larger caliber donor nerve allows a greater margin for error in achieving a successful graft-to-distal stump anastomosis. Prior to the apical dissection and pedicle dissections, the distal and proximal nerve stumps are identified using the CaverMap stimulator *(26,27)*. Prior to transection, the proximal nerve stump is marked with a 4-0 Prolene™ suture for identification later. The distal end may be marked with a 4-0 Prolene™ suture or double small clips to distinguish from a bleeding vessel at the time of transection, with these removed at the time of neural anastomosis (Fig. 1 and Color Plate 3, following p. 264). The prostate is removed, the bladder neck is matured, and the urethral anastomotic sutures are placed and protected. Final hemostasis is secured. The nerve graft is then performed (Fig. 2 and Color Plate 4, following p. 264). If the nerve stumps cannot be adequately identified, the nerve graft procedure is omitted

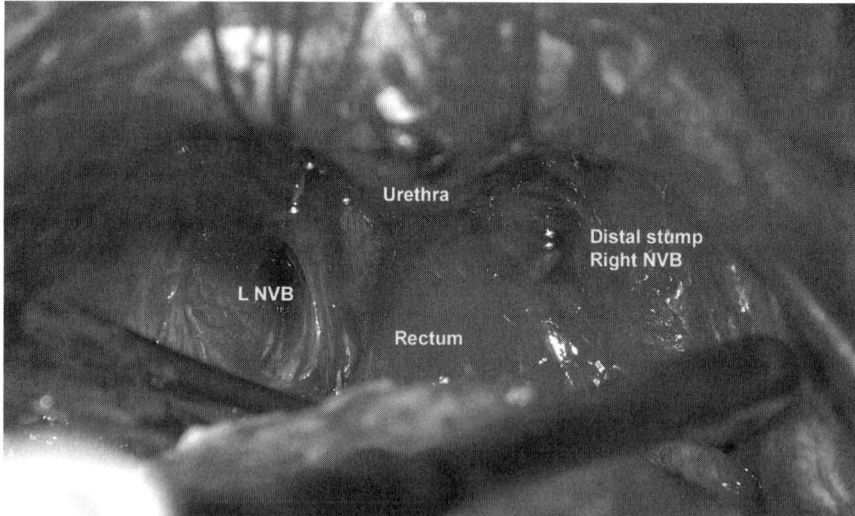

Fig. 1 Intraoperative photograph showing the right distal neurovascular bundle stump with double clips to distinguish it from a bleeding vessel. These are removed at the time of neural anastomosis (*See* Color Plate 3, following p. 264)

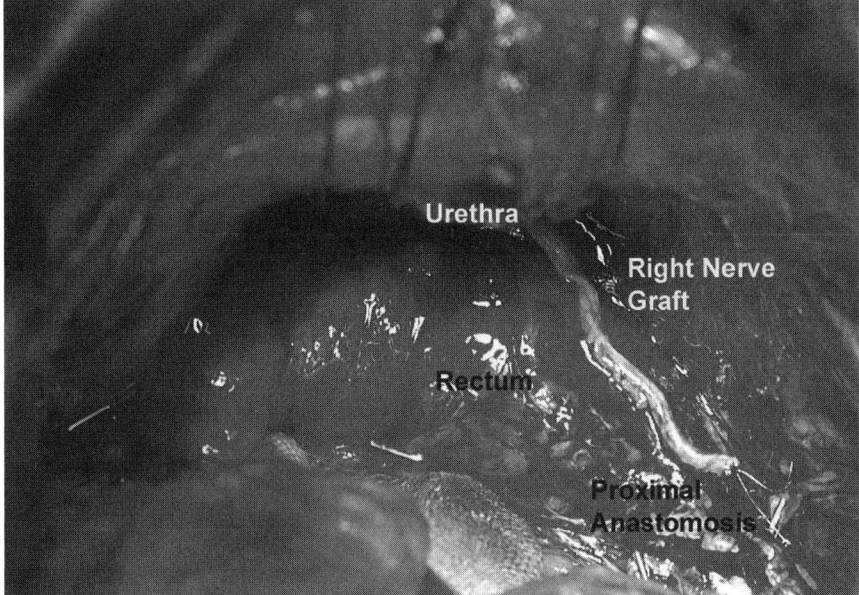

Fig. 2 Intraoperative photograph showing the completed right cavernous nerve graft (*See* Color Plate 4, following p. 264)

as close apposition of nerve endings is essential for graft success. Muneuchi et al. *(28)* have commented on their early experience with nerve grafting, reporting that sural nerve grafting was more difficult than expected with visualization of the distal end sometimes difficult and the ends of the recipient nerve not always fresh, highlighting the importance of having an experienced plastic surgical team. The gap is measured between the nerve stumps, and an appropriate length of nerve, approximately 20% longer than the gap, is then resected so as to perform a tension-free anastomosis. If the sural nerve is used, a curvilinear incision is made superior and posterior to the lateral malleolus and up to 30 cm of sural nerve is harvested *(10)*. When the sural nerve is harvested, the proximal and distal sural nerve stumps are thoroughly cauterized to prevent neuroma, then buried deeply within the gastrocnemius muscle. The grafts are trimmed to the appropriate length and anastomosed to the nerve stumps using 7-0 Prolene interrupted sutures through the epineurium with the orientation of the donor nerve reversed to avoid blind ending nerve fascicles. At this point, 2.5–3.5× loupe magnification are mandatory to optimally identify the nerves in the neurovascular bundle. Upon completion of the neural anastomosis, suction is used sparingly to avoid disruption of the graft anastomosis with a trap placed on the suction tubing. The bladder neck closure and vesicourethral anastomosis is then completed, drains are placed, and the abdomen is closed. In the event of unilateral nerve grafting, a single Jackson–Pratt drain is placed in the contralateral obturator fossa and in the event of bilateral nerve grafting, bilateral Penrose drains are placed. There are no special postoperative considerations except foot elevation when the sural nerve is harvested with no restrictions on postoperative ambulation.

Laparoscopic and robot-assisted nerve graft procedures have been described *(29–32),* but the long-term efficacy is not yet established.

CaverMap™ nerve stimulation is controversial in terms of ultimate erectile outcome prediction, but it has been shown to have excellent sensitivity for identifying the neurovascular bundles. In a multi-institutional trial, Klotz et al. *(27)* reported improved erectile function at 12 months as measured by RigiScan and Sexual Function Inventory Questionnaire. Walsh and coworkers *(33)* found that the CaverMap™ device was able to identify the neurovascular bundle with a sensitivity and specificity of 88 and 54%, respectively, while Kim and colleagues *(34)* reported a sensitivity of 77%. Rabbani et al. have reported that the degree of response to intraoperative stimulation was associated with erectile function recovery *(35)*.

Based on cadaveric studies, Takenaka et al. *(36)* have recently suggested that the pelvic splanchnic nerve fibers may join the neurovascular bundle as the cavernous nerve distal to the vesicoprostatic junction, the most usual place that the proximal stump is located and anastomosed during nerve grafting. These authors showed a "spray-like" distribution of nerve fibers entering the neurovascular bundle at various points along its course. They suggested that nerve stimulation be conducted at the presacral and pararectal regions in addition to the proximal and distal neurovascular stumps to identify the areas of best stimulation so that the nerve graft will perform most effectively.

Graft-related complications are rare *(7,8,37,38)*. They include neuroma, mild paresthesia, along the nerve distribution, and sympathetic dystrophy in the ipsilateral lower limb.

5 Results

Bilateral nerve grafting was first reported by Kim et al. *(10)* using sural nerve grafts for cavernous nerve interruption during RRP in humans, reporting that 1/9 patients had return of medically unassisted erections adequate for intercourse, and two additional patients had erections just below the normal threshold established by the International Index of Erectile Function (IIEF) *(39)*. In a later update with a minimum of 12 months of follow-up, Kim and colleagues reported on 23 patients that 6/23 (26%) had medically unassisted erections *(40)*. An additional four patients were able to have intercourse using sildenafil, yielding a total of 43% with return of sexual function in their series, and providing proof of concept. Functional return did not start until 5 months and plateaued by 18 months postoperatively. There were no graft-related complications, but both operative time and blood loss were higher in the grafted cohort. Chang et al. studied 30 patients with locally advanced prostate cancer who underwent RRP with bilateral wide neurovascular bundle excision with sural nerve grafting *(8)*. The authors used penile rehabilitation starting 6 weeks postoperatively with RigiScan testing to document erectile function. They found that 13/30 (43%) were eventually able to have intercourse, and 7/13 were able to do so without medical assistance.

More recent data do not appear to be as promising as earlier reports. Secin et al. *(41)* reported that 34% of bilaterally nerve-grafted patients had recovered erections sufficient for penetration at 5 years, and only 11% of the cohort were able to consistently obtain erections adequate for intercourse. These inferior results may be due to less stringent selection criteria, differing degrees of patient motivation, and potential differences between genitofemoral and sural nerve grafting success due to the difference in the caliber of the nerves.

While bilateral nerve grafting clearly may have some benefit, some have questioned the efficacy of unilateral nerve grafting. In a recent editorial, Kim and Scardino *(37)* argued that since approximately 30% of patients with unilateral nerve-sparing were able to have medically unassisted intercourse compared to 55% of those who received unilateral nerve grafts, unilateral nerve grafting essentially has the same results as bilateral nerve-sparing surgery. At Memorial Sloan Kettering Cancer Center between 1998 and 2002, 108 patients underwent unilateral nerve grafting after unilateral nerve resection and were compared with patients undergoing bilateral nerve-sparing and with a historical cohort of patients undergoing unilateral nerve resection without grafting. At 4 years, 40% of unilateral graft patients had return of erections by IEFF erectile function (EF) domain score > 17, compared to 80% with bilateral nerve-sparing, and 25% with unilateral nerve-sparing without grafting *(42)*. Canto et al. *(43)* have reported that 12/41 patients with unilateral sural nerve grafts regained potency compared with 3/34 with unilateral nerve-sparing without grafting when erectile function was defined as greater than or equal to 17 on the IEFF-EF domain score. Saito et al. *(44)* found that the postoperative sexual function score of unilaterally grafted patients showed an intermediate level of recovery between those of men with bilateral nerve-sparing and unilateral nerve resection without grafting at 12 months and reached the same level as the score at 12 months of the bilateral nerve-sparing group at 18 months postoperatively. The difference in the sexual function score between the grafted and non-grafted men with unilateral nerve resection began to appear after 6 months postoperatively and increased with time. As this study was not randomized, the grafted men were younger with better preoperative erectile function than non-grafted men, possibly accounting for the difference in results seen in men with and without grafts.

Some authors have postulated that nerve grafting may also aid in recovery of continence. Singh and coworkers *(38)* compared the urinary functional outcomes of 40 unilateral nerve graft patients to that of 40 unilateral nerve-sparing patients who did not undergo grafting. They defined continence as completely dry or occasional leakage of a few drops, and noted that 95% of patients with unilateral nerve grafting were continent at 12 months compared to 58% without grafts. Additionally, the authors found the UCLA Prostate Cancer Index (PCI) score as being better; the median score was almost tenfold higher for patients receiving unilateral nerve grafting compared to those who had unilateral nerve-sparing with no nerve graft and only one nerve bundle spared, even when age was entered into the model as a covariate.

Important limitations exist in human studies of cavernosal nerve grafting. To date, most series have been modestly powered, retrospective single institution experiences. Interim analysis of a randomized phase II trial of unilateral nerve grafting versus no grafting in men undergoing unilateral nerve-sparing prostatectomy has revealed no statistical difference between the two arms at 2 years (44% potency rate for nerve grafting versus 43% for no grafting, $p = 0.974$) *(44)*. Nocturnal penile tumescence testing with RigiScan revealed no difference in either group at 8, 12 or 16 months compared to the baseline measurements taken at 4 months *(45)*. Also, there was no difference in recovery of penile length between the two groups *(45)*. Patient selection for unilateral nerve grafting may account for much of the reported potency recovery advantages *(46)*. These patients tend to be young and sexually active preoperatively, and may be more motivated toward penile rehabilitation following RRP.

6 Conclusions

Bilateral cavernosal nerve grafting appears to have some benefit in preservation of potency and potentially urinary continence in patients undergoing wide neurovascular resection at prostatectomy for locally advanced prostate cancer. The use of unilateral nerve grafting, while technically feasible, is controversial, but may potentially have an impact on erectile and urinary function recovery although a recent randomized trial showed no improvement in recovery of erectile function. More recent studies have shown inferior results compared to earlier pilot studies, possibly due to less stringent patient selection as well as possible differences between sural and genitofemoral nerves being used as the donor nerve. Ultimately, randomized trials are necessary to determine the role of nerve grafting. In the future, possible use of adjuncts such as neurotrophic growth factors may augment nerve grafts.

References

1. Walsh, P.C., and Donker, P.J. (1982) Impotence following radical prostatectomy: insight into etiology and prevention. *J. Urol.* **128**, 492.
2. Walsh, P.C., Lepor, H., and Eggleston, J.C. (1983) Radical prostatectomy with preservation of sexual function: anatomical and pathological considerations. *Prostate* **4**, 473.
3. Walsh, P.C., and Schlegel, P.N. (1988) Radical pelvic surgery with preservation of sexual function. *Ann. Surg.* **208**, 391.
4. Rabbani, F., Stapleton, A.M., Kattan, M.W., Wheeler, T.M., and Scardino, P.T. (2000) Factors predicting recovery of erections after radical prostatectomy. *J. Urol.* **164**, 1929.
5. Catalona, W.J., Carvalhal, G.F., Mager, D.E., and Smith, D.S. (1999) Potency, continence and complication rates in 1,870 consecutive radical retropubic prostatectomies. *J. Urol.* **162**, 433.
6. Quinlan, D.M., Epstein, J.I., Carter, B.S., and Walsh, P.C. (1991) Sexual function following radical prostatectomy: influence of preservation of neurovascular bundles. *J. Urol.* **145**, 998.
7. Kim, E.D., Nath, R., Kadmon, D., Lipshultz, L.I., Miles, B.J., Slawin, K.M., et al. (2001) Bilateral nerve graft during radical retropubic prostatectomy: 1-year follow up. *J. Urol.* **165**, 1950.
8. Chang, D.W., Wood, C.G., Kroll, S.S., Youssef, A.A., and Babaian, R.J. (2003) Cavernous nerve reconstruction to preserve erectile function following non-nerve-sparing radical retropubic prostatectomy: a prospective study. *Plast. Reconstr. Surg.* **111**, 1174.
9. Quinlan, D.M., Nelson, R.J., and Walsh, P.C. (1991) Cavernous nerve grafts restore erectile function in denervated rats. *J. Urol.* **145**, 380.

10. Kim, E.D., Scardino, P.T., Hampel, O., Mills, N.L., Wheeler, T.M., and Nath, R.K. (1999) Interposition of sural nerve restores function of cavernous nerves resected during radical prostatectomy. *J. Urol.* **161,** 188.

11. Syme, D.B., Corcoran, N.M., Bouchier-Hayes, D.M., and Costello, A.J. (2006) Hope springs eternal: cavernosal nerve regeneration. *BJU Int.* **97,** 17.

12. Schmidt, C.E., and Leach, J.B. (2003) Neural tissue engineering: strategies for repair and regeneration. *Annu. Rev. Biomed. Eng.* **5,** 293.

13. Abernethy, D.A., Rud, A., and Thomas, P.K. (1992) Neurotropic influence of the distal stump of transected peripheral nerve on axonal regeneration: absence of topographic specificity in adult nerve. *J. Anat.* **180**(Pt 3), 395.

14. Reynolds, M.L., and Woolf, C.J. (1993) Reciprocal Schwann cell-axon interactions. *Curr. Opin. Neurobiol.* **3,** 683.

15. Ide, C. (1996) Peripheral nerve regeneration. *Neurosci. Res.* **25,** 101.

16. Burgers, J.K., Nelson, R.J., Quinlan, D.M., and Walsh, P.C. (1991) Nerve growth factor, nerve grafts and amniotic membrane grafts restore erectile function in rats. *J. Urol.* **146,** 463.

17. Ball, R.A., Lipton, S.A., Dreyer, E.B., Richie, J.P., and Vickers, M.A. (1992) Entubulization repair of severed cavernous nerves in the rat resulting in return of erectile function. *J. Urol.* **148,** 211.

18. May, F., Weidner, N., Matiasek, K., Caspers, C., Mrva, T., Vroemen, M., et al. (2004) Schwann cell seeded guidance tubes restore erectile function after ablation of cavernous nerves in rats. *J. Urol.* **172,** 374.

19. Lowe, J.B., III, Hunter, D.A., Talcott, M.R., and Mackinnon, S.E. (2006) The effects of cavernous nerve grafting following surgically induced loss of erectile function in a large-animal model. *Plast. Reconstr. Surg.* **118,** 69.

20. Crumley, R.L. (1984) Selective reinnervation of vocal cord adductors in unilateral vocal cord paralysis. *Ann. Otol. Rhinol. Laryngol.* **93,** 351.

21. Tio, R.A., Reyners, A.K., van Veldhuisen, D.J., van den Berg, M.P., Brouwer, R.M., Haaksma, J., et al. (1997) Evidence for differential sympathetic and parasympathetic reinnervation after heart transplantation in humans. *J. Auton. Nerv. Syst.* **67,** 176.

22. Stephenson, A.J., Scardino, P.T., Eastham, J.A., Bianco, F.J., Jr., Dotan, Z.A., DiBlasio, C.J., et al. (2005) Postoperative nomogram predicting the 10-year probability of prostate cancer recurrence after radical prostatectomy. *J. Clin. Oncol.* **23,** 7005.

23. Ohori, M., Kattan, M.W., Koh, H., Maru, N., Slawin, K.M., Shariat, S., et al. (2004) Predicting the presence and side of extracapsular extension: a nomogram for staging prostate cancer. *J. Urol.* **171,** 1844.

24. Yu, K.K.K., Hricak, H.H., Alagappan, R.R., Chernoff, D.D.M., Bacchetti, P.P., and Zaloudek, C.C.J. (1997) Detection of extracapsular extension of prostate carcinoma with endorectal and phased-array coil MR imaging: multivariate feature analysis. *Radiology* **202,** 697.

25. Eastham, J.A., and Scardino, P.T. (2006) Radical prostatectomy for clinical stage T1 and T2 prostate cancer. In: Vogelzang, N.J., Scardino, P.T., Shipley, W.U., Debruyne, F.M.J., and Linehan, W.M., eds. *Comprehensive Textbook of Genitourinary Oncology*, 3rd edn. Philadelphia: Lippincott Williams & Wilkins, pp. 166–188.

26. Klotz, L. (2004) Cavernosal nerve mapping: current data and applications. *BJU Int.* **93,** 9.

27. Klotz, L., Heaton, J., Jewett, M., Chin, J., Fleshner, N., Goldenberg, L., et al. (2000) A randomized phase 3 study of intraoperative cavernous nerve stimulation with penile tumescence monitoring to improve nerve sparing during radical prostatectomy. *J. Urol.* **164,** 1573.

28. Muneuchi, G., Kuwata, Y., Taketa, S., Inui, M., Tsukuda, F., Shimada, O., et al. (2005) Cavernous nerve reconstruction during radical prostatectomy by sural nerve grafting: surgical technique in nerve harvesting and grafting. *J. Reconstr. Microsurg.* **21,** 525.

29. Porpiglia, F., Ragni, F., Terrone, C., Renard, J., Musso, F., Grande, S., et al. (2005) Is laparoscopic unilateral sural nerve grafting during radical prostatectomy effective in retaining sexual potency? *BJU Int.* **95,** 1267.

30. Turk, I.A., Deger, S., Morgan, W.R., Davis, J.W., Schellhammer, P.F., and Loening, S.A. (2002) Sural nerve graft during laparoscopic radical prostatectomy. Initial experience. *Urol. Oncol.* **7,** 191.

31. Mikhail, A., Song, D., Orvieto, M., Stockton, B., Gong, E., Billatos, E., et al. (2006) *Sural Nerve Grafting During Robotic Assisted Laparoscopic Radical Prostatectomy (Abstract).* Presented at the American Urologic Association Annual Conference, Atlantal, GA.

32. Uchio, E., Kishinevsky, A., Hwang, J., and Narayan, D. (2006) *Minimally Invasive Sural Nerve Harvest for Cavernous Nerve Reconstruction in Non-Nerve-Sparing Radical Retropubic Prostatectomy.* Presented at the American Urologic Association Annual Conference, Atlanta, GA.

33. Walsh, P.C., Marschke, P., Catalona, W.J., Lepor, H., Martin, S., Myers, R.P., et al. (2001) Efficacy of first-generation Cavermap to verify location and function of cavernous nerves during radical prostatectomy: a multi-institutional evaluation by experienced surgeons. *Urology* **57,** 491.

34. Kim, H.L., Stoffel, D.S., Mhoon, D.A., and Brendler, C.B. (2000) A positive caver map response poorly predicts recovery of potency after radical prostatectomy. *Urology* **56,** 561.

35. Rabbani, F., Cozzi, P., and Scardino, P. (2002) Quantitative assessment of the response to CaverMap nerve stimulation at radical prostatectomy [Abstract]. *J. Urol.* **167,** 356.

36. Takenaka, A., Murakami, G., Soga, H., Han, S.H., Arai, Y., and Fujisawa, M. (2004) Anatomical analysis of the neurovascular bundle supplying penile cavernous tissue to ensure a reliable nerve graft after radical prostatectomy. *J. Urol.* **172,** 1032.

37. Scardino, P.T., and Kim, E.D. (2001) Rationale for and results of nerve grafting during radical prostatectomy. *Urology* **57,** 1016.

38. Singh, H., Karakiewicz, P., Shariat, S.F., Canto, E.I., Nath, R.K., Kattan, M.W., et al. (2004) Impact of unilateral interposition sural nerve grafting on recovery of urinary function after radical prostatectomy. *Urology* **63,** 1122.

39. Rosen, R.C., Riley, A., Wagner, G., Osterloh, I.H., Kirkpatrick, J., and Mishra, A. (1997) The international index of erectile function (IIEF): a multidimensional scale for assessment of erectile dysfunction. *Urology* **49,** 822.

40. Kim, E.D., Nath, R., Slawin, K.M., Kadmon, D., Miles, B.J., and Scardino, P.T. (2001) Bilateral nerve grafting during radical retropubic prostatectomy: extended follow-up. *Urology* **58,** 983.

41. Secin, F., Koppie, T., Patel, M., Kuroiwa, K., Bianco, F., Eastham, J., et al. (2006) Determinants of success of bilateral cavernous nerve interposition grafting during radical retropubic prostatectomy (abstract). Presented at the American Urologic Association Annual Meeting, Atlanta, GA.

42. Patel, M., Rabbani, F., Disa, J., McKiernan, J., Cozzi, P., and Scardino, P. (2004) Recovery of potency after cavernous nerve graft reconstruction at radical prostatectomy: The MSKCC Experience [Abstract]. *J. Urol.* **171,** 213.

43. Canto, E.I., Nath, R.K., and Slawin, K.M. (2001) Cavermap-assisted sural nerve interposition graft during radical prostatectomy. *Urol. Clin. North Am.* **28,** 839.

44. Wood, C.G., Chang, D., Wang, R., Shen, Y., Pettaway, C.A., Pisters, L.L., et al. (2007) A randomized phase II trial evaluating the importance of early erectile dysfunction rehabilitation and unilateral autologous sural nerve grafting in patients undergoing a unilateral cavernous nerve sparing radical prostatectomy for clinically localized PR [Abstract]. *J. Urol.* **177,** 461.

45. Pham, D.Q., Wood, C.G., Wen, S., Sotelo, T., Shen, Y., Babaian, R.J., et al. (2007) Penile rehabilitation after unilateral nerve sparing radical prostatectomy with or without sural nerve grafting: results of a prospective randomized trial [Abstract]. *J. Urol.* **177,** 311.

46. Saito, S., Namiki, S., Numahata, K., Satoh, M., Ishidoya, S., Ito, A., et al. (2007) Impact of unilateral interposition sural nerve graft on the recovery of sexual function after radical prostatectomy in Japanese men: a preliminary study. *Int. J. Urol.* **14,** 133.

Chapter 10
Erectile Function Preservation and Rehabilitation

Alexander Müller and John P. Mulhall

Abstract Despite modified surgical techniques including nerve-sparing procedures radical prostatectomy (RP) is a significant source of long-term erectile function impairment which can be caused by cavernous nerve trauma, insufficient arterial inflow, hypoxia-related and neuropraxia-associated damage to erectile tissue resulting in veno-occlusive dysfunction. An increasing understanding of the pathophysiological mechanisms leading to post-RP erectile dysfunction (ED) has provided concepts for prophylaxis and rehabilitation of erectile function. Penile rehabilitation is the term given to the concept that we can use medications to prevent the structural damage that erectile tissue undergoes after radical pelvic surgery, while nerve recovery occurs. Rehabilitation revolves around two strategies, regular phosphodiesterase type 5 inhibitor (PDE5i) use and early postoperative erectile regeneration. The reason and the logical background to use the PDE5i drug category as prophylaxis for erectile function preservation after RP are not fully understood yet. Supported by experimental and clinical data the postulate is that PDE5i might have a positive effect on endothelial protection, neurogenesis, and cavernosal smooth muscle pro-

From: *Current Clinical Urology* Series, *Sexual Function in the Prostate Cancer Patient*
Edited by John P. Mulhall, DOI 10.1007/978-1-60327-555-2_10,
© Humana Press, a part of Springer Science+Business Media, LLC 2009

tection involving neuronal and endothelial regeneration, lowering apoptosis, and recovery of nocturnal erections thus inducing cavernosal oxygenation in an effort to protect the erectile tissue. The current literature also sustains data that an early postoperative erection may optimize the functional rehabilitation by improving cavernosal oxygenation and preventing hypoxia-induced corporal fibrosis. Besides the oral use of PDE5i alternatives are available including transurethral suppositories, vacuum erection devices, and intracavernosal injections complementing the rehabilitation strategies. Based on the current evidence from human and animal studies there is a strong signal for a positive effect of a prophylactic penile rehabilitation after RP which may translate into greater preservation of erectile function. However, a formal analysis of what the optimal rehabilitation program represents, remains unsettled to date. Large prospective multi-center, randomized, placebo-controlled studies in the future will hopefully be able to answer question about an optimal dosing, a time frame for the application, duration and form of the use, and maybe differences between the different medications. Further, supportive managements including cavernous nerve reconstruction and neuroprotection stratagems are under investigation finding their place of value in the future. Comprehensively, for a sufficient erectile rehabilitation after RP it needs a well-informed patient who is highly motivated to follow a medical regimen and is willing to pay for it to maintain sexual quality of life after a potential curative cancer treatment.

Keywords Penile rehabilitation; cavernosal oxygenation; phosphodiesterase type 5 inhibitor; post-radical prostatectomy erectile dysfunction; endothelial protection; neurogenesis; cavernosal smooth muscle protection.

1   Introduction

Prostate cancer is the leading cancer in men older than 50 years of age. Curative treatment options include a surgical approach in form of a radical prostatectomy (RP) or radiation. With regards to PSA-free survival and long-term survival overall, radical prostatectomy (RP) appears to be the "gold standard" for prostate cancer therapy *(1)*. Of all men presenting with erectile dysfunction (ED) it is estimated that 10% suffer this condition as a result of pelvic surgery *(2)*. Despite modified surgical techniques for RP and the advent of nerve-sparing procedures a significant percentage of men continue to suffer from ED following RP. According to the literature a major discrepancy exists regarding postoperative potency rates citing the occurrence of spontaneous erectile function rates between approximately 20 and 90% *(3)*. RP is a significant source of long-term incontinence and erectile function impairment.

2 Pathophysiology of Erectile Dysfunction After Radical Prostatectomy

Generally, post-RP ED can be caused by cavernous nerve trauma, insufficient arterial inflow, hypoxia-related and neuropraxia-associated damage to erectile tissue resulting in veno-occlusive dysfunction. Finally, a small group of men have long-term ED that is predominantly psychogenic in nature.

2.1 Neural Trauma

A major factor for the development of postoperative ED is neural insufficiency due to surgical manipulation during the operation (4). The time interval for erectile function (EF) recovery is individual and depends on the severity of the intraoperative trauma to the neurovascular bundle (5). Due to the hypothesis that the neural trauma is generally not complete and irreparable, improvement of erectile function may be expected up to 24 months after surgery (6). Mild trauma by handling the nerve fibers may lead to a neuropraxia, which may recover within months. However, more severe damage will not heal at all or may need much longer time to regenerate. Even neuropraxia may result in structural changes in the corporal bodies influencing the potential revitalization of the erectile tissue (7–9). In a rat cavernous nerve trauma model, even nerve exposure alone without any direct manipulation has been shown to result in a significant reduction in intracavernous pressure generation in response to cavernous nerve stimulation (10). This suggests that there are mechanisms other than direct handling or stretching of the nerves that play a role in ED development, perhaps reactive oxygen species, inflammatory mediators, and/or peri-neural scarring. Supported by strong data from the literature the greater the volume of nerve tissue preserved the better the spontaneous EF recovery and the better the response to oral pharmacotherapy (11–13). An important factor is the patient's age. Men younger than 60 years of age appear to have a faster recovery of the neuromuscular function because of their better biological neuroplasticity (14–16).

Neural injury in the penis has been shown to result in three distinct penis-threatening events: (i) smooth muscle and endothelial apoptosis, (ii) an increase in the production of fibrogenic cytokines especially TGF-β, and (iii) collagen deposition. In pioneer work, Klein et al. were able to document a significant increase in inter-nucleosomal DNA fragmentation as a marker for apoptosis in the denervated penile erectile tissue of the rat after bilateral CN neurotomy compared to sham animals (17). The finding of increased penile smooth muscle apoptosis induced by neural CN injury was confirmed by several other working groups. Using a bilateral CN crush injury model in rats, Mulhall and Mueller et al. documented a more than sixfold reduction in smooth muscle–collagen ratio and a significant increase in apoptosis (10% in sham vs. 63% in nerve crush, $p < 0.001$) within the corporal tissue at 28 days after CN injury (18).

In a similar animal model User et al. showed that a bilateral CN neurotomy induced significant apoptosis, while unilateral surgery caused significantly less apoptosis *(7)*. The apoptosis occurred mostly in smooth muscle cells and showed an apoptotic clustering just beneath the tunica albuginea. The authors concluded from their findings that the sub-tunical location of apoptotic smooth muscle cells was a mechanism for veno-occlusive dysfunction observed after radical prostate-ctomy. At 45 days in rats after bilateral CN resection, Ferrini et al. demonstrated veno-occlusive dysfunction measured by the drop rate during dynamic infusion cav-ernosometry as well as a 60% reduction in the smooth muscle–collagen ratio, and a threefold increase in intracorporeal apoptosis compared to sham animals *(19)*. Furthermore neural damage by bilateral CN incision 3 months later resulted in hypoxia and fibrosis in rat corpora cavernosal *(8)*. Leungwattanakij et al. demon-strated in the neurotomy group compared to sham animals an increase in transform-ing growth factor-β_1, hypoxia-inducible factor-1alpha, and collagen III synthesis using Western blot analysis and immunohistochemical staining in rat caver-nosal smooth musculature concluding that cavernous fibrosis may be reduced by vasoactive drugs or strategies to augment corporal oxygenation during the postoperative period.

2.2 Arteriogenic ED

The primary rationale for post-RP arteriogenic ED lies in injury to accessory puden-dal arteries *(20)*. The term "accessory pudendal artery" refers to any artery that arises from a source above the levator ani and travels toward the penis infrapubi-cally. The supradiaphragmatic location of APAs puts them at risk of injury during extirpation of the prostate. They typically originate from the obturator, vesical, and femoral arteries, among others. Those originating from extrapelvic arteries, like the femoral arteries, have been described in cadaveric dissection studies. Intrapelvic APAs are identified in the periprostatic region running parallel to the dorsal vascu-lar complex and extending caudally toward the pubic symphysis (Fig. 1 and Color Plate 5, following p. 264). The arteries traveling with the cavernous nerves and corona mortis (an anatomic variant—if present, it is an anastomotic branch between the inferior epigastric or external iliac artery and the obturator artery) *(21,22)*, and the artery/ies running the depth of the dorsal vascular complex (retrograde branch of the pudendal artery that irrigates the anterior surface of the prostate and bladder neck) *(23)* are not considered APAs.

A review of the relevant literature suggests that the prevalence of these APAs varies from 4 to 75%, depending on how the arteries were identified at the time of open or laparoscopic prostatectomy; angiographically during internal pudendal or internal iliac artery flush; or during cadaveric dissection *(24–33)* (Table 1).

Gray et al. performed angiographies of the iliopudendal vascular tree for the evaluation of impotence in 73 patients *(28)*. Accessory arteries were present unilat-erally in 14% and bilaterally in 7% of the patients. Rosen et al. performed selective

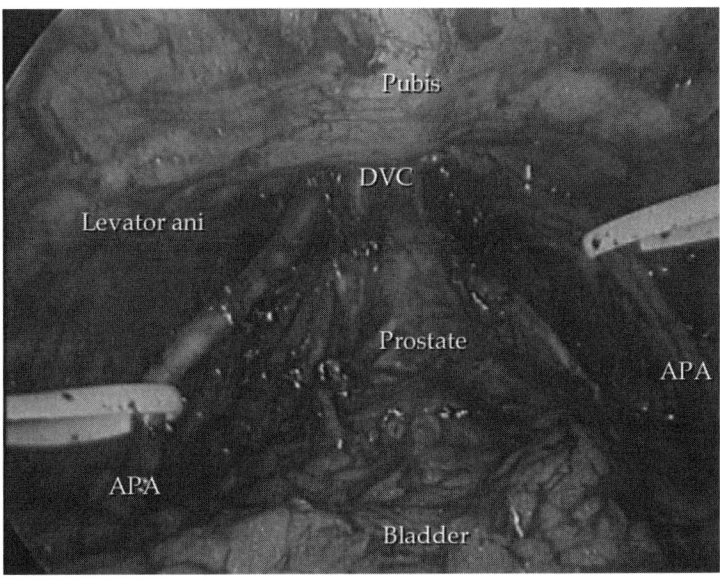

Fig. 1 Intra-operative photograph taken during laparoscopic radical prostatectomy demonstrating bilateral accessory pudendal arteries (*See* Color Plate 5, following p. 264)

Table 1 Accessory Pudendal Arteries (APAs)

Author	Year	No. of patients	Incidence of APA (%)	APA preserved (%)	Type of study
Matin *(26)*	2006	70	26	78	Laparoscopic radical prostatectomy
Secin *(25)*	2005	325	30	83	Laparoscopic radical prostatectomy
Rogers *(33)*	2004	2,399	4	100	Radical retropubic prostatectomy
Polascik *(32)*	1995	835	4	79	Radical retropubic prostatectomy
Droupy *(29)*	1999	12	75	NR	Transrectal color Doppler ultrasound
Rosen *(27)*	1990	195	7	NR	Angiography
Gray *(28)*	1982	73	21	NR	Angiography
Benoit *(30)*	1999	85	70	NR	Cadaveric dissection
Breza *(31)*	1989	10	70	NR	Cadaver dissection

NR: not reported.

bilateral internal pudendal angiography in 195 men who were suspected of having arteriogenic impotence *(27)*. The researchers found substantial variation in the origin of the internal pudendal artery, with APAs recognized in 7% of the patients. In all cases, APAs provided the main blood supply to the penile artery.

Cadaveric dissections have rendered much higher APA identification rates. Breza et al. dissected the pelvic vasculature in ten cadavers and found APAs present in seven of them *(31)*. In four of the cases, the APAs were found to be a major source of arterial inflow to the corpora cavernosa, and in one of the subjects the APA was the sole source of erectile arterial inflow.

Similarly, Benoit et al. reported a 70% incidence of intrapelvic APAs based on cadaveric dissections *(30)*. They identified 33 APAs in 20 cadavers, including at least 1 APA in 17 of the 20 (not all of them intrapelvic). In eight cadavers, only one accessory pudendal artery was present, but in nine of the cadavers APAs were present bilaterally (two arteries in five, three in one, and four in three cases). The APAs originated from the inferior vesical artery in 46% of cases, from the obturator in 36%, and from the external pudendal artery in 18%. In 15% of cases the penile arterial inflow originated exclusively from APAs.

Intrapelvic APAs have been identified in 26–30% of patients undergoing LRP, and 4% of patients undergoing open retropubic radical prostatectomy *(25,26,32)*. Of the 30% of patients undergoing LRP who had APAs, it is possible to preserve 83% of the arteries, with 89% preservation rate for lateral APAs and 79% for apical arteries. The side-specific incidence of positive surgical margins was 3% when APAs were preserved and 6% when not preserved ($p = 0.5$) *(25)*. Droupy et al. performed preoperative transrectal color Doppler ultrasound on 12 patients with normal erectile function who were undergoing radical pelvic surgery to assess APA presence and function *(27)*. APAs were identified in 75% of the patients. Pharmacologically induced erections performed concurrently demonstrated that the hemodynamic changes in the APAs were similar to those described in the cavernous arteries, supporting the concept that APAs play a functional role in penile erection. However, those authors were unable to make decisive functional conclusions because they could not preserve any of the nine APAs during the open RP ($n = 10$) or radical cystoprostatectomy ($n = 2$). They stated that "it was impossible to over-sew effectively the distal part of the dorsal venous complex without damaging the accessory pudendal artery."

It is likely that the magnification permitted by the laparoscope has contributed to the difference in APA identification rates between open and laparoscopic surgery. It is also probable that angiography defines APAs that are not readily visible to the naked eye or laparoscope. And without the need for hemostasis, cadaveric dissection is not hampered by the usual concerns that affect intraoperative visualization.

Between 1987 and 1994, the research group at Johns Hopkins found APAs in only 4% of 835 patients undergoing RP *(32)*. After development of the surgical technique, preservation of APAs was possible in 19 of 24 patients (79%). On assessment of EF, there was little difference between those who had APAs preserved (67%, $n = 12$) and those who did not (50%, $n = 10$). At the time, the authors concluded that APA presence was rare; that although preservation was possible in the majority of patients, it was associated with excessive dorsal vein complex bleeding; and that because no significant difference in erectile function was seen with preservation, routine APA preservation may not be productive. Nine years later, the same group compared EF outcomes between patients who underwent nerve-sparing RP without APA preservation and those who underwent nerve-sparing surgery with simultaneous preservation of APAs *(33)*. They cited a trend toward a statistically significant difference in EF recovery in those who had APA preservation (93%) compared with those who did not (70%). In a control group of patients without APAs, EF recovery was seen in 81%.

The accumulating evidence supports the concept that APA preservation plays a role in EF recovery post-RP. The difficulty lies in deciding which arteries should be preserved and which can be sacrificed. Thus, defining that the role of APAs in EF recovery will require an intraoperative analysis of the functional role of these vessels (we are using intraoperative penile Doppler before and after APA clamping to evaluate their contribution to penile irrigation), which is currently ongoing in our institution. Mulhall et al. *(19)* in a study that included preoperative and serial postoperative erectile hemodynamic assessment demonstrated that 60% of postoperative impotent men with normal preoperative erectile vascular status demonstrated postoperative bilateral arterial insufficiency, and 40% had venous leak *(34)*. Further, they showed that these vascular abnormalities did not improve over the 24 months after surgery. In a later analysis using vascular testing of men presenting after bilateral nerve-sparing RP, 96 men with a mean age of 54 years were studied *(35)*. Patients were divided into four groups according to the timing of their postoperative vascular studies (<4, 4–8, 9–12, >12 months). Normal vascular status was diagnosed in 35% of the study participants; arterial insufficiency was present in 59%, and venous leak in 26%. No difference in incidence of arterial insufficiency was noted between the four groups. However, there was a significant association between postoperative time and the incidence of venous leak: 14% experienced venous leak less than 4 months after surgery, and 35% after the eighth postoperative month. The correlation between vascular diagnosis and return of functional erections was even more pronounced: 47% of the patients with normal hemodynamics were capable of having sexual intercourse postoperatively without the assistance of an erectogenic medication, versus 31% of those with arterial insufficiency and only 9% of patients with venous leak.

Montorsi et al. in a randomized, controlled study assessing the utility of early postoperative intracavernosal injections demonstrated that 33% of those in the treatment arm and 80% of those in the control arm failed to recover erectile function at 6 months post-RP *(36)*. The majority of failures had venous leak on duplex Doppler ultrasound. More recently, a study (also using duplex Doppler ultrasound) of 111 men with postoperative EF found that 71% had abnormal erectile hemodynamics and 15% of the total had venous leak *(37)*. At 18 months post-RP there were significant differences between those with normal and those with abnormal hemodynamics in relation to self-reported erectile rigidity and International Index of Erectile Function (IIEF) EF domain scores. The study also demonstrated that there was a strong correlation not only between peak systolic velocity and EF domain score ($r = 0.48$, $p = 0.018$) but also between end diastolic velocity and EF domain score ($r = 0.36$, $p = 0.025$).

Thus, given the accumulating evidence in favor of arterial insufficiency as a contributor to ED in patients after RP, renewed attention has been focused on accessory pudendal arteries.

2.3 The Concept of Cavernosal Oxygenation

During erection increasing arterial inflow of oxygen rich blood leads to an increase of penis pressure and volume. This expansion of the erectile tissue leads finally to an occlusion of the subtunical venules resulting in a firm erection *(38)*. During the cavernous blood pooling there is a shift from venous pO_2 (25–40 mmHg) in the flaccid state to arterial pO_2 (70–100 mmHg) under full erection *(39)*. Inducing a receptor-mediated cascade prostaglandin E_1 (PGE_1) leads to smooth muscle relaxation via the second messenger cyclic adenosine-monophosphate (cAMP). Both pathways seem to be modulated by oxygen saturation of the corpora cavernosa. This has led to the hypothesis that nocturnal tumescence is protective for erectile function preservation. Experimental (in vitro) data have shown that a one time activation of the PGE_1 cascade mediated by cAMP was able to suppress the induction of collagen synthesis by repressing transforming growth factor-beta 1 (TGF-β_1) activity sufficiently *(40)*. The development of corporal fibrosis may be dependent on intracavernosal pO_2 levels. Hypoxic conditions led to increased TGF-β_1 production, which is presumed to result in collagenization of the corporal smooth muscle *(41–43)*. These data are supported by the finding of an increase in hypoxia inducible factor-1 (HIF-1α) and TGF-β_1 as well as increase in cavernous tissue collagen synthesis after cavernous nerve injury in a rat model *(8)*.

2.4 Corporo-venoocclusive Dysfunction

Appropriate corporal smooth muscle expandability guarantees a functional veno-occlusive mechanism with a sufficient occlusion of the subtunical venules against the tunica albuginea *(44)*. Malfunction of the smooth muscle due to structural alterations of the erectile tissue results in veno-occlusive dysfunction or venous leak. Structural changes are likely based upon corporal smooth muscle collagenization and fibrosis which seem most likely due to either apoptosis associated with neural injury, and/or disuse atrophy of the erectile tissue possibly related to the absence of cavernosal oxygenation *(7)*. The occurrence of venous leak development post-RP appears to be time-dependent. The incidence of venous leak after RP in patients with good preoperative erectile function who did not receive any post-operative pharmacotherapy was 14% < 4 months and 35% between 9 and 12 months postoperatively *(35)*. More recent data indicate that the post-RP penile vascular status is predictive of return of spontaneous erections, degree of erectile rigidity, and response to sildenafil whereby in the presence of abnormal end diastolic velocity values the prognosis seems poor for the return of functional erections *(37)*. A sufficient veno-occlusive apparatus is a major determinant of successful use of vasoactive therapeutics.

2.5 *Psychogenic Mechanisms*

Among all other potential reasons for post-RP ED psychogenic mechanisms have received little attention *(45,46)*. However, there is a subpopulation of patients post-RP who suffer long-term erectile function changes after 24 months that are related to the erosion of confidence a man experiences over the course of 12–24 months of ED. This is likely one of the reasons for the continued improvement seen in erectile function between 24 and 48 months after surgery. The classic scenario is a man 24 months after RP who complains of no erection in the bedroom during attempted relations, however, he experiences excellent nocturnal erections. The discrepancy between the two erections is adrenaline-mediated and this has the potential to improve with time and confidence restoration.

3 Penile Rehabilitation of the Erectile Function After Radical Prostatectomy

An increasing understanding of pathophysiological mechanisms leading to post-RP ED despite nerve-sparing surgery has provided concepts for prophylaxis and rehabilitation of erectile function *(47)*. The concept of corporal damage caused by a lack of oxygenation to the erectile tissue has motivated the introduction of medical support to improve an early post-RP blood supply to the penis. Penile rehabilitation is the term given to the concept that we can use medications to prevent the structural damage that erectile tissue undergoes after radical pelvic surgery, while nerve recovery occurs. Rehabilitation revolves around two strategies, regular PDE5 inhibitor use and early postoperative erection generation (with oral, transurethral, or intracavernosal agents).

3.1 *Data Supporting the Concept of PDE5 Inhibitor Rehabilitation*

The introduction of phosphodiesterase type 5 (PDE5) inhibitors has revolutionized the management of ED in general. The efficacy of PDE5 inhibitors for the treatment of post-RP ED has recently been studied. At present three PDE5 inhibitors are in clinical use worldwide including sildenafil (Viagra^{TM}), vardenafil (Levitra^{TM}), and tadalafil (Cialis^{TM}). The reason and the logical background to use this drug category as prophylaxis for erectile function preservation after RP are not fully understood yet. The postulate is that PDE5 inhibitors might improve neuronal and endothelial regeneration, lower apoptosis, and recover nocturnal erections and thus induce cavernosal oxygenation in an effort to protect the erectile tissue.

For an effective use of the PDE5 inhibitors, neuronal and endothelial nitric oxide (NO) release is necessary which makes the presence and preservation of cavernous nerve fibers essential. However, it is not clear whether such nerve function is required for the myoprotection that PDE5i appear to accomplish. Thus, only patients who have undergone a nerve-sparing procedure are expected to respond to these agents with a functional erection at least early after surgery. Sexual stimulation leads to NO release from intracorporeal cavernous nerve terminals and from the endothelium. NO diffuses into the smooth muscle cells and activates the enzyme guanylate cyclase, which catalyzes the reaction from guanosine triphosphate to cyclic guanosine monophosphate (cGMP). cGMP as a second messenger activates specific protein kinases leading after further intracellular cascades to a reduction of intracellular calcium which finally results in smooth muscle cell relaxation. cGMP is under the influence of the enzyme phosphodiesterase type 5 which usually degrades cGMP.

3.2   Endothelial Protection

One of the first indications that PDE5 inhibition may have a positive impact on endothelial function is the fact that the incidence of myocardial infarction was lower in sildenafil arms of the phase II–IV trials compared to the placebo arms (0.56/100 patient-years vs. 0.84/100 patient-years). Desouza et al. in 2002 published data that unequivocally demonstrated the positive effect of sildenafil on endothelial function *(48)*. In 14 patients with ED and type 2 diabetes, the acute and chronic effect of sildenafil on flow-mediated dilation (FMD) was investigated. All patients received both sildenafil and placebo in a staggered fashion. Baseline FMD was measured and then 1 h after administration of placebo or 25 mg of sildenafil, FMD was re-measured and significant improvement in brachial artery diameter was seen in the sildenafil arm (15% vs. 8%; pre-treatment was 8%). In the chronic phase of the study, patients received 14 nights of sildenafil 25 mg or placebo (all patients received both agents at different times) and 24 h after the last dose had FMD measured again. Once again sildenafil resulted in significant changes in FMD (14% vs. 9%; pre-treatment was 8%). Thus, sildenafil appears to have a significant effect on endothelium even at a time point beyond its duration of action (half-life of 4 h; present in serum for 4–5 half-lives). This has been confirmed at the basic level by our laboratory and others by demonstration that sildenafil administration results in the activation of the PI3/AKT/eNOS pathway, a key regulator of endothelial function *(49)*. More recently, Rosano et al. evaluated 32 men with increased cardiovascular risk (men with ED with more than 2 risk factors for coronary artery disease causing a 10-year CV risk >20%) using FMD who were randomized to either tadalafil 20 mg every other day or placebo *(50)*. At 4 weeks tadalafil significantly improved FMD from 4 to 9% (change between pre- and post-occlusion brachial artery diameters). The improvements with tadalafil were sustained at 6 weeks, i.e., 2 weeks after cessation of the medication. These data mirror the sildenafil in that significant improvements were seen in endothelial function (approximately a doubling of degree of vasodilatation) even beyond the survival of the drug within the body. These findings suggest that the impact of PDE5 inhibitors on endothelium at the cellular level may be self-sustaining long after the drug has been metabolized.

The RhoA/Rho-kinase pathway plays a supportive role in the modulation of the contractile smooth muscle tone in the flaccid penis and it seems that this pathway might represent a promising alternative therapeutic target for ED treatment. The RhoA/Rho-kinase pathway supports the noradrenergic dominance of smooth muscle contraction in the flaccid state of the penis through phosphorylated inhibition of the myosin phosphatase leading to increased sensitization of myofilaments to basal cytoplasmic Ca ion concentration *(51)*. In vivo Rho-kinase inhibition stimulates rat penile erection independently of NO and causes relaxation in vitro *(52)*. Molecular studies in human corpora cavernosa have documented a high expression of RhoA contributing to the RhoA-mediated Ca sensitization in the flaccid state of the penis *(53)*. Mulhall and Muller et al. documented in a bilateral CN crush injury model in rats an endothelial protective effect in the tissue of the corpora cavernosa with daily use of sildenafil. Using immunohistochemical staining for endothelial factors including the antibodies for CD31 and eNOS both staining levels were significantly reduced by CN injury compared to sham animals ($p < 0.05$). Thus, daily sildenafil treatment resulted in a restoration of CD31 and eNOS staining levels to that of sham animals (no statistical differences between sham and both treatment groups). Furthermore, these findings have been supported by the immunoblotting results documenting a significant increase in activated (phosphorylated) AKT and eNOS compared to non-phosphorylated forms in both sildenafil treatment groups. These results have been supported by prior observation of Musicki et al. reporting on an extended erectile response after cavernous nerve stimulation with a prolonged detumescence time and an increased expression of phosphorylated eNOS and Akt in aged rats (19-month-old) after long-term administration of sildenafil for 3 weeks *(54)*. They concluded that patients with impaired erectile function may benefit from a long-term use of sildenafil by enhancing Akt-dependent eNOS phosphorylation.

The second potential mechanism is the concept that PDE5 inhibitors promote the generation of endothelial progenitor cells (EPCs) from the bone marrow. Circulating EPCs originate from hematopoietic stem cells in bone marrow, migrate into peripheral circulation, and differentiate into mature endothelial cells, thus providing a circulating pool of cells that may contribute to ongoing endothelia repair. It has been demonstrated that the injured endothelial monolayer is regenerated by circulating bone marrow-derived EPCs *(55)*. Patients affected with erectile dysfunction with or without cardiovascular risk factors have a decreased number of circulating EPCs *(56)*. An essential role for the functional activity of hematopoietic stem cells and progenitor cells has been shown for endothelial nitric oxide synthase (eNOS) in mice, which produces NO *(57)*. It has been demonstrated that NO may induce an increase in the number of circulation EPCs, and that a lack of eNOS induces defective hematopoietic recovery and progenitor mobilization *(58)*. Foresta et al. showed an increase in circulating EPCs after treatment with vardenafil as well as after tadalafil treatment *(59,60)*. They observed a significant increase in endothelial function, related to flow-mediated dilatation, and circulating progenitor cells after 3-month treatment with tadalafil, postulating that the improvement in the number of progenitor cells results in effective vasculoprotection preventing the initiation and progression of endothelial dysfunction.

3.3 PDE5 Inhibitor-Induced Neurogenesis

In a study conducted in a rat model of stroke (middle cerebral artery occlusion), the administration of sildenafil to rats resulted in up-regulation of neural progenitor cells in the brain and led to an improvement in functional recovery at 21 days after induction of stroke. Thus there may be pathways outside of erection induction and cavernosal oxygenation by which such a regimen may affect amelioration of long-term erectile function *(61)*. Also tadalafil, administered orally every 48 h for 6 consecutive days commencing 24 h after embolic middle cerebral artery occlusion in a rat model, resulted in significantly improved neurological functional recovery compared with control rats treated with saline *(62)*. The improved functional recovery after ischemic stroke with tadalafil was associated with increases in brain cGMP levels and enhancement of angiogenesis and neurogenesis.

4 Cavernosal Smooth Muscle Protection

In a rat animal study carried out by Mulhall and Muller, the daily use of sildenafil subcutaneously (sc) demonstrated a restoration of functional and structural changes after bilateral cavernous nerve crush injury *(18)*. In both treatment groups using 10 and 20 mg/kg sildenafil sc an improvement in erectile function reported as maximal intracavernosal pressure–mean arterial blood pressure ratio during electrical cavernous nerve stimulation was observable compared to the control group which had untreated bilateral CN crush injury. The functional and structural protection appeared in a dose- and time-dependent manner with maximization of erectile function recovery occurring with daily 20 mg/kg at the 28-day time-point. The pharmacological effect on erectile function recovery appeared to be mediated by preserving smooth muscle content, endothelial integrity, and reducing apoptosis. Looking at penile mid-shaft cross-sections using Masson's trichrome staining the control animals showed 28 days after bilateral CN crush injury a more than 6 times decrease of smooth muscle–collagen ratio compared to sham animals ($p < 0.05$). The daily administration of 20 mg/kg sildenafil citrate sc resulted in a significant preservation of smooth muscle content which was nearly three times higher than for the control group ($p < 0.05$). Additionally at 28 days both sildenafil dosing regimens demonstrated a highly significant reduction in apoptosis of the corporal body tissue compared to the control group ($p < 0.001$). This was the first animal evidence supporting the findings of the human nightly post-RP sildenafil study carried out by

Padma-Nathan et al., which demonstrated a signal that regular sildenafil use after radical prostatectomy was of some benefit in the preservation of erectile function *(63)*. It has now been shown that all three PDE5 inhibitors sildenafil, vardenafil, and tadalafil are able to protect erectile smooth muscle content and reduce apoptosis after CN damage in the animal model. Assessing functional and structural data 45 days after bilateral CN resection in the rat daily administration of 30 mg/L vardenafil in the drinking water showed a normalization of the dynamic infusion cavernosometry drop rate and penile smooth muscle–collagen ratio *(19)*. Animals with bilateral CN resection demonstrated a 60% reduction in the smooth muscle–collagen ratio and a threefold increase in intracorporeal apoptosis compared with the sham group. Congruent with sildenafil findings in the CN injury model the authors concluded that long-term treatment with vardenafil may prevent corporal veno-occlusive dysfunction after radical prostatectomy by preserving smooth muscle content and inhibiting corporal fibrosis possibly by its effect on inducible nitric oxide synthase (iNOS) which was increased by vardenafil.

Also daily retrolingually administration of tadalafil 5 mg/kg for 45 days after CN damage resulted in prevention of corporal veno-occlusive dysfunction and the underlying corporal fibrosis in the rat through a cGMP-related mechanism that appeared to be independent of inducible nitric oxide synthase induction *(64)*. Using immunohistochemistry, histochemistry, and Western blotting daily tadalafil treatment prevented corporal collagenization, preserved the smooth muscle cell content, and decreased the apoptotic index in the rat penile tissue after unilateral or bilateral CN resection. There were no effects of tadalafil on increased transforming growth factor beta1 or inducible nitric oxide synthase.

Furthermore Mulhall and Muller et al. showed in their CN crush injury study that immunohistochemistry staining for endothelial parameter expression (CD31 and eNOS) was significantly preserved within the cavernosal tissue for sildenafil compared to control ($p < 0.05$) supporting the hypothesis of endothelial protection by sildenafil *(18)*. It appears that the endothelial protection afforded by sildenafil is mediated, at least in part, by phosphorylation of AKT and eNOS. The clinical implications of these data are obvious.

Muller et al. using the identical cavernous nerve crush injury model in rats showed with PDE5 inhibitor pre-treatment administering 20 mg/kg sildenafil daily starting 3 days prior to bilateral CN injury the highest erectile function recovery after 28 days which was significant improved compared to commencing sildenafil at the same day or 3 days after nerve injury *(65)*. These data are consistent with the experiments demonstrating the pharmacological preconditioning effect of sildenafil against ischemia/reperfusion injury in the heart when administering the drug prior to the injury *(66)*. The mechanism of action of sildenafil is through phosphodiesterase type 5 (PDE5) inhibition resulting in the accumulation of intracellular cyclic GMP. While the effects on vascular smooth muscle relaxation are well-appreciated, other effects on apoptosis and endothelial integrity are less well-appreciated. Based on several recent basic and clinical studies it emerges that clinically approved phosphodiesterase type 5 inhibitors may be developed for several conditions besides the treatment of ED, especially for cardiovascular indications including endothelial dysfunction, ischemia/reperfusion injury, myocardial infarction, ventricular remodeling, and heart failure *(67)*. Phosphodiesterase-5 (PDE5) inhibitors including sildenafil and vardenafil induce powerful preconditioning-like cardioprotective effect against ischemia/reperfusion injury through opening of mitochondrial K(ATP) channels in the heart. Recently, Salloum et al. demonstrated that both sildenafil and vardenafil reduced the area of cardiac necrosis in a rabbit model of cardiac ischaemia–reperfusion *(68,69)*. After an ischemia induction by 30 min of coronary artery occlusion followed by 3 h of reperfusion infarct size was reduced in sildenafil as well as vardenafil intravenously treated groups as compared to control. Both sildenafil and vardenafil protected the ischemic myocardium against reperfusion injury through a mechanism dependent on mitochondrial K(ATP) channel opening. In a prior study Das et al. using mouse cardiac myocyte cells exposed to hypoxia and re-oxygenation showed that sildenafil treated cells demonstrated less necrosis and apoptosis than control cells *(70)*. The authors also showed increased expression of eNOS in the sildenafil treated groups, along with an increase in the ratio of the anti-apoptotic protein Bcl-2 compared to the pro-apoptotic protein Bax.

In a study carried out by Schwartz et al. of men with bilateral nerve-sparing RP, randomized to 50 mg or 100 mg sildenafil every other night for 6 months beginning the day of catheter removal the content of smooth muscle within the corpora cavernosa was determined by biopsy before and 6 months after RP *(71)*. With 50 mg sildenafil a preservation of smooth muscle content was observed and with 100 mg a significant increase in intracorporeal smooth muscle content was documented ($p < 0.05$). Despite the limitations of this study including low power with 11 and 10 patients, respectively, in each group and a lower smooth muscle content at base line in the 100 mg group maintaining important pro-erectile ultrastructure seems to be essential for rehabilitating post-RP erectile function *(71)*. It is now established that after radical prostatectomy erectile tissue undergoes progressive fibrosis. In a study by Iacono et al. 19 patients of 57–69 years of age with reported preoperative normal erectile function underwent corpora cavernosal biopsy before radical prostatectomy for prostate cancer, 2 and 12 months after surgery *(72)*. Using immunostaining and computerized morphometric imaging, trabecular elastic fibers ($p < 0.0003$) and smooth muscle fibers were decreased and collagen content was significantly increased ($p < 0.0003$) compared with preoperative biopsies. One year after surgery elastic fibers ($p < 0.0003$) and smooth muscle fibers were decreased and collagen content was significantly increased ($p < 0.0003$) compared with the first postoperative biopsy. Moreover, organized collagen and trabecular protocollagen deposits were increased.

In another clinical study, in 95% of patients undergoing nerve-sparing RP, it was possible to demonstrate a spontaneous nocturnal erectile activity in the night after catheter removal after nerve-sparing RP in comparison to no activity within the patient's group with no nerve-sparing surgery, which the authors suggest makes the effective use of PDE5 inhibitors in the first group more likely *(73)*. The same working group looked at erectile function recovery in patients after either unilateral or bilateral nerve-sparing radical prostatectomy for prostate cancer with nightly low-dose sildenafil compared to control patients *(74)*. In 23 patients with preserved spontaneous erections measured by nocturnal penile tumescence and rigidity in the first night after catheter removal daily sildenafil 25 mg starting immediately was introduced. A control group of 18 patients underwent follow-up without PDE5 inhibitor. Both groups showed a nadir of the International Index of Erectile Function (IIEF) 5 Domain Score at 6 weeks follow-up which was in the daily sildenafil group from preoperative 20.8 mean score to 3.6 and for the control group from preoperative 21.2 mean score to 2.4. Statistical evaluation showed a significant difference in IIEF-5 score and time to recover of erectile function between the group on daily 25 mg sildenafil and control ($p < 0.05$). The mean IIEF 5 score at 78 weeks after surgery was 19.3 for the sildenafil group and 13.2 for the control group. The authors concluded that these findings might be important for an appropriate choice of pharmacotherapy for an optimal recover of erectile function after nerve-sparing radical prostatectomy.

In the first prospective study in preoperatively potent men the daily use of sildenafil at bedtime (50 mg or 100 mg) compared to placebo after bilateral nerve-sparing RP might have a benefit. After a post-RP therapy duration of 9 months 27% of the sildenafil group had recovered erectile rigidity to the preoperative level and only 4% in the placebo group ($p = 0.0156$) *(63)*. Recent literature implies a beneficial effect of regular PDE5 inhibitor administration on the improvement of erectile function by rehabilitation of vascular endothelium *(75)*. Results from recent studies suggest that regular treatment with PDE5 inhibitor may lead to enhanced erectile function beyond that observed with on-demand usage, possibly through improvement of endothelial function which can be considered as rehabilitation of damaged erectile tissue.

4.1 Data Supporting the Concept of Early Postoperative Erection as Rehabilitation

In a non-randomized study in which patients with preoperative functional erections underwent RP and complied with an erectogenic pharmacotherapy regimen for 18 months either with oral sildenafil 100 mg or intracavernosal injection therapy three times a week showed that 52% were capable of having medication-unassisted intercourse compared to 19% of men who did not use any rehabilitation ($p < 0.001$) *(76)*. From the same study population a logistic regression analysis demonstrated statistically significant predictors of failure to respond to sildenafil post-RP that is represented in Table 2 *(77)*. Intracorporeal injection therapy with alprostadil (prostaglandin E1) alone is effective in the majority of post-RP ED patients regardless of the status of their cavernosal nerves *(78)*. In 1997 Montorsi et al. assessed in a prospective study, men after bilateral nerve-sparing retropubic RP with the use of intracavernosal injection of alprostadil on a regular basis over a period of 12 weeks *(36)*. He demonstrated improved spontaneous erection frequency compared to the observation group alone. Starting with 5 µg alprostadil within the first week after surgery the men used the ICI three times a week independent of sexual activity. Sixty-seven percent of the 12 men who completed the treatment had erections good

Table 2 Predictors of Failure for Erectile Function Recovery After RP

Predictor	RR	[95%] CI	P value
Age > 60 years	1.3	1.1–2.4	< 0.05
Non-bilateral nerve-sparing	1.6	1.2–4.4	< 0.01
≥ 2 vascular co-morbidities	2.1	1.4–4.5	< 0.01
Commencement of rehabilitation >6 m after RP	2.8	1.6–6.8	< 0.01
Sildenafil failure at 12 m post-RP	4.5	1.8–8.2	< 0.01
Use of trimix dose > 50 Units	8.1	2.3–14.7	< 0.001

RP: radical prostatectomy; m: month; RR: [95%] CI: 95% confidence interval.

enough for intercourse which was statistically significant better compared to 20% of the control group ($p < 0.01$). The conclusion of this study was that nocturnal erection supplies the cavernosal tissue with oxygen that might protect it from developing fibrotic changes during the period of ED following nerve-sparing RP. This landmark study is to date the only evidence-based medicine for the role of penile rehabilitation with intracavernosal injections after RP.

The early beginning of the rehabilitation may improve cavernosal oxygenation and prevent hypoxia-induced corporal fibrosis. An improvement of penile hemodynamics and return of spontaneous erections were shown after long-term use of alprostadil in patients with arteriogenic ED *(79)*. In a clinical study looking for the optimal timing of ICI after non-nerve-sparing RP, the patient compliance was much higher with a later commencement of therapy *(80)*. However, injections given in the first postoperative month gave the best response rate but with poor compliance. Simply, from a preventive standpoint the erectile rehabilitation should be started as soon as possible to preserve erectile tissue which otherwise undergoes structural changes with the loss of function over time *(35)*. The iatrogenic trauma during surgery to the cavernous nerves may cause a release of mediators which can cause a hypersensitivity of nocireceptors. Intracavernosal injections of alprostadil alone may cause significant pain because of this, resulting in an early cessation of therapy by patients. This can be minimized by the use of combination agents that permit reduction in alprostadil dose *(80)*. The use of a combination including alprostadil, papaverine, and phentolamine (trimix) for intracavernosal injection therapy obtains a very high response rate in patients with ED and a dramatically reduced rate of penile pain *(81)*. Patients using the trimix combination of papaverine, phentolamine and PGE1 for post-RP ED treatment reported an efficacy rate of almost 95% with the intracavernosal self-injection therapy *(82)*.

5   Alternative Rehabilitation Strategies

5.1   *Intra-urethral Alprostadil Suppositories*

The intra-urethral administration of alprostadil (prostaglandin E1) was first introduced in 1997 with an overall efficacy rate of 44% for ED treatment in patients after RP *(83)*. In a retrospective study of 27 patients with post-RP ED-treated with intra-urethral alprostadil after a mean duration of 2.2 years, a 48% rate of significant improvement in all domains of the Sexual Health Inventory for Men (SHIM) was reported *(84)*. However, very few men had recovery of their pre-operative scores, and 52% ceased the use of intra-urethral alprostadil after a mean of 8 months mainly due to inadequate response or side effects. Only 51% of patients who had a rigid erection in an office-test were able to achieve a consistent response at home *(85)*.

Recently, studies have explored intra-urethral alprostadil in combination with oral sildenafil, in monotherapy failures *(86,87)*. An enhancement of sexual satisfaction with this combination therapy in sildenafil failures was demonstrated in the post-RP population *(88)*.

Might there be some intrinsic value to the use of prostaglandin? We are aware that PGE1 may modulate TGF-β production in cavernosal smooth muscle. This has not yet been fully studied. In a prospective controlled study of 91 sexually active men (mean age 59 years) who underwent nerve-sparing radical prostatectomy for prostate cancer the early administration of intra-urethral alprostadil in form of MUSE (Medicated Urethral System for Erection (MUSE^{TM}, Vivus Inc., Mountain View, CA, USA) starting 3 weeks after surgery seems to shorten the recovery time to regaining erectile function *(86)*. Fifty-six patients were treated with MUSE 125 or 250 μg three times per week for 6 months while the remaining 35 had no erectogenic aids, except as necessary when attempting sexual activity. With a compliance rate of 68% patients reported a significant improvement in all domains of the Sexual Health Inventory for Men (SHIM) questionnaire after using MUSE. At the end of 6 months 74% of the patients *who remained on MUSE* were able to have successful vaginal intercourse with a mean SHIM score of 18.9 compared to 37% of the untreated control group who regained erections sufficient for vaginal intercourse with a mean SHIM score of 15.8. The role of MUSE in penile rehabilitation is unclear but there are ongoing studies assessing this role. It is conceivable that the future of penile rehabilitation will involve multi-modal therapy with MUSE being one of those strategies.

5.2 Vacuum Erection Devices (VED)

VED is a manual device and is one of the oldest treatments for ED. In times when oral pharmacological ED therapy was not available, reports documented a long-term efficacy and high-satisfaction rate for patients and partners with a VED *(89)*. Though, discontinuation rates of 65% were reported whereby most of the patients stopped use of the VED use within a mean time period of 4 months *(90)*. Literature on the subject of VED in the post-RP population is almost lacking. In a prospective, randomized trial assessing the efficacy of VED following RP, 60/74 patients successfully used their VED with a constriction ring for vaginal intercourse twice a week and achieved an overall partner satisfaction rate of 58% (33/60) *(91)*. After a mean duration of 3 months 18% (14/74) terminated the VED use. In another prospective trial, a total of 28 patients were randomized after retropubic RP sparing at least one neurovascular bundle to an early group using a VED after 1-month post-surgery or to a control group starting the VED 6 months after RP *(92)*. Using the VED without a constriction ring for 10 min daily the International Index of Erectile Function score was significantly higher in group 1 than group 2 at 3 months and at 6 months ($p < 0.05$) concluding an improved sexual function by an early introduction of a VED after RP. It has also been reported that the combination of sildenafil with VED improved sexual satisfaction and penile rigidity in 77% (24/31) patients dissatisfied with VED alone after radical prostatectomy *(93)*. Might there be some intrinsic value to penile stretching as occurs with the VED in the post-RP population? However, given that VEDs do not oxygenate the penis well, without animal data to off a scientific rationale, and in the absence of large, randomized-controlled trials looking at VED post-RP, conclusions are difficult to arrive at. Future data may permit us to better define the role of VED post-RP.

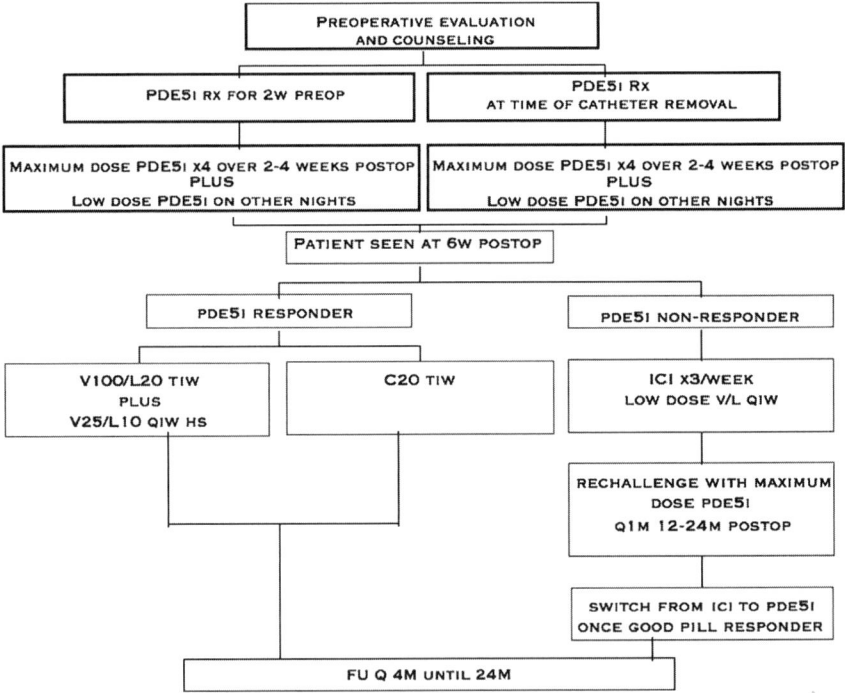

Fig. 2 The Memorial Sloan Kettering Penile Rehabilitation after Algorithm

6 Rehabilitation Regimens

To date, there has been no formal analysis of what represents the optimal rehabilitation program and thus giving the reader formal guidelines is difficult. Figure 2 represents the current approach at Memorial Sloan-Kettering Cancer Center, although this is not to say that this is the only approach. The algorithm is based on the animal and human data at this time highlighting the idea that there is probably a value to erections in the early period after RP and that there is probably an adjunctive value to regular PDE5 inhibitor use.

7 Conclusion

Initiation of prostate cancer screening programs the mean age of patients with prostate cancer is declining more and more which goes hand in hand with the demand for optimal quality of life after RP. Following the newest surgical guidelines a nerve-sparing RP seems to be a meaningful procedure in a carefully selected patient population respecting the oncological standard as the highest priority a nerve-sparing RP seems to be a meaningful procedure in a carefully selected patient population following precisely the newest surgical guidelines. Based on the current literature the little above-mentioned data from human and animal evidence gives a strong signal that there might be a positive effect of a prophylactic penile rehabilitation after RP using intracavernosal injection therapy or PDE5 inhibitors on a regular base which may translate into greater preservation of erectile function. However, many questions about the mechanisms for the development of ED after RP and about the potential therapy options remain open and investigational. Large prospective multi-center, randomized, placebo-controlled studies in the future will hopefully be able to answer questions about an optimal dosing, a time frame for the application, duration and form of the use, and maybe about differences between the different medications. Further supportive managements including cavernous nerve reconstruction and neuroprotection stratagems are under investigation finding their place of value in the future. Under a socio-economic standpoint the patient usually has to pay for such a rehabilitation program because the insurances do not cover these expenses. For a sufficient erectile rehabilitation after RP it needs a well-informed patient who is highly motivated to follow a medical regimen and is willing to pay for it to maintain quality of life after a potential curative cancer treatment.

References

1. Van der Horst, C., Martinez-Portillo, F.J., and Jünemann, K.P. (2005) Pathophysiology and Rehabilitation der erektilen Dysfunktion nach nervenhalternder radikaler Prostatektomie. *Urologe A* **44,** 667–673.

2. Lue, T.F. (1990) Impotence after prostatectomy. *Urol. Clin. North Am.* **17**, 613.
3. Talcott, J.A., Rieker, P., Propert, K.J., et al. (1997) Patient-reported impotence and incontinence after nerve-sparing radical prostatectomy. *J. Natl. Cancer Inst.* **89**, 1117.
4. Burnett, A.L. (2003) Neuroprotection and nerve grafts in the treatment of neurogenic erectile dysfunction. *J. Urol.* **170**, 31–34.
5. Michl, U., Graefen, M., Noldus, J., Eggert, T., and Huland, H. (2003) Functional results of various surgical techniques for radical prostatectomy. *Urologe A* **42**, 1196–1202.
6. Walsh, P.C., Marschke, P., Riecker, D., et al. (2000) Patient-reported urinary continence and sexual function after anatomic radical prostatectomy. *Urology* **55**, 58.
7. User, H.M., Hairstron, J.H., Helner, D.J., et al. (2003) Penile weight and cell subtype specific changes in a post-radical prostatectomy model of erectile dysfunction. *J. Urol.* **169**, 1175.
8. Leungwattanakij, S., Bivalacqua, T.J., Usta, M.F., et al. (2003) Cavernous neurotomy causes hypoxia and fibrosis in rat corpus cavernosum. *J. Androl.* **24**, 239.
9. Carrier, S., Zvara, P., Nunes, L., et al. (1995) Regeneration of nitric oxide synthase-containing nerves after cavernous nerve neurotomy in the rat. *J. Urol.* **195**, 1722.
10. Mullerad, M., Donohue, J.F., Li, P.S., Scardino, P.T., and Mulhall, J.P. (2006) Functional sequelae of cavernous nerve injury in the rat: model dependency. *J. Sex. Med.* **3**, 77–83.
11. Muhall, J., and Glina, S. (2006) Radical pelvic surgery-associated sexual dysfunction. In: Porst, H., and Buvat, J., eds. *Standard Practice in Sexual Medicine*, 1st edn. Massachusetts: Blackwell Publishing, pp. 210–224.
12. Begg, C.B., Riedel, E.R., Bach, P.B., Kattan, M.W., Schrag, D., Warren, J.L., and Scardino, P.T. (2002) Variations in morbidity after radical prostatectomy. *N. Engl. J. Med.* **346**, 1138.
13. Standord, J.L., Feng, Z., Hamilton, A.S., et al. (2000) Urinary and sexual function after radical prostatectomy for clinically localized prostate cancer. The prostate cancer outcome study. *JAMA* **283**, 354.
14. Flanigan, K.M, Lauria, G., Griffin, J.W., and Kuncl, R.W. (1998) Age-related biology and diseases of muscle and nerve. *Neurol. Clin.* **16**, 659–669.
15. Burnett, A.L. (2003) Strategies to promote recovery of cavernous nerve function after radical prostatectomy. *World J. Urol.* **20**, 337–342.
16. Quinlan, D.M., Epstein, J.I., Carter, B.S., and Walsh, P.C. (1991) Sexual function following radical prostatectomy: influence of preservation of neurovascular bundles. *J. Urol.* **145**, 998–1002.
17. Klein, L.T., Miller, H.I., Buttyan, R., Raffo, A.J., Burchard, M., Deviris, G., Cao, Y.C., Olsson, C., and Shabsigh, R. (1997) Apoptosis in the rat penis after penile denervation. *J. Urol.* **158**, 626–630.
18. Mulhall, J.P., Muller, A., Donohue, J.F., Mullerad, M., Tal, R., Kobylarz, K., Paduch, D., Li, P.S., and Scardino, P. (2008) The functional and structural consequences of cavernous nerve injury are ameliorated by sildenafil citrate. *J. Sex. Med.* **5**, 1126–36.
19. Ferrini, M.G., Davila, H.H., Kovanecz, I., Sanchez, S.P., Gonzalez-Cadavid, N.F., and Rajfer, J. (2006) Vardenafil prevents fibrosis and loss of corporal smooth muscle that occurs after bilateral cavernosal nerve resection in the rat. *Urology* **68**, 429–435.
20. Aboseif, S., Shinohar, K., Breza, J., et al. (1994) Role of penile vascular injury in erectile dysfunction after radical prostatectomy. *Br. J. Urol.* **89**, 75.
21. Darmanis, S., Lewis, A., Mansoor, A., and Bircher, M. (2007) Corona mortis: an anatomical study with clinical implications in approaches to the pelvis and acetabulum. *Clin. Anat.* **20**, 433–439.
22. Okcu, G., Erkan, S., Yercan, H.S., and Ozic, U. (2004) The incidence and location of corona mortis: a study on 75 cadavers. *Acta. Orthop. Scand.* **75**, 53.
23. Testut, L., and Latarget, A. (1983) In: *Tratado de Anatomia Humana*, 9th edn. Edited and published by Salvat: Barcelona, Spain, Vol. **4**, pp. 325–350.
24. Secin, F.P., Karanikolas, N., Tourijer, A.K., Salamanca, J.I., Vickers, A.J., and Guillonneau, B. (2005) Anatomy of accessory pudendal arteries in laparoscopic radical prostatectomy. *J. Urol.* **174**, 523.

25. Secin, F.P., Karanikolas, N., Kuroiwa, K., Vickers, A., Touijer, K., and Guillonneau, B. (2005) Positive surgical margins and accessory pudendal artery preservation during laparoscopic radical prostatectomy. *Eur. Urol.* 48: 786.

26. Matin, S.F. (2006) Recognition and preservation of accessory pudendal arteries during laparoscopic radical prostatectomy. *Urology* **67**: 1012.

27. Rosen, M.P., Greenfield, A.J., Walker, T.G., Grant, P., Guben, J.K., Dubrow, J., Bettmann, M.A., Goldstein, I. (1990) Arteriogenic impotence: findings in 195 impotent men examined with selective internal pudendal angiography. *Young Investigators's Award. Radiol.* **174,** 1043.

28. Gray, R.R., Keresteci, A.G., St. Louis, E.L., Grosman, H., Jewett, M.A., Rankin, J.T., and Provan, J.L. (1982) Investigation of impotence by internal pudendal angiography: experience with 73 cases. *Radiology* **144,** 773.

29. Droupy, S., Hessel, A., Benoit, G., Blanceht, P., Jardin, A., and Giuliano, F. (1999) Assessment of the functional role of accessory pudendal arteries in erection by transrectal color Doppler ultrasound. *J. Urol.* **162,** 1987.

30. Benoit, G., Droupy, S., Qullard, J.,Paradis, V., and Giuliano, F. (1999) Supra and infralevator neurovascular pathways to the penile corpora cavernosa. *J. Anat.* **195,** 605.

31. Breza, J., Aboseif, S.R., Orvis, B.R., Lue, T.F., and Tanogho, E.A. (1989) Detailed anatomy of penile neurovascular structures: surgical significance. *J. Urol.* **141,** 437.

32. Polascick, T.J., and Walsh, P.C. (1995) Radical retropubic prostatectomy: the influence of accessory pudendal arteries on the recovery of sexual function. *J. Urol.* **154,** 150.

33. Rogers, C.G., Trock, B.P., and Walsh, P.C. (2004) Preservation of accessory pudendal arteries during radical retropubic prostatectomy: surgical technique and results. *Urology* **64,** 148.

34. Mulhall, J.P., and Graydon, R.J. (1996) The hemodynamics of erectile dysfunction following nerve-sparing radical retropubic prostatectomy. *Int. J. Impot. Res.* **8,** 91.

35. Mulhall, J.P., Slovick, R., Hotaling, J., Aviv, N., Valenzuela, R., Waters, W.B., and Flanigan, R.C. (2002) Erectile dysfunction after radical prostatectomy: hemodynamic profiles and their correlation with the recovery of erectile function. *J. Urol.* **167,** 1371.

36. Montorsi, F., Guazzoni, G., Strambi, L.F., Da Pozzo, L.F., Nava, L., Barbieri, L., Rigatti, P., Pizzini, G., and Miani, A. (1997) Recovery of spontaneous erectile function after nerve-sparing radical retropubic prostatectomy with and without early intracavernous injections of alprostadil: results of a prospective, randomized trial. *J. Urol.* **158,** 1408.

37. Ohebshalom, M., Parker, M., and Mulhall, J.P. *Erectile Hemodynamic Status Following Radical Prostatectomy Correlates with Erectile Function Outcomes.* Abstract presented at SMSNA Annual Meeting, NY, November 2005.

38. Junemann, K.P., Luo, J.A., Lue, T.F., and Tanagho, E.A. (1986) Further evidence of venous outflow restriction during erection. *Br. J. Urol.* **58,** 320–324.

39. Kim, N., Vardi, Y., Padma Nathan, H., Daley, J., Goldstein, I., and Saenz de Tejada, I. (1993) Oxygen tension regulates the nitric oxide pathway. Physiological role in penile erection. *J. Clin. Invest.* **91,** 437–442.

40. Moreland, R.B., Traish, A., McMillin, M.A., Smith, B., Goldstein, I., and Saenz de Tejada, I. (1995) PGE1 suppresses the induction of collagen synthesis by transforming growth factor-beta 1 in human corpus cavernosum smooth muscle. *J. Urol.* **153,** 826–834.

41. Moreland, R.B., Albadawi, H., Bratton, C., et al. (2001) O_2-dependent prostanoid synthesis activates functional PGE receptors on corpus cavernosum smooth muscle. *Am. J. Physiol. Heart Circ. Physiol.* **281,** H552.

42. Moreland, R.B., Watkins, M.T., and Nehra, A. (1998) Oxygen tension modulates transforming growth factor-beta1 expression and PGE production in human corpus cavernosum smooth muscle cells. *Mol. Rol.* **2,** 41–47.

43. Moreland, R.B., Gupta, S., Goldstein, I., and Traish, A. (1998) Cyclic AMP modulates TGF-beta 1-induced fibrillar collagen synthesis in cultured human corpus cavernosum smooth muscle cells. *Int. J. Impot. Res.* **10,** 159–163.

44. Lue, T.F. (2000) Erectile dysfunction. *N. Engl. J. Med.* **342,** 1802.

45. Canada, A.L., Neese, L.E., Sui, D., et al. (2005) Pilot intervention to enhance sexual rehabilitation for couples after treatment for localized prostate carcinoma. *Cancer* **104,** 2689.
46. Schover, L.R., Fouladi, R.T., Warneke, C.L., et al. (2004) Seeking help for erectile dysfunction after treatment for prostate cancer. *Arch. Sex. Behav.* **33,** 443.
47. Montorsi, F., Briganti, A., Salonia, A., Rigatti, P., and Burnett, A.L. (2004) Current and future strategies for preventing and managing erectile dysfunction following radical prostatectomy. *Eur. Urol.* **45,** 123–133.
48. Desouza, C., Parulkar A., Lumpkin, D., Akers, D., and Fonseca, V.A. (2002) Acute and prolonged effects of sildenafil on brachial artery flow-mediated dilation in type 2 diabetes. *Diabetes Care* **25,** 1336–1339.
49. Musicki, B., Dramer, M.F., Becker, R.E., and Burnett, A.L. (2005) Inactivation of phosphorylated endothelial nitric oxide synthase (Ser-1177) by O-GlcNAc in diabetes-associated erectile dysfunction. *Proc. Natl. Acad. Sci. USA* **102,** 11870–11875.
50. Rosano, G.M., Aversa, A., Vitale, C., Fabbri, A., Fini, M., and Spera, G. (2005) Chronic treatment with tadalafil improves endothelial function in men with increased cardiovascular risk. *Eur. Urol.* **47,** 214–220.
51. Somlyo, A.P., and Somlyo, A.. (2000) Signal transduction by G-proteins, rho-kinase and protein phosphatase to smooth muscle and non-muscle myosin II. *J. Physiol.* **522,** 177–185.
52. Chitaley, K., Wingard, C.J., Clinton Webb, R., Branam, H., Stopper, V.S., Lewis, R.W., and Millis, T.M. (2001) Antagonism of Rho-kinase stimulates rat penile erection via a nitric oxide-independent pathway. *Nat. Med.* **7,** 119–122.
53. Wang, H., Eto, M., Steers, W.D., Somlyo, A.P., and Somlyo, A.V. (2002) RhoA-mediated Ca^{2+} sensitization in erectile function. *J. Biol. Chem.* **277,** 30614-30621,..
54. Musicki, B., Champion, H.C., Bekcer, R.E., Liu, T., Kramer, M.F., and Burnett, A.L. (2005) Erection capability is potentiated by long-term sildenafil treatment: role of blood flow-induced endothelial nitric-oxide synthase phosphorylation. *Mol. Pharmacol.* **68,** 226–232.
55. Asahara, T., et al. (1997) Isolation of putative progenitor endothelial cells for angiogenesis. *Science* **275,** 964–967.
56. Foresta, C., Caretta, N., Lana, A., Cabrelle, A., Palù, G., and Ferlin, A. (2005) Circulating endothelial progenitor cells in subjects with erectile dysfunction. *Int. J. Impot. Res.* **17,** 288–290.
57. Aicher, A., Heeschen, C., and Dimmeler, S. (2004) The role of NOS3 in stem cell mobilization. *Trends Mol. Med.* **10,** 421–425.
58. Aicher, A., et al. (2003) Essential role of endothelial nitric oxide synthase for mobilization of stem and progenitor cells. *Nat. Med.* **9,** 1370–1376.
59. Foresta, C., Lana, A., Cabrelle, A., Ferigo, M., Caretta, N., Garolla, A., et al. (2005) PDE-5 inhibitor, Vardenafil, increases circulating progenitor cells in humans. *Int. J. Impot. Res.* **17,** 377–380.
60. Foresta, C., Ferlin, A., De Toni, L., Lana, A., Vinanzi, C., Galan, A., and Caretta, N. (2006) Circulating endothelial progenitor cells and endothelial function after chronic tadalafil treatment in subjects with erectile dysfunction. *Int. J. Impot. Res.* **18,** 484–488.
61. Zhang, R., Wang, Y., Zhang, L., Zhang, Z., Tsang, W., Lu, M., Zhang, L., and Chopp, M. (2002) Sildenafil induces neurogenesis and promotes functional recovery after stroke in rats. *Stroke* **33,** 2675–2680.
62. Zhang, L., Zhang, Z., Zhang, R.L., Cui, Y., LaPointe, M.C., Silver, B., and Chopp, M. (2006) Tadalafil, a long-acting type 5 phosphodiesterase isoenzyme inhibitor improves neurological functional recovery in a rat model of embolic stroke. *Brain Res.* **1118,** 192–198.
63. Padma-Nathan, E., McCullough, A.R., Giulionao, F., Toler, S.M., Wohlhuter, C., and Shpinsky, A.B. (2003) Postoperative nightly administration of sildenafil citrate significantly improves the return of nightly spontaneous erectile function after bilateral nerve-sparing radical prostatectomy. *J. Urol.* **4**(Suppl), 375.
64. Kovanecz, I., Rambhatla, A., Rerrini, M.G., Vernet, D., Sanchez, S., Rajfer, J., and Gonzalez-Cadavid, N. (2007) Chronic daily tadalafil prevents the corporal fibrosis and

veno-occlusive dysfunction that occurs after cavernosal nerve resection. *BJU Int.* [Epub ahead of print].

65. Donohue, J.F., Tal, R., Akin-Olugbade, Y., Muller, A., Bennett, N.E., Kobylarz, K., Paduch, D., Scardino, P.T., and Mulhall, J.P. (2006) Sildenafil and cavernous nerve injury in the rat: defining the optimal dosing and timing regimen. *J. Urol.* (Suppl), AUA, Atlanta (Abstract #10017).

66. Kukreja, R.C., Salloum, F., Das, A., Ockaili, R., Yin, C., Bremer, Y.A., Fisher, P.W., Wittkamp, M., Hawkins, J., Chou, E., Kukreja, A.K., Wang, X., Marwaha, V.R., and Xi, L. (2005) Pharmacological preconditioning with sildenafil: basic mechanisms and clinical implications. *Vascul. Pharmacol.* **42**, 219–232.

67. Kukrajy, R.C. (2007) Cardiovascular protection with sildenafil following chronic inhibition of nitric oxide synthase. *Br. J. Pharmacol.* **150**, 538–540.

68. Salloum, F.N., Ockaili, R.A., Wittkamp, M., Marwaha, V.R., and Kukreja, R.C. (2006) Vardenafil: a novel type 5 phosphodiesterase inhibitor reduces myocardial infarct size following ischemia/reperfusion injury via opening of mitochondrial K(ATP) channels in rabbits. *J. Mol. Cell. Cardiol.* **40**, 405–411.

69. Salloum, F.N., Takenoshita, Y., Ockaili, R.A., Daoud, V.P., Chou, E., Yoshida, K., and Kukreja, R.C. (2007) Sildenafil and vardenafil but not nitroglycerin limit myocardial infarction through opening of mitochondrial K(ATP) channels when administered at reperfusion following ischemia in rabbits. *J. Mol. Cell Cardiol.* **42**, 453–458.

70. Das, A., Xi, L., and Kukreja, R.C. (2005) Phosphodiesterase-5 inhibitor sildenafil preconditions adult cardiac myocytes against necrosis and apoptosis. Essential role of nitric oxide signaling. *J. Biol. Chem.* **280**, 12944–12955.

71. Schwartz, E.J., Wong, P., and Graydon, R.J. (2004) Sildenafil preserves intracorporeal smooth muscle after radical retropubic prostatectomy. *J. Urol.* **171**, 771–774.

72. Iacono, F., Giannella, R., Somma, P., Manno G., Fusco, F., and Mirone, V. (2005) Histological alterations in cavernous tissue after radical prostatectomy. *J. Urol.* **173**, 1673–1676.

73. Bannowsky, A., Schulze, H., van der Horst, C., Seif, C., Braun, P.M., and Jünemann, K.P. (2006) A parameter for postoperative erectile integrity after nerve sparing radical prostatectomy. *J. Urol.* **175**, 2214–2217.

74. Bannowsky, A., Schulze, H., van der Horst, C., Hautmann, S., and Juenemann, K.P. (2007) *Improved Recovery of Erectile Function with Nightly Low Dose Sildenafil – 18 Month Follow-Up After Nerve-Sparing Radical Prostatectomy.* Presented at the annual meeting of the American Urology Association, Abstract number 1172, May 19–24, Anaheim, CA, USA.

75. Sommer, F., and Schulze, W. (2005) Treating erectile dysfunction by endothelial rehabilitation with phosphodiesterase 5 inhibitors. *World J. Urol.* **23**, 385–392.

76. Mulhall, J., Land, S., Parker, M., Waters, W.B., and Falnigan, R.C. (2005) The use of an erectogenic pharmacotherapy regimen following radical prostatectomy improves recovery of spontaneous erectile function. *J. Sex. Med.* **2**, 532–542.

77. Muller, A., Parker, M., Waters, B.W., Glanigan, R.C., and Mulhall, J.P. (2006) Analysis of predictors of outcomes with pharmacological penile rehabilitation following radical prostatectomy. *J. Urol.* (Suppl), AUA, Atlanta.

78. Briganti, A., Salonia, A., Zanni, G., Fabbri, F., Sacca, A., Bertinii, R., et al. (2004) Erectile dysfunction and radical prostatectomy: an update. *EAU Update Series* **2**, 84.

79. Brock, G., Tu, L.M., and Linet, O.I. (2001) Return of spontaneous erection during long-term intracavernosal alprostadil (Caverject) treatment. *Urolgy* **57**, 536–541.

80. Gontero, P., Fontana, F., Gagnasacco, A., Panell, M., Kocjanicic, E., Pretti, G., and Frea, B. (2003) Is there an optimal time for intracavernous prostaglandin E1 rehabilitation following nonnerve sparing radical prostatectomy? Results from a hemodynamic prospective study. *J. Urol.* **169**, 2166–2169.

81. Montorsi, F., Guazzoni, G., Bergamaschi, F., Dodensini, A., Rigatti, P., Pizzini, G., et al. (1993) Effectiveness and safety of multidrug intracavernous therapy for vasculogenic impotence. *Urology* **42**, 554–558.

82. Claro, A., de Aboim, J.E., Marringolo, M., Andrade, E., Aguiar, W., Nogueira, M., et al. (2001) Intracavernous injection in the treatment of erectile dysfunction after radical prostatectomy: an observational study. *Sao Paulo Med. J.* **5,** 135.

83. Padma-Nathan, H., Hellstrom, W.J., Kaiser, F.E., Laboasky, R.F., Lue, T.F., Nolten, W.E., Norwwod, P.C., Peterson, C.A., Shabsigh, R., and Tam, P.Y. (1997) Treatment of men with erectile dysfunction with transurethral alprostadil. Medicated Urethral System for Erection (MUSE) Study Group. *N. Engl. J. Med.* **336,** 1–7.

84. Raina, R., Agarwal, A., and Zippe, C.D. (2005) Management of erectile dysfunction after radical prostatectomy. *Urology* **66,** 923.

85. Mulhall, J.P., Jahoda, A.E., Ahmed, A., and Parker, M. (2001) Analysis of the consistency of intraurethral prostaglandin E(1) (MUSE) during at-home use. *Urology* **58,** 262–266.

86. Raina, R., Pahlajanie, G., Agarwal, A., and Zippe, C.D. (2007) The early use of transurethral alprostadil after radical prostatectomy potentially facilitates an earlier return of erectile function and successful sexual activity. *BJU Int.* **100,** 1317–1321.

87. Nehra, A., Blute, M.L., Barrett, D.M., and Moreland, R.B. (2002) Rational for combination therapy of intraurethral prostaglandin E(1) and sildenafil in the salvage of erectile dysfunction patients desiring noninvasive therapy. *Int. J. Impot. Res.* **14**(Suppl 1), S38–S42.

88. Raina, R., Nandipati, K.C., Agarwal, A., Mansour, D., Kaelber, D.C., and Zippe, C.D. (2005) Combination therapy: medicated urethral system for erection enhances sexual satisfaction in sildenafil citrate failures following nerve-sparing radical prostatectomy. *J. Androl.* **26,** 757–760.

89. Cookson, M.D., and Nadig, P.W. (1993) Long term results with vacuum constriction device. *J. Urol.* 149: 200.

90. Dutta, T.C., and Eid, J.F. (1999) Vacuum constriction devices for erectile dysfunction: a long-term, prospective study of patients with mild, moderate, and severe dysfunction. *Urology* **54,** 891.

91. Raina, R., Agarwal, A., Ausmundson, S., Lakin, M., Nandipati, K.C., Montague, D.K., et al. (2006) Early use of vacuum constriction device following radical prostatectomy facilitates early sexual activity and potentially earlier return of erectile function. *Int. J. Impot. Res.* **18,** 77.

92. Köhler, T.S., Pedro, R., hendlin, K., Utz, W., Ugarte, R., Reddy, P., Makhlouf, A., Ryndin, I., Canales, B.K., Weiland, D., Nakib, N., Ramani, A., Anderson, J.K., and Monga, M. (2007) A pilot study on the early use of the vacuum erection device after radical retropubic prostatectomy. *BJU Int.* **100,** 858–862.

93. Raina, R., Agarwal, A., Allamaneni, S.S., Lakin, M.M., and Zippe, C.D. (2005) Sildenafil citrate and vacuum constriction device combination enhances sexual satisfaction in erectile dysfunction alter radical prostatectomy. *Urology* **65,** 360–364.

Chapter 11
Impact of Androgen Deprivation on Male Sexual Function

Ricardo Munarriz and Abdul Traish

Abstract *Introduction:* The role of androgens in sexual function and in particular in erectile physiology remains controversial. The aim of this chapter is to review the preclinical and clinical data on the impact of androgen deprivation in male sexual functioning since androgen ablation is the main treatment option for men with advanced prostate cancer and a critical component of radiation therapy for localized prostate cancer.

Methods: Review of preclinical and clinical evidence on the role of androgens in sexual function.

Results: Preclinical data show that androgens regulate penile development, smooth muscle and neural integrity, fibroelastic properties, adipocyte accumulation and distribution, expression and activity of NOS and PDE5 resulting in a dose–response relationship between testosterone and erectile function. Clinical evidence documents the negative impact of androgen ablation on sexual desire and activity, nocturnal erections, and erectile function in a dose–response relationship. In addition, androgen replacement in men improves the effectiveness of PDE 5 inhibitors.

Conclusions: The literature supports that androgen ablation results in a decrease of sexual desire, nocturnal erections, erectile function, and overall sexual satisfaction. These observations are particularly important in men with prostate cancer, since androgen ablation is the main treatment option for men with advanced prostate cancer and a critical component of radiation therapy for localized prostate cancer.

Keywords Androgens; androgen ablation; NOS; PDE; adipocyte; erectile dysfunction.

From: *Current Clinical Urology* Series, *Sexual Function in the Prostate Cancer Patient*
Edited by John P. Mulhall, DOI 10.1007/978-1-60327-555-2_11,

1   Introduction

It is generally accepted that androgens are critical for gender differentiation, development of male sexual characteristics, and maintenance of bone density and muscle to fat ratio. However, their role in sexual function and in particular in erectile physiology remains controversial. The role of androgens in male sexual function is particularly important in men with prostate cancer, since androgen ablation is the main treatment option for men with advanced prostate cancer and a critical component of radiation therapy for localized prostate cancer. In addition, many men after successful treatment for localized prostate cancer are severely crippled by an androgen insufficiency state.

Traish and Kim in a very elegant review of the physiological role of androgens in penile erection postulated that the changes in penile erectile function in the castrated animal model may be due to (i) reduced synthesis of paracrine growth factors that are necessary to maintain the structural and functional integrity of the smooth muscle, endothelium, and nerves; (ii) upregulation of paracrine factors, such as connective tissue growth factors, which increases expression of connective tissue proteins; and (iii) dysregulation of metalloproteinases resulting in increased extracellular matrix deposition. They also suggested that these alterations may change tissue fibroelastic properties that impede cavernosal expandability resulting in significant changes in the inflow and outflow (veno-occlusion) mechanisms leading to erectile dysfunction *(1)*.

The aim of this chapter is to review the preclinical and clinical data on the impact of androgen deprivation in male sexual functioning.

2   Penile Erectile Physiology

Penile erection follows relaxation of arterial and trabecular smooth muscle *(2)*. Dilation of the cavernosal and helicine arteries increases blood flow into the lacunar spaces. Relaxation of the trabecular smooth muscle dilates the lacunar spaces, accommodating a larger volume of blood and thus engorging the penis. The expansion of the relaxed trabecular walls against the tunica albuginea compresses the plexus of subtunical venules *(3–5)*. These result in increased resistance to the outflow of blood with increased lacunar space pressure, making the penis rigid. The reduction of venous outflow by the mechanical compression of subtunical venules is known as the corporal veno-occlusive mechanism. The parasympathetic nerves, originating in the intermediolateral nuclei of the S2–S4 spinal cord segments, provide the major excitatory input to the penile erectile tissue and are responsible for vasodilation of the penile vasculature and subsequent erection. The primary mediator of NANC parasympathetic input is nitric oxide (NO). The ability of NO, a highly reactive and unstable gas, to regulate a wide array of physiologic functions in mammals has become evident only within the last two decades. Along with carbon monoxide, NO is a unique primary effector molecule with the characteristics of an intracellular second messenger that defies previous classification schemes. NO, produced by nitric oxide synthase (NOS), directly activates guanylate cyclase, which regulates the intracellular events, leading to relaxation of trabecular smooth muscle. The levels of cGMP are also regulated by phosphodiesterases (PDEs), which break down cGMP and terminate signaling. Inhibition of this enzyme leads to an increase in levels of intracellular cGMP and enhancement of the relaxation of smooth muscle in response to stimuli that activates the NO/cGMP pathway. This activity explains the success of potent, selective, and reversible PDE type 5 inhibitors in the treatment of male erectile dysfunction *(6)*.

3   Preclinical Evidence on the Role of Androgens in Male Sexual Function

1. **Androgens and Penile Development:** It is well-accepted that androgens modulate penile development and growth *(7,8)*. Gonzalez-Cavadid et al. and Lugget et al. suggested that 5α-dihydrotestosterone (5α-DHT) and not testosterone is responsible for penile growth and development in the rat model *(9,10)*. This hypothesis is supported by the observation that the administration of testosterone and 5α-reductase inhibitor did not prevent decline in erectile function in orchiectomized rats while administration of testosterone or 5α-DHT did *(11)*. Furthermore, clinical studies have shown that administration of 5α-DHT to infants and children with micropenis promotes penile growth *(12,13)* (Table 1).

2. **Androgens and Penile Smooth Muscle Integrity**: It is well-accepted that penile trabecular smooth muscle regulates erectile function *(14)*. Traish et al. have shown in the animal model that surgical or medical castration results in a significant reduction of trabecular smooth muscle content and intracavernosal pressure after pelvic nerve stimulation *(15,16)*. In addition, ultrastructural studies using electron microscopy have shown that trabecular smooth muscle from castrated animals appears disorganized, with large number of cytoplasmatic vacuoles and decreased amounts of cytoplasmatic myofilaments *(17)*. It is also believed that some of these changes are due to the activation of programmed cell death. However, the role on androgens in programmed cell death has not been investigated in penile trabecular smooth muscle.

3. **Androgens and Penile Neural Integrity:** It has been shown that androgens modulate structure and function on pelvic ganglions *(18,19)*. However, the role of androgens on penile neural integrity and synthesis/distribution of neurotransmitters has been poorly investigated. Giuliano et al. suggested that androgens modulate erectile function by acting on postganglionic parasympathetic neurons *(20)*. In addition, Rogers et al. showed that the ultrastructure of the dorsal nerve is altered in castrated rats *(17)*. They also showed that testosterone treatment restores dorsal nerve integrity. Finally, androgens are important in maintaining

Table 1 Role of Androgens in Male Sexual Function: Preclinical Evidence

Penile development *(9,10)*	• T is responsible for penile growth and development. Administration of T and 5-ARI does not prevent decline in EF in orchiectomized rats while administration of T or 5α-DHT does *(11)*.
Trabecular smooth muscle *(15–17)*	• Androgen ablation results in a reduction of TSM content.
Penile neural integrity *(18–21)*	• Androgens modulate structure and function of pelvic ganglions. • The ultrastructure of the dorsal nerve is altered in castrated rats. • Androgens maintain anatomical integrity of NADPH diaphorase-stained cavernosal nerve fibers.
Penile fibroelastic properties *(15,16,23–25)*	• Castration results in a marked decrease in muscle to collagen ratio. • Androgens modulate the extracellular matrix through growth factors.
Adipocyte accumulation *(26–28)*	• Castration results in accumulation of adipocytes in the corpora cavernosa. • Androgens may favor differentiation of pluripotent cells into smooth muscle and inhibit differentiation into adipocytes.
NOS isoforms *(11,30–40)*	• Androgens regulate expression of NOS in penile tissues. • Supplementing T restores NOS enzymatic activity.
PDE5 expression *(15,43,44)*	• Castration results in decreased expression and activity of PDE5. • Testosterone upregulates PDE5 activity.
Testosterone and erectile function *(45)*	• There may be a threshold testosterone value below which erectile function correlates with testosterone in a dose-dependent fashion.

anatomical integrity of NADPH diaphorase-stained dorsal and cavernosal nerve fibers in the rat model *(21)*. Shabsigh et al. showed in a randomized, placebo-controlled, double-blind, multicenter study that testosterone-treated subjects had greater improvement in orgasmic function compared to those who received placebo *(22)*.

4. **Androgens and Penile Fibroelastic Properties:** The penile extracellular matrix consists of a network of fibrillar collagen types I and III that provides support and regulates penile trabecular smooth muscle. Androgen ablation in the animal model results in a marked decrease of the smooth muscle to extracellular matrix ratio *(23–25)*, which alters penile compliance and hemodynamics resulting in erectile dysfunction *(15,16)*. In other cell lines, several investigators have shown that androgens modulate the extracellular matrix through growth factors. However, these findings have not been investigated in penile tissues.

5. **Androgens and Adipocyte Accumulation and Distribution in Penile Tissues:** In addition to the previously described changes in penile extracellular matrix and smooth muscle content and ultrastructure, androgen deprivation in the animal model results in the accumulation of adipocytes in penile tissues, particularly in the subtunical region *(26)*. Interestingly, testosterone replacement restores normal cavernosal appearance (unpublished observations by Traish et al.). Since these tissue alterations are accompanied by decreased intracavernosal pressures following pelvic nerve stimulation, it has been postulated that deposition of adipocytes may lead to corporo-occlusive dysfunction. The mechanisms by which androgens regulate penile tissue growth and differentiation are poorly understood. However, Bashin et al. suggested that androgens may favor differentiation of pluripotent cells into trabecular smooth muscle and inhibit differentiation into adipocytes *(27)*. This hypothesis is supported by the findings of Singh et al. who showed that differentiation of pluripotent cells is androgen dependent *(28)*. Other investigators have suggested that androgen deficiency may lead to dedifferentiation into other phenotypes *(29)*. However, there are no data in dedifferentiation of penile smooth muscle.

6. **Androgens and NOS Isoforms:** The parasympathetic nerves (S2–S4) provide the major excitatory input to the penile erectile tissue and are responsible for the vasodilation of the penile vasculature and subsequent erection. The primary mediator of NANC parasympathetic input is NO. It is apparently synthesized on demand with little or no storage and it directly activates a soluble enzyme (guanylate cyclase) rather than a 'traditional' receptor molecule. Nitric oxide is produced by nitric oxide synthase (NOS), which utilizes the amino acid L-arginine and molecular oxygen as substrates to produce NO and L-citrulline. Nitric oxide can readily cross plasma membranes to enter target cells, where it binds the heme component of soluble guanylate cyclase. This activation of guanylate cyclase stimulates the production of cyclic guanosine monophosphate (cGMP), with the resulting activation of the cGMP-dependent protein kinase, which regulates the intracellular events, leading to relaxation of trabecular smooth muscle. Several investigators have reported that androgens regulate the expression of NOS in penile tissues *(30,11,31–40)*. Castration in the animal model results in a 50% reduction of the activity of penile neural and endothelial NOS and testosterone treatment restores NOS enzymatic activity *(35,37,41)*. However, in aging rats, enzymatic and Western blot assays showed no difference in NOS activity or levels between testosterone-treated and not treated aged rats *(33)*.

7. **Androgens Control the Expression and Activity of PDE5:** The intracellular levels of cGMP are regulated by phosphodiesterases (PDEs), which break down cGMP and terminate signaling. Phosphodiesterase type 5 (PDE5) is the major enzyme responsible for cGMP hydrolysis in penile erectile tissue *(42)*. Inhibition of this enzyme leads to an increase in levels of intracellular cGMP and enhancement of the relaxation of smooth muscle in response to stimuli that activate the NO/cGMP pathway. Traish et al. not only showed that castration in the animal model results in decreased expression and activity of PDE5, but also that

testosterone treatment upregulates PDE5 activity *(15)*. These observations have been confirmed by Morelli et al. using real-time RT-PCR and Western blot analysis *(43,44)*. In addition, Traish et al. reported that PDE5 administration to castrated animals did not significantly increase intracavernosal pressure following pelvic nerve stimulation *(16)*. Such findings were corroborated by studies from Magi and co-workers *(45)* (Fig. 1).

8. **Dose–Response Relationship Between Testosterone and Erectile Function:** The relationship between serum testosterone levels and erectile function remains unclear. However, a recent study by Armagan et al. suggested that there is a

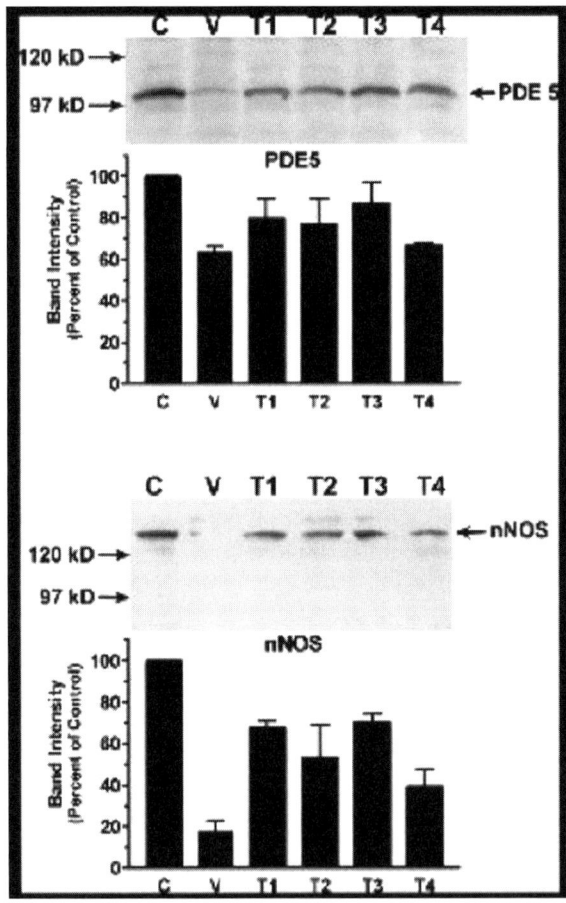

Fig. 1 Effect of testosterone on neural nitric oxide synthase (nNOS) and phosphodiesterase type 5 (PDE5) in rat penile tissue. Penile tissue from intact control rats (C) and surgically castrated rats infused with vehicle (V) or varying doses of testosterone (T1 440 mg/d, T2 220 mg/d, T3 88 mg/d, T4 44 mg/d) were pooled according to treatment group

testosterone threshold value (one-tenth of the normal range), below which erectile physiology correlates with testosterone in a dose-dependent fashion *(46)*.

4 Clinical Evidence on the Role of Androgens in Male Sexual Function

A recent meta-analysis of 656 subjects by Isisdori et al. showed that androgen replacement in men with testosterone levels below 12 nmol/L, moderately improved the number of nocturnal erections, desire, frequency of successful intercourses, erectile function, and overall sexual satisfaction *(47)*.

1. **Androgen Ablation and Erectile Function:** Several investigators have suggested that androgen ablation results in erectile dysfunction (Table 2). Peters and Walsh showed that the use of nafarelin acetate, a potent luteinizing-hormone releasing hormone (LHRH) agonists, in patients with benign prostatic hyperplasia (BPH) causes ED in most of the patients. Interestingly, only half of them regained their erectile function *(48)*. Eri et al. also showed that approximately 50% of patients with BPH treated with bicalutamine (anti-androgen) developed some degree of ED when compared to placebo. They also showed that the use of leuprolide (GnRH agonist) in patients with BPH resulted in decreased erectile function *(49,50)*. In addition, Rousseau et al. reported that the use of anti-androgens in patients with prostate cancer was associated with an inability to initiate an erection (57%) and inability to maintain an erection during sexual activity (71%) *(51)*. Greenstein et al. showed that castration in the management of prostate cancer resulted in erectile dysfunction in 75% of patients when free testosterone was significantly reduced (0.628 pg/mL) *(57)*.

2. **Androgen Ablation and Sexual Desire and Activity:** It is generally accepted that castration results in loss of sexual desire (Table 2). However, Eri et al. in a double-blind randomized, placebo-controlled study of 50 men with BPH showed that leuprolide resulted in loss of sexual activity while libido was partially maintained *(49)*. The same investigators also found that the use of bicalutamide (anti-androgen) in men with BPH resulted in reduced sexual activity despite a well-maintained libido when compared to placebo *(49)*. On the other

Table 2 Role of Androgen Insufficiency in Male Sexual Function: Clinical Evidence

Erectile function *(47–49,50,56)*	• Use of LHRH agonists causes ED.
	• Anti-androgens result in some degree of ED.
Sexual desire *(48–50,56)*	• Patients using LHRH agonists may have some degree of desire preservation.
	• Anti-androgens reduce sexual activity, although some patients will maintain some libido.
Nocturnal erections *(51–53)*	• LHRH agonist use results in a significant reduction in the frequency, duration, and rigidity of nocturnal erections.

hand, Rousseau et al. reported that approximately 70% of men with prostate cancer using anti-androgens experienced a significant reduction in their sexual desire *(51)*. In addition, Greenstein et al. reported that sexual desire and activity decreased following castration in men with prostate cancer *(57)*. Finally, Marumo et al. reported that in sexual active patients with prostate cancer treated with LHRH agonist, sexual desire, interest, and activity were significantly reduced *(52)*.

3. **Androgen Ablation and Nocturnal Erections (NPT):** Nocturnal erections in healthy men are common events (Table 2). However, aging and hypogonadal states have been associated with a decreased nocturnal erections. The mechanisms by which androgens modulate NPT activity are poorly understood. Marumo et al. reported that men with prostate cancer treated with LHRH agonists experienced a significant reduction in the frequency, duration, and rigidity of their nocturnal erections *(53)*. Kumamoto et al. reported a decrease in NPT in all patients treated with anti-androgens *(52)*. Finally, Betocchi et al. suggested that nocturnal erections are androgen dependent *(54)*.

4. **Androgen Replacement and Erectile Function:** Several investigators have suggested that testosterone treatment of hypogonadal men provides short-term or no improvement in erectile function *(55,56)* (Table 3). In addition, Christ-Crain et al. found no correlation between hypogonadal symptoms and testosterone levels *(58)*. However, Ojumo and Dobs suggested that ED is a common symptom in hypogonadal men and testosterone treatment improved erectile responses *(59)*. Kratzik et al. reported that patients with very low androgen levels (bioavailable testosterone <1 ng/mL) had 3 times the risk of severe ED when compared to men with bioavailable testosterone greater than 1 ng/mL *(60)*. Svartberg et al. reported that testosterone administration in men with COPD was associated with better erectile function and quality of life *(61)*. More importantly, Albrecht-Betancourt et al. suggested that testosterone treatment of hypogonadal men with ED is effective, especially in younger and healthier men *(62)*.

5. **Androgen Replacement and Nocturnal Erections:** Carani et al. reported that hypogonadal men treated with testosterone experienced a significant increase in NPT activity while Foresta et al. reported normalization of NPT activity after testosterone treatment *(63,64)* (Table 3). Schiavi et al. investigated the relationship between hormones (LH, estradiol, prolactin, total testosterone) and NPT activity in healthy aging men and found that only bioavailable testosterone correlated with NPT activity *(65)*.

6. **Androgen Replacement in Men with ED Refractory to PDE5 Inhibitors:** Aversa et al. studied 52 men with erectile dysfunction free of cardiovascular risk factors and found that resistive index values during penile duplex Doppler correlated with free testosterone suggesting that testosterone modulates smooth muscle relaxation and erectile function *(66)* (Table 3). More interestingly, Aversa et al. in a subsequent study found that testosterone replacement in men with ED who failed sildenafil treatment (100 mg on 6 consecutive attempts) was able to improve erectile function *(67)*. These findings have been further verified by other investigators *(68,69)*. Guay et al. reported that decreasing levels of testosterone

Table 3 Role of Androgen Replacement in Male Sexual Function: Clinical Evidence

Erectile function *(46,58–61)*	• ED is a common event in men with hypogonadism.
	• Testosterone improves some aspects of erectile function.
	• T replacement in hypogonadal men improves desire, frequency of successful intercourse, and overall sexual satisfaction.
Nocturnal erections *(62–64)*	• Hypogonadal men treated with testosterone experience increased NPT activity.
PDE5 inhibitor-refractory patients *(22,65–69)*	• There may be a correlation between testosterone levels and erectile hemodynamic parameters.
	• Testosterone supplementation of hypogonadal men who have failed PDE5i results in improved response.
	• Decreasing levels of testosterone negatively predict response to PDE5 inhibitors.

negatively predict response to PDE5 inhibitors *(70)*. These clinical data correlate with Traish et al. findings in preclinical studies *(15)*.

7. **Dose–Response Relationship Between Testosterone and Erectile Function:** A recent clinical study by Zitzmann et al. reported that a threshold for androgen exists for the various androgen dependent functions *(71)*. It was clearly demonstrated that erectile function requires the lowest threshold among all others.

5 Conclusions

The literature supports that androgen ablation results in a decrease of sexual desire, nocturnal erections, erectile function, and overall sexual satisfaction. More importantly, androgen therapy results in a moderate improvement in sexual function. These observations are particularly important in men with prostate cancer, since androgen ablation is the main treatment option for men with advanced prostate cancer and a critical component of radiation therapy for localized prostate cancer. In addition, many men after successful treatment for localized prostate cancer are severely crippled by an androgen insufficiency state.

References

1. Traish, A., and Kim, N. (2005 Nov) The physiological role of androgens in penile erection: regulation of corpus cavernosum structure and function. *J. Sex. Med.* **2**(6), 759–70.
2. Saenz de Tejada, I., Goldstein, I., Blanco, R., et al. (1985) Smooth muscle of the corpora cavernosae: role in penile erection. *Surg. Forum.* **36,** 623–624.
3. de Groat, W.C., and Steers, W.D. (1988) Neuroanatomy and neurophysiology of penile erection. In: Tanagho, E.A., Lue, T.F., and McClue, R.D., eds. *Contemporary Management of Impotence and Infertility.* Baltimore: Williams & Wilkins, pp. 3–27.

4. Blanco, R., Saenz de Tejada, I., Goldstein, I., et al. (1988) Cholinergic neurotransmission in human corpus cavernosum. II. Acetylcholine synthesis. *Am. J. Physiol.* **254,** H468–H472.
5. Ignarro, L.J., Bush, P.A., Buga, G.M., et al. (1990) Nitric oxide and cyclic GMP formation upon electrical field stimulation cause relaxation of corpus cavernosum smooth muscle. *Biochem. Biophys. Res. Comm.* **170,** 843–850.
6. Goldstein, I., Lue, T.F., Padma-Nathan, H. et al. (1998) Oral sildenafil in the treatment of erectile dysfunction. Sildenafil Study Group. *N. Engl. J. Med.* **338,** 1397–1404.
7. Dorfman, R.I., and Shipley, R.A. (1956) *Androgens: Biochemistry, Physiology, and Clinical Significance.* New York: John Wiley & Sons, Inc.
8. Shen, R., Lin, M.C., Sadeghi, F., Swerdloff, R.S., Rajfer, J., and Gonzalez-Cadavid, N.F. (1996) Androgens are not major down-regulators of androgen receptor levels during growth of the immature rat penis. *J. Steroid Biochem. Mol. Biol.* **57,** 301–313.
9. Gonzalez-Cadavid, N., Vernet, D., Fuentes, N.A., Rodriguez, J.A., Swerdloff, R.S., and Rajfer, J. (1993) Up-regulation of the levels of androgen receptor and its mRNA by androgens in smooth-muscle cells from rat penis. *Mol. Cell Endocrinol.* **90,** 219–229.
10. Lugg, J.A., Rajfer, J., and Gonzalez-Cadavid, N.F. (1995) Dihydrotestosterone is the active androgen in the maintenance of nitric oxide-mediated penile erection in the rat. *Endocrinology* **136,** 1495–1501.
11. Seo, S.I., Kim, S.W., and Paick, J.S. (1999) The effects of androgen on penile reflex, erectile response to electrical stimulation and penile NOS activity in the rat. *Asian J. Androl.* **1,** 169–174.
12. Choi, S.K., Han, S.W., Kim, D.H., and de Lignieres, B. (1993) Transdermal dihydrotestosterone therapy and its effects on patients with microphallus. *J. Urol.* **150,** 657–660.
13. Charmandari, E., Dattani, M.T., Perry, L.A., Hindmarsh, P.C., and Brook, C.G. (2001) Kinetics and effect of percutaneous administration of dihydrotestosterone in children. *Horm. Res.* **56,** 177–181.
14. Saenz de Tejada I. (2002) Molecular mechanisms for the regulation of penile smooth muscle contractility. *Int. J. Impot. Res.* **14**(Suppl 1):S6–S10.
15. Traish, A.M., Park, K., Dhir, V., Kim, N.N., Moreland, R.B., and Goldstein, I. (1999) Effects of castration and androgen replacement on erectile function in a rabbit model. *Endocrinology* **140,** 1861–1868.
16. Traish, A.M., Munarriz, R., O'Connell, L., Choi, S., Kim, S.W., Kim, N.N., Huang, Y.H., and Goldstein, I. (2003) Effects of medical and surgical castration on erectile function in an animal model. *J. Androl.* **24,** 381–387.
17. Rogers, R.S., Graziottin, T.M., Lin, C.M., Kan, Y.W., and Lue, T. (2003) Intracavernosal vascular endothelial growth factor (VEGF) injection and adeno-associated virus- mediated VEGF gene therapy prevent and reverse venogenic erectile dysfunction in rats. *Int. J. Impot. Res.* **15,** 26–37.
18. Meusburger, S.M., and Keast, J.R. (2001) Testosterone and nerve growth factor have distinct but interacting effects on structure and neurotransmitter expression of adult pelvic ganglion cells in vitro. *Neuroscience* **108,** 331–340.
19. Keast, J.R., Gleeson, R.J., Shulkes, A., and Morris, M.J. (2002) Maturational and maintenance effects of testosterone on terminal axon density and neuropeptide expression in the rat vas deferens. *Neuroscience* **112,** 391–398.
20. Giuliano, F., Tostain, J., and Rossi, D. (2004) Testosterone and male sexuality: basic research and clinical data. *Prog. Urol.* **14,** 783–790.
21. Baba, K., Yajima, M., Carrier, S., Akkus, E., Reman, J., Nunes, L., Lue, T.F., and Iwamoto, T. (2000a) Effect of testosterone on the number of NADPH diaphorase-stained nerve fibers in the rat corpus cavernosum and dorsal nerve. *Urology* **56,** 533–538.
22. Shabsigh, R., Kaufman, J.M., Steidle, C., and Padma-Nathan, H. (2004 Aug) Randomized study of testosterone gel as adjunctive therapy to sildenafil in hypogonadal men with erectile dysfunction who do not respond to sildenafil alone. *J. Urol.* **172**(2), 658–663.
23. Jevtich, M., Khawand, N.Y., and Vidic, B. (1990) Clinical significance of ultrastructural findings in the corpus cavernosa of normal and impotent men. *J. Urol.* **143,** 289–293.

24. Nehra, A., Goldstein, I., Pabby, A., Nugent, M., Huang, Y.H., de las Morenas, A., Krane, R.J., Udelson, D., Saenz de Tejada, I., and Moreland, R.B. (1996) Mechanisms of venous leakage: a prospective clinicopathological correlation of corporeal function and structure. *J. Urol.* **156,** 1320–1329.

25. Wespes, E., Schiffmann, S., Depierreux, M., Vanderhaegan, J.J., and Schulman, C.C. (1990) Is cavernovenous leakage related to a reduction of intracavernous smooth muscle fibers? *Int. J. Impot. Res.* **2,** 30.

26. Traish, A.M., Toselli, P., Jeong, S.J., and Kim, N.N. (2005) Adipocyte accumulation in penile corpus cavernosum of the orchiectomized rabbit: a potential mechanism for veno-occlusive dysfunction in androgen deficiency. *J. Androl.* **26,** 242–248.

27. Bhasin, S., Taylor, W.E., Singh, R., Artaza, J., Sinha-Hikim, I., Jasuja, R., Choi, H., and Gonzalez-Cadavid, N.F. (2003) The mechanisms of androgen effects on body composition: mesenchymal pluripotent cell as the target of androgen action. *J. Gerontol.* **58A,** 1103–1110.

28. Singh, R., Artaza, J.N., Taylor, W.E., Gonzalez-Cadavid, N.F., and Bhasin, S. (2003) Androgens stimulate myogenic differentiation and inhibit adipogenesis in C3H 10T1/2 pluripotent cells through an androgen receptor-mediated pathway. *Endocrinology* **144,** 5081–5088.

29. Corradi, L.S., Goes, R.M., Carvalho, H.F., and Taboga, S.R. (2004) Inhibition of 5a-reductase activity induces stromal remodeling and smooth muscle de-differentiation in adult gerbil ventral prostate. *Differentiation* **72,** 198–208.

30. Baba, K., Yajima, M., Carrier, S., Morgan, D.M., Nunes, L., Lue, T.F., and Iwamoto, T. (2000) Delayed testosterone replacement restores nitric oxide synthase-containing nerve fibers and the erectile response in rat penis. *BJU Int.* **85,** 953–958.

31. Lugg, J., Ng, C., Rajfer, J., and Gonzalez-Cadavid, N. (1996) Cavernosal nerve stimulation in the rat reverses castration-induced decrease in penile NOS activity. *Am. J. Physiol.* **271,** E354–E361.

32. Zvara, P., Sioufi, R., Schipper, H.M., Begin, L.R., and Brock, G.B. (1995) Nitric oxide mediated erectile activity is a testosterone dependent event: A rat erection model. *Int. J. Impot. Res.* **7,** 209–219.

33. Garban, H., Marquez, D., Cai, L., Rajfer, J., and Gonzalez-Cadavid, N.F. (1995) Restoration of normal adult penile erectile response in aged rats by long-term treatment with androgens. *Biol. Reprod.* **53,** 1365–1372.

34. Penson, D.F., Ng, C., Cai, L., Rajfer, J., and Gonzalez-Cadavid, N.F. (1996) Androgen and pituitary control of penile nitric oxide synthase and erectile function in the rat. *Biol. Reprod.* **55,** 567–574.

35. Penson, D.F., Ng, C., Rajfer, J., and Gonzalez-Cadavid, N.F. (1997) Adrenal control of erectile function and nitric oxide synthase in the rat penis. *Endocrinology* **138,** 3925–3932.

36. Shen, Z., Chen, Z., Lu, Y., Chen, F., and Chen, Z. (2000) Relationship between gene expression of nitric oxide synthase and androgens in rat corpus cavernosum. *Chin. Med. J. (Engl)* **113,** 1092–1095.

37. Marin, R., Escrig, A., Abreu, P., and Mas, M. (1999) Androgen dependent nitric oxide release in rat penis correlates with levels of constitutive nitric oxide synthase isoenzymes. *Biol. Reprod.* **61,** 1012–1016.

38. Reilly, C.M., Zamorano, P., Stopper, V.S., and Mills, T.M. (1997) Androgenic regulation of NO availability in rat penile erection. *J. Androl.* **18,** 110–115.

39. Schirar, A., Bonnefond, C., Meusnier, C., and Devinoy, E. (1997) Androgens modulate nitric oxide synthase messenger ribonucleic acid expression in neurons of the major pelvic ganglion in the rat. *Endocrinology* **138,** 3093–3102.

40. Park, K.H., Kim, S.W., Kim, K.D., and Paick, J.S. (1999) Effects of androgens on the expression of nitric oxide synthase mRNAs in rat corpus cavernosum. *BJU Int.* **83,** 327–333.

41. Reilly, C.M., Stopper, V.S., and Mills, T.M. (1997) Androgens modulate the alpha-adrenergic responsiveness of vascular smooth muscle in the corpus cavernosum. *J. Androl.* **18,** 26–31.

42. Moreland, R.B., Goldstein, I., Kim, N.N., et al. (1999) Sildenafil citrate, a selective phospho-diesterase type 5 inhibitor: research and clinical implications in erectile dysfunction. *Trends Endocrinol. Metab.* **10**, 97–104.

43. Morelli, A., Filippi, S., Mancina, R., Luconi, M., Vignozzi, L., Marini, M., Orlando, C., Van-nelli, G.B., Aversa, A., Natali, A., Forti, G., Giorgi, M., Jannini, E.A., Ledda, F., and Maggi, M. (2004) Androgens regulate phosphodiesterase type 5 expression and functional activity in corpora cavernosa. *Endocrinology* **145**, 2253–2263.

44. Zhang, X.H., Morelli, A., Luconi, M., Vignozzi, L., Filippi, S., Marini, M., Vannelli, G.B., Mancina, R., Forti, G., and Maggi, M. (2005) Testosterone regulates PDE5 expression and in vivo responsiveness to tadalafil in rat corpus cavernosum. *Eur. Urol.* **47**, 409–416.

45. Zhang, X.H., Morelli, A., Luconi, M., Vignozzi, L., Filippi, S., Marini, M., Vannelli, G.B., Mancina, R., Forti, G., and Maggi, M. (2005 Mar) Testosterone regulates PDE5 expres-sion and in vivo responsiveness to tadalafil in rat corpus cavernosum. *Eur. Urol.* **47**(3), 409–416.

46. Armagan, A., Kim, N.N., Goldstein, I., and Traish, A.M. (2006 Jul–Aug) Dose-response rela-tionship between testosterone and erectile function: evidence for the existence of a critical threshold. *J. Androl.* **27**(4), 517–526.

47. Isidori, A.M., Giannetta, E., Gianfrilli, D., Greco, E.A., Bonifacio, V., Aversa, A., Isidori, A., Fabbri, A., and Lenzi, A. (2005 Oct) Effects of testosterone on sexual function in men: results of a meta-analysis. *Clin. Endocrinol. (Oxford)* **63**(4), 381–394.

48. Peters, C.A., and Walsh, P.C. (1987) The effect of nafarelin acetate, a luteinizing-hormone-releasing hormone agonist, on benign prostatic hyperplasia. *N. Engl. J. Med.* **317**, 599–604.

49. Eri, L.M., and Tveter, K.J. (1994) Safety, side effects and patient acceptance of the luteinizing hormone releasing hormone agonist leuprolide in treatment of benign prostatic hyperplasia. *J. Urol.* **152**, 448–452.

50. Eri, L.M., and Tveter, K.J. (1994) Safety, side effects and patient acceptance of the antiandro-gen Casodex in the treatment of benign prostatic hyperplasia. *Eur. Urol.* **26**, 219–226.

51. Rousseau, L., Dupont, A., Labrie, F., and Couture, M. (1988) Sexuality changes in prostate cancer patients receiving antihormonal therapy combining the antiandrogen flutamide with medical (LHRH agonist) or surgical castration. *Arch. Sex. Behav.* **17**, 87–98.

52. Marumo, K., Baba, S., and Murai, M. (1999) Erectile function and nocturnal penile tumescence in patients with prostate cancer undergoing luteinizing hormone-releasing hormone agonist therapy. *Int. J. Urol.* **6**, 19–23.

53. Kumamoto, Y., Yamaguchi, Y., Sato, Y., Suzuki, R., Tanda, H., Kato, S., Mori, K., Matsumoto, H., Maki, A., Kadono, M., et al. (1990) [Effects of anti-androgens on sexual function. Double-blind comparative studies on allylestrenol and chlormadinone acetate Part I: Nocturnal penile tumescence monitoring]. *Hinyokika Kiyo.* **36**, 213–226.

54. Bettocchi, C., Palumbo, F., Cormio, L., Ditonno, P., Battaglia, M., and Selvaggi, F.P. (2004) The effects of androgen depletion on human erectile function: a prospective study in male-to-female transsexuals. *Int. J. Impot. Res.* **16**, 544–546.

55. Handelsman, D.J., and Zajac, J.D. (2004) Androgen deficiency and replacement therapy in men. *Med. J. Aust.* **180**, 529–535.

56. Mulhall, J.P., Valenzuela, R., Aviv, N., and Parker, M. (2004) Effect of testosterone supplemen-tation on sexual function in hypogonadal men with erectile dysfunction. *Urology* **63**, 348–353.

57. Greenstein, A., Plymate, S.R., and Katz, P.G. (1995) Visually stimulated erection in castrated men. *J. Urol.* **153**, 650–652.

58. Christ-Crain, M., Mueller, B., Gasswer, T.C., Kraenzlin, M., Trummler, M., Huber, P., Meier, C. (2004) Is there a clinical relevance of partial androgen deficiency of the aging male? *J. Urol.* **172**, 624–627.

59. Ojumu, A., and Dobs, A.S. (2003) Is hypogonadism a risk factor for sexual dysfunction. *J. Androl.* **24**, S46-S51.

60. Kratzik, C.W., Schatzl, G., Lunglmayr, G., Rucklinger, E., and Huber, J. (2005) The impact of age, body mass index and testosterone on erectile dysfunction. *J. Urol.* **174**, 240–243.

61. Svartberg, J. (2005) Should older men be treated with testosterone? *Tidsskr. Nor. Laegeforen.* **125,** 879–882.
62. Albrecht-Betancourt, M., Hijazi, R.A., and Cunningham, G.R. (2004) Androgen replacement in men with hypogonadism and erectile dysfunction. *Endocrine* **23,** 143–148.
63. Carani, C., Granata, A.R., Bancroft, J., and Marrama, P. (1995) The effects of testosterone replacement on nocturnal penile tumescence and rigidity and erectile response to visual erotic stimuli in hypogonadal men. *Psychoneuroendocrinology* **20,** 743–753.
64. Foresta, C., Coretta, N., Rosatto, M., Garolla, A., and Ferlin, A. (2004) Role of androgens in erectile function. *J. Urol.* **171,** 2358–2362.
65. Schiavi, R.C., White, D., Mandeli, J., and Schreiner-Engel, P. (1993) Hormones and nocturnal penile tumescence in healthy aging men. *Arch. Sex. Behav.* **22,** 207–215.
66. Aversa, A., Isidori, A.M., De Martino, M.U., Caprio, M., Fabbrini, E., Rocchietti-March, M., Frajese, G., and Fabbri, A. (2000) Androgens and penile erection: evidence for a direct relationship between free testosterone and cavernous vasodilation in men with erectile dysfunction. *Clin. Endocrinol. (Oxford)* **53,** 517–522.
67. Aversa, A., Isidori, A.M., Spera, G., Lenzi, A., and Fabri, A. (2003) Androgens improve cavernous vasodilatation and response to sildenafil in patients with erectile dysfunction. *Clin. Endo.* **58,** 632–638.
68. Amar, E., Grivel, T., Hamidi, K., Lemaire, A., and Giuliano, F. (2005) Ageing men's sexual functions decline and the erectile dysfunction (ED) increase. *Prog. Urol.* **15,** 6–9.
69. Shamloul, R., Ghanem, H., Fahmy, I., El-Meleigy, A., Ashoor, S., Elnashaar, A., Kamel, I. (2005) Testosterone therapy can enhance erectile function response to sildenafil in patients with PADAM: a pilot study. J. Sex. Med. **2,** 559–564.
70. Guay, A.T., Perez, J.B., Jacobson, J., and Newton, R.A. (2001) Efficacy and safety of sildenafil citrate for treatment of erectile dysfunction in a population with associated organic risk factors. *J. Androl.* **22,** 793–797.
71. Zitzmann, M., Faber, S., and Nieschlag, E. (2006) Association of specific symptoms and metabolic risks with serum testosterone in older men. *J. Clin. Endocrinol. Metab.* **91,** 4335–4343.

Chapter 12
The Utility of PDE5 Inhibitors After Radical Prostatectomy

Andrea Salonia, Alberto Briganti, Andrea Gallina, and Francesco Montorsi

Abstract Radical prostatectomy of any form (open, laparoscopic, or robotic) has become a widely performed procedure for patients with clinically localized prostate cancer. This procedure may be associated with treatment-specific sequelae affecting health-related quality of life, with urinary incontinence and erectile dysfunction being the most prevalent. The importance of postoperative erectile dysfunction has assumed greater importance in recent years, because the diagnosis of prostate cancer is becoming ever more frequent in younger patients, who are motivated to preserve their sexual function and the couple's sexual health. Phosphodiesterase type 5 inhibitor therapy is the most frequently used first-line, on-demand treatment for patients who have undergone radical prostatectomy, reaching the highest effectiveness in patients younger than 65 years of age who were preoperatively objectively fully potent and surgically treated with a nerve-sparing anatomic approach to ensure preservation of at least one neurovascular bundle. Although recent evidence suggests the presence of residual erectile function as early as the first night after catheter removal when a nerve-sparing procedure has been done, data have also suggested that some time after radical prostatectomy is needed for the best response to on-demand phosphodiesterase type 5 inhibitors. Pharmacological prophylaxis with phosphodiesterase type 5 inhibitors may have a significantly expanding role in future strategies aimed at preserving postoperative erectile function.

We used Ovid and PubMed (updated April 2007) to conduct an electronic literature search on Medline that included peer-reviewed English-language studies of phosphodiesterase type 5 inhibitor use for either the recovery of erectile function or the treatment of postoperative erectile dysfunction in patients who underwent radical prostatectomy.

From: *Current Clinical Urology* Series, *Sexual Function in the Prostate Cancer Patient*
Edited by John P. Mulhall, DOI 10.1007/978-1-60327-555-2_12,
© Humana Press, a part of Springer Science+Business Media, LLC 2009

Keywords Erectile dysfunction; radical prostatectomy; sildenafil; tadalafil; vardenafil.

1 Introduction

Radical prostatectomy (RP) is a widely performed procedure for patients with clinically localized prostate cancer (pCa) and a life expectancy of at least 10 years *(1–6)*. This procedure may be associated with treatment-specific sequelae affecting health-related quality of life *(7,8)*, which is increasingly important because the diagnosis of pCa is becoming ever more frequent in younger patients. Such patients are motivated to preserve their sexual function and the couple's sexual health and, therefore, are candidates for a bilateral nerve-sparing (BNS) procedure. Research in post-RP recovery indicates that approximately 25–75% of men experience postoperative erectile dysfunction (ED) *(9–14)*. This broad range of postoperative erectile function (EF) impairment can be attributed to several study design factors, including differences in baseline tumor and sexual health sample characteristics, surgical technique, surgeons' surgical volumes, length of follow-up (FU) from surgery, and the quality of study methodologies in assessing both prevalence and severity of male ED *(9,15–17)*.

The pioneering work by Walsh and Donker *(18)* significantly contributed to the understanding of the functional and surgical anatomy of the prostate and still represents the cornerstone for the subsequent development of the anatomic RP technique. This technique promotes optimal cancer removal while preserving the integrity of the anatomical structures that form the basis of urinary continence and EF *(19–24)*.

Historically, patients complaining of postoperative ED had options that increased the likelihood of obtaining valid erections for satisfactory sexual intercourse, including intracavernous injections, urethral microsuppository, vacuum device therapy, and penile implants. However, the advent of the phosphodiesterase type 5 inhibitors (PDE5i), given their demonstrated efficacy, ease of use, good tolerability, excellent safety, and positive impact on patients' quality of life, has clearly revolutionized the management of this medical condition. At present, PDE5i represent the first-line oral pharmacotherapy for the treatment of post-RP ED in patients who underwent either a unilateral nerve-sparing (UNS) or BNS surgical approach. Not surprisingly patients and their partners prefer this least invasive option for treating post-RP ED *(25)*. PDE5i have the greatest effectiveness in patients who have undergone a rigorous NS procedure.

We used Ovid and PubMed (updated April 2007) to conduct an electronic literature search on Medline that included peer-reviewed English-language articles. We analyzed those studies that investigated the use of PDE5i for the recovery of EF and the treatment of ED in patients who underwent RP. This review critically evaluates the use of the three PDE5i in this challenging ED population: sildenafil, the first FDA- and EMEA-approved PDE5i launched on the market; tadalafil; and vardenafil. We also evaluate data suggesting the role of the three compounds for the treatment and prophylaxis of post-RP ED. Due to the substantial heterogeneity of outcome measures and FU intervals in case studies, we did not apply meta-analytic techniques to the data.

1.1 Sildenafil

Sildenafil citrate is a highly potent, orally active cyclic guanosine monophosphate (cGMP)-specific PDE5i, which acts as a peripheral conditioner treatment of ED of broad-spectrum etiology *(26,27)*.

Phosphodiesterases catalyze the hydrolysis of the second messengers, cyclic adenosine monophosphate (cAMP) and cGMP, which are involved in the signal pathways of cavernous smooth muscle (SM). The accumulation of cGMP sets in motion a cascade of events at the intracellular level that induces the loss of contractile tone of the vessels at the penile level. Many neurotransmitters activate guanylate cyclase, which catalyzes the conversion of guanosine triphosphate (GTP) to cGMP and subsequently triggers relaxation by lowering cytosolic Ca^{2+}. Thus, SM relaxation derives from the resumption of a precontractile state accomplished by lowering cytosolic Ca^{2+} or decreasing the sensitivity of the contractile machinery to Ca^{2+} *(27)*. Phosphodiesterase type 5 constitutes the majority of the cGMP hydrolytic activity in corpora cavernosa (CC) SM cells and, functionally, the two isoforms PDE3A and PDE5A seem to be the most important *(24)*. Therefore, as a class of agents, PDE5i act within the SM cells by inhibiting PDE5, finally providing SM relaxation and an erection by allowing the CC to be filled by blood for an adequate time span. In both animal models and in humans, many in vivo and in vitro studies have demonstrated an essential role for nitric oxide (NO) in promoting the formation of cGMP and other pathways finally attaining erection of the penis *(24)*.

1.1.1 Pharmacology and Pharmacokinetics

After oral administration, sildenafil is rapidly absorbed with an absolute bioavailability of 40%. Time to peak plasma concentration (T_{max}) after oral absorption in the fasting state ranges between 30 and 120 min (median, 60 min), but a high-fat meal increases the T_{max} by 60 min and reduces the peak plasma concentration by about 30%. Otherwise, from a clinical point of view the onset of efficacy frequently is optimal if sildenafil is taken on an empty stomach *(27)*. The terminal half-life ($T_{1/2}$) of sildenafil is 3–5 h. Sildenafil is metabolized predominantly at the hepatic level by four cytochromes: CYP3A4, -2C9, -2C19, and -2D6 *(27)*. Inherent to its pharmacology, the coadministration of sildenafil and CYP3A4 inhibitors may lead to increased plasma concentrations of the compound. This may, in turn, lead to enhanced pharmacological and adverse events (AEs) commonly associated with sildenafil, such as headache, flushing, dyspepsia, and visual changes *(27)*.

1.1.2 Sildenafil as an On-Demand Treatment Compound: Efficacy in Post-RP Patients

Post-RP patients represent a challenging category for urologists. Indeed, even patients undergoing BNS RP often experience impairment of erections in the early postoperative period. This outcome has been related to the development of neuropraxia, which appears to be caused by some damage to the cavernosal nerves, which inevitably occurs during the excision of the prostate, even in the hands of the highest-volume surgeons. Absence of early postoperative erections is associated with poor corporeal oxygenation, which may facilitate the development of corporeal fibrosis, ultimately leading to veno-occlusive dysfunction *(28,29)*. The role of SM apoptosis also has been considered in the pathophysiology of post-RP ED *(30)*. Preliminary findings have also suggested postoperative arterial insufficiency to the CC as a significant etiological cofactor in post-RP ED *(31–35)*. In support of the role of an adequate arterial inflow as a key factor in preserving a sufficient post-RP EF, Rogers et al. *(36)* highlighted the importance of preserving accessory pudendal arteries while performing a BNS RP to shorten the interval to recovery after RP.

As mentioned earlier, the release of NO is necessary to allow sildenafil to exert its action. Because NO is mainly released from cavernosal nerve terminals, a beneficial effect of sildenafil should be expected only in patients treated with some degree of NS RP. Since its introduction in 1998, several studies have shown that sildenafil is significantly efficacious in patients who have undergone an NS procedure, and several success predictors have been clearly outlined *(14,27,28,37–44)*. Historically, these include patient's age (i.e., the younger the patient the better the response to sildenafil, with the < 60 years age group responding the best) and rigorous preservation of the neurovascular bundles *(44,45)*. Clinically, those men who report some degree of spontaneous penile tumescence after an NS RP are the most likely to respond to sildenafil. A more recent report by Raina et al. *(46)* emphasized these former criteria and identified several factors that are significantly associated with a successful outcome of on-demand sildenafil therapy after RP, including age < 65 years, the surgical preservation of at least one neurovascular bundle, an adequate interval from surgery to sildenafil use (i.e., more than 6 months), and good EF preoperatively (i.e., a Sexual Health Inventory for Men [SHIM] score ≥ 15). We consider preoperative EF a fundamental matter in assessing postoperative response to oral compounds, having recently demonstrated that a subjective, self-reported preoperative full potency is not equal to an objective assessment with validated instruments, thus potentially reducing the final response rates to PDE5i *(15–17)*. Moreover, in their univariate and multivariate logistic regression analyses, Wille et al. *(47)* identified preoperative EF (as assessed with the SHIM) as a significant predictor even of postoperative urinary incontinence in patients who underwent a retropubic RP (RRP); however, age and NS RP did not predict postoperative urinary incontinence.

Raina et al. reported the long-term results of sildenafil use in post-RP ED patients *(46)*. Their study enrolled 91 patients stratified according to the type of RP procedure (53 BNS, 12 UNS, and 26 non-NS). At least 3 months after surgery, all patients were prescribed sildenafil at the recommended, user-friendly starting dose of 50 mg, which was up-titrated to 100 mg if participants did not obtain a satisfactory response. At the 12-month assessment performed by means of the SHIM and Erectile Dysfunction Inventory of Treatment Satisfaction (EDITS) *(48)* questionnaires, 53% of all patients reported having achieved successful vaginal intercourse, and this value was 72% in those patients treated with a BNS approach. Moreover, at the 3-year FU assessment, 31 (72%) of the 43 patients who returned the questionnaires were still using sildenafil for sexual intercourse, with a variable degree of spontaneous partial erections. When the responses were stratified according to the neurovascular bundle status, the magnitude of improvement in SHIM score over time was greater in the BNS group than in the UNS and non-NS groups. These data supported the idea that most patients affected by post-RP ED who initially respond to sildenafil continue to do so and are satisfied with the treatment regimen.

Although largely accepted by the vast majority of the researchers across the world, these findings are not unequivocal. Shimizu et al. *(49)* retrospectively evaluated the postoperative rate of EF and the 25–100 mg sildenafil effectiveness rate in 48 post-NS RP Japanese men, according to their preoperative potency as defined by a validated questionnaire. As expected, they reported that the overall estimated recovery rates of spontaneous erection of any degree improved over time, being 51% at the 36-month FU and 94% at the 60-month assessment; sufficient erection to penetrate was registered only in BNS RP men. However, Shimizu et al. reported that for those men achieving any degree of erection, there was no significant difference between BNS RP and UNS RP. Sildenafil was reported to be effective in 69% of those patients without spontaneous erection, and thus classified as postoperative ED men. Sildenafil was effective regardless of the type of NS procedure, being effective in both the UNS and BNS RP patients. Surprisingly, sildenafil was also effective in 75% of those patients who reported preoperative ED. Based on their results, Shimizu et al. suggested that sildenafil may have been effective in those patients because their preoperative ED was mild and with a good response to the PDE5i even prior to the surgery. Moreover, they also hypothesized that if sildenafil was effective in ED men before RP, then an NS procedure becomes mandatory in order to maintain sildenafil effectiveness postoperatively, even in the UNS RP group *(49)*.

Studies have suggested that some time after surgery is needed to observe the best response to sildenafil *(19,40,42,46)*. Typically the response rate to sildenafil has been shown to increase as time passes after the procedure, with the best results seen from 12 to 24 months postoperatively *(14,19,40,42,45,46)*. In their very elegant prospective study, Hong et al. gathered data on patient satisfaction across time in a cohort of preoperatively fully potent PDE5i-naïve men, most of whom underwent a BNS RP and postoperatively used sildenafil *(40)*. The study group was stratified into five subgroups according to the length of time between surgery and the beginning of sildenafil treatment. Sildenafil promoted a significant improvement in EF, and overall 41% of men were very or somewhat satisfied with the oral compound as defined by the EDITS questionnaire. In addition, the subgroup analysis revealed a significant increase in the patient satisfaction rate with increasing time from surgery *(40)*.

The 100-mg dose is usually necessary in this particular patient group. In their cohort of post-RP patients treated with sildenafil, Zippe et al. *(44)* confirmed the significant role of NS surgery. In their study, the ability to achieve vaginal penetration (72% of the cases) was directly correlated with the spousal satisfaction rate (66%). Among the positive responders, 29% required only a 50-mg dose, but the remaining 71% required the maximum 100-mg dose for achieving valid erections *(44)*. More recently, we reported the functional outcome results in 42 patients undergoing a technical modification of the Walsh's anatomic open retropubic BNS RP *(20)*. As expected, participants regained normal EF (i.e., IIEF-EF domain score ≥ 26 *(50)*) linearly with time, reaching the greatest prevalence (52%) at the 6-month FU. All patients used PDE5i throughout the first 6 months postoperatively; 64% used PDE5i at the maximum dose (including 100 mg sildenafil) only on-demand prior to any sexual intercourse *(20)*. We also studied a sample of 51 selected PDE5i-naïve BNS RRP patients (mean age ± SD, 57.2 ± 4.3 years) *(51)*. Each subject was provided with eight 100-mg tablets and comprehensively instructed to use this maximum 100-mg dose on-demand at least 1 h prior to sexual intercourse for the first 4 months after surgery. Complete data were collected from 44 (86%) of the original patients; mean duration of the treatment was 35 days, with an average number of pill intake of 5.2 tablets (Table 1). No significant ($p = 0.057$) differences in terms of IIEF-EF domain scores were found between the preoperative and postoperative periods in this cohort of patients treated with 100 mg sildenafil. However, 3 (6%) of the 51 patients prematurely discontinued sildenafil because of AEs. Similarly, in their 3-year FU study, Raina et al. *(46)* reported that 72% of the original 43 patients were still using sildenafil, having been classified as "sildenafil-dependent," with a variable degree of partial erections. In addition, 31% of the sildenafil users up-titrated their dose to 100 mg, with no correlation between the frequency of use and the need to increase the dose. In the same long-term FU analysis, Raina et al. reported a dropout rate of 27%, mainly due to the return of natural erections sufficient for vaginal intercourse in 50% of the discontinuers, while lack of effectiveness was the reason for discontinuation in 5/12 men.

Therefore, the 100-mg dose is usually necessary in post-RP patients, although it has been suggested that the use of the off-label 150- and 200-mg doses of sildenafil might salvage patients not responding to the approved maximum dose *(52,53)*. This reinforces the absolute need for extensive patient counseling with regard to all the available therapies for ED.

Montorsi and McCullough *(54)* reported the results of a meta-analysis of English-language articles in Medline and Cancerlit published between 1998 and January 2004 and regarding primary, discrete data sets of post-RP patients with ED treated with sildenafil monotherapy. Eleven studies fulfilled the inclusion criteria; sample sizes ranged from 13 to 198 (mean age, 61 ± 3 years). Treatment durations were from 4 weeks (or more than four doses) to 12 months, and sildenafil dosing was in the recommended range (25–100 mg). The results of these studies demonstrated that in more than one-third of post-RP patients using sildenafil an erection sufficient for intercourse was achieved. Seven of the analyzed studies reported a response rate ranging from 14 to 53% for an end point consistent with the primary meta-analysis outcome (i.e., erection sufficient for vaginal intercourse), which corresponds to a 35% (95% CI, 24–48%) of combined estimated probability of response. Overall,

Table 1 PDE5i Response Rates in Patients Who Have Undergone Radical Prostatectomy

References	No. of pts	Drug	Nerve-sparing	Time from surgery (months)	Response rate	Method of assessment
(37)	18	Sildenafil 100 mg	Bilateral	N.D.	67% (intercourse)	The Cleveland Clinic post-prostatectomy questionnaire
(39)	84	Sildenafil 50–100 mg	Bilateral Unilateral	25 years	53% improved erection 40% improved ability for intercourse	IIEF SEP-3 SEP 4
(41)	170	Sildenafil 50–150 mg	Bilateral Unilateral	3–18	Overall 29% Age <55 (BNSRRP): 80% Age <55 (UNSRRP): 40%	Viagra (sildenafil citrate) questionnaire
(43)	69	Sildenafil 25–100 mg	Monthly non-NS	1.5–2.5	20%	Not validated questionnaire
(49)	13	Sildenafil 25–100	Bilateral Unilateral	27	69.2%	Not validated questionnaire
(20)	202	Tadalafil 20 mg	Bilateral	12–48	Successful penetration attempts 54% Successful intercourse attempts 41%.	IIEF SEP
(75)	287	Vardenafil 10–20 mg	Bilateral Unilateral	6–60	74% in men with mild to moderate ED 28% in men with severe ED	IIEF SEP-2 SEP-3 GAQ

the meta-analysis confirmed that there was strong evidence for a lower response rate after non-NS (range, 0–15%) versus NS procedures (range, 35–75%; combined OR, 12.1; 95% CI, 5.5–26.6). The odds of responding improved 12-fold with preservation of at least one neurovascular bundle. However, there was not sufficiently strong data to support a difference between response rates in patients who underwent UNS RP (range, 10–80%) and BNS RP (range, 46–72%; combined OR, 2.21; 95% CI, 0.75–6.54). Confirming the previously reported experiences of single centers, the meta-analysis showed that early treatment failure does not necessarily imply lack of subsequent efficacy after having waited a sufficient length of time after RP.

1.1.3   Safety of Sildenafil in Post-RP Patients

Safety and tolerability of sildenafil have been clearly demonstrated in multiple studies. AEs are usually transitory and of minor intensity; the discontinuation of sildenafil therapy due to AEs is very low in the broad-spectrum etiology ED population *(55)*. The most common AEs are headache, flushing (due to vasodilation), and dyspepsia (due to relaxation of the SM of the gastroesophageal sphincter with reflux). Transient visual symptoms, mainly disturbances of color vision, were reported predominantly at the 100-mg dose and temporally related to the time of peak plasma levels. The visual symptoms are due to transient inhibition of cGMP-specific PDE6, which is present in rods and cones of the retina. The safety profile results were also excellent in post-RP patients. Zippe et al. *(44)* reported that the most common drug-related AEs were transient headaches (29%), flushing (22%), dizziness (9%), dyspepsia (6%), and nasal congestion (5%), with an increased incidence of headache observed at the higher dose ($p = 0.04$). None of the patients in their series suffered from any serious cardiovascular effects. Similarly, the 3-year FU analysis of Raina et al. *(46)* showed that the most common AEs at that long-term assessment were headaches (12%), flushing (10%), and blue or blurred vision (2%). No patient dropped out because of AEs at the 3-year FU.

1.1.4   Sildenafil as a Prophylactic Treatment: Efficacy in Post-RP Patients

As previously detailed in this chapter, different pathophysiological theories of postoperative ED are currently being explored, including the concept of neuropraxia, impaired arterial inflow, and—probably even more important—tissue damage consequent to cavernous nerve injury and poor postoperative corporeal oxygenation. All these findings have clearly supported the application of prophylactic pharmacological regimens aimed at improving an earlier corporeal blood filling with consequent EF protection, i.e., preservation and rehabilitation *(14,56,57)*. Although the rationale for the use of the different treatment compounds as prophylaxis still is not completely understood and an optimal therapeutic regimen has not yet been established, the concept has been applied to PDE5i, which may be administered in a continuous regimen (i.e., either daily or ≥ 2 times weekly for rehabilitative treatment).

Recently, several studies have elucidated some mechanisms potentially involved in the activity of sildenafil (57–62), with postoperative preservation of intracorporeal SM content underlying all these studies. Schwartz et al. demonstrated that the early use of a high dose of sildenafil after RP was associated with preservation of SM content within human CC (58). The study enrolled 40 potent patients who underwent RRP and were subsequently treated either with daily 50 mg (group 1) or 100 mg (group 2) sildenafil for 6 months, starting from the day of catheter removal. Patients underwent percutaneous penile biopsy both preoperatively and 6 months after surgery. Although in group 1 there was no statistically significant change in the mean intracavernosal SM content between the pre- and postoperative measurements (51% and 53%, respectively), a statistically significant increase (43% vs. 57%; $p < 0.05$) was observed in group 2. Experimental data about the mechanisms underlying the chronic use of sildenafil have also been published (59). The effect of an 8-week treatment with 60 mg/kg/day sc sildenafil in male rats was assessed on electrically induced erectile response in vivo before and after an acute injection of sildenafil (0.3 mg/kg iv). Endothelial-dependent and endothelial-independent relaxation of strips of corpus cavernosum was examined in vitro and compared to cavernosal strips of untreated rats. The acetylcholine-induced endothelial relaxation was significantly enhanced in chronically sildenafil-treated rats as compared with the untreated animals. Behr-Roussel et al. speculated that chronic sildenafil administration might be able to up-regulate either muscarinic receptors or the transduction mechanisms leading to the activation of endothelial NO synthase (59). Moreover, functional in vivo evaluations showed that chronic administration of sildenafil significantly enhanced frequency-dependent erectile response and was associated with greater response to an acute injection of sildenafil in treated rats as compared with controls; this finding allowed researchers to exclude the presence of tachyphylaxis in chronically treated animals.

All of these findings support the rationale for using sildenafil chronically in BNS RP men. The administration of PDE5i at bedtime might facilitate the occurrence of nocturnal erections, which, in turn, are believed to have a natural protective role on the structural and functional properties of the CC (60). As previously debated, however, the recovery of EF can take up to 24 months after surgery (19). At the same time, it is important not to wait inactively until spontaneous erections are regained, as the lack of oxygenation of the CC can lead to further involutional atrophy as a consequence of increased SM fibrosis (29,56). In this context, Mulhall et al. (62) reported the results of a nonrandomized, prospective trial to assess the ability of postoperative early use of an erectogenic medication program to improve long-term spontaneous EF in a similar set of patients. Complete data were available for 58 men with preoperative functional erections who were challenged early postoperatively with oral sildenafil. Nonresponders were switched to intracavernosal injection therapy, and patients were instructed to inject three times a week. Data from men who were committed to rehabilitation were compared with those of 74 men of comparable age, comorbidity profile, intraoperative NS status, and postoperative erectile hemodynamics who did not follow the protocol but continued to be serially followed after RP. At 18 months post-RP, there were statistically significant differences between the two groups in the percentage of patients who were capable of having drug-free intercourse ($p < 0.001$), the mean erectile rigidity ($p < 0.01$), the mean IIEF-EF domain scores ($p < 0.01$), the percentage of patients with IIEF-EF ≥ 26 ($p < 0.01$), the percentage of patients responding to sildenafil ($p < 0.001$), and the time to become a sildenafil responder (9 ± 4 vs. 13 ± 3 months; $p = 0.02$).

To assess the organic penile integrity in 27 preoperatively sexually potent (as objectively assessed by the IIEF-5) patients, Bannowsky et al. *(57)* prospectively recorded nocturnal penile tumescence and rigidity during the acute phase (i.e., during the first night after removal of the catheter) after either UNS or BNS RP. On the night following catheter removal (i.e., postoperative days 7–14) a nocturnal penile tumescence and rigidity recording was made using the RigiScan device. Twenty-five (93%) patients showed one to five nocturnal erection events of greater than 70% for at least 10 min, which was significantly different than a control group of men submitted to a non-NS RP, for whom no nocturnal erections were recorded. These results demonstrated the presence of residual EF as early as the first night after catheter removal when a NS procedure was done.

In this context, Padma-Nathan et al. *(61)* reported on the prospective administration of daily bedtime 50 or 100 mg sildenafil, as compared with placebo, in preoperatively fully potent men undergoing BNS RP. Inclusion criteria included having a score of 8 on Q3 and Q4 of the IIEF combined. Four weeks after surgery patients were randomized to sildenafil or placebo, which was carried on nightly for 36 weeks. Eight weeks after cessation of the intervention (sildenafil vs. placebo), patients' spontaneous EF was assessed in a variety of ways including IIEF. Among other end points, a responder status required maintenance of the score of 8 on Q3 and Q4 of the IIEF combined. Of the participants receiving sildenafil 27% were responders versus only 4% ($p = 0.0156$) in the placebo group. Postoperative nocturnal penile tumescence and rigidity assessments confirmed that continuous sildenafil exposure promoted a higher rate being a responder compared to placebo. Although similar data are not yet available for tadalafil and vardenafil, we believe that there is no reason not to expect similar results with other PDE5i. Moreover, Padma-Nathan's unpublished preliminary experience provides the important message that daily PDE5i administration after NS RP may improve every surgeon's baseline results.

Despite the enthusiasm engendered by the above-mentioned results, the benefit induced by a continuous rehabilitative approach compared with an on-demand PDE5i treatment has not been confirmed. To this end, we prospectively studied a cohort of 80 patients submitted to BNS RRP with 12-month postoperative EF data *(63)*. Patients were selectively assigned to four groups: (1) no erection therapy; (2) on-demand intracavernosal injection therapy; (3) on-demand PDE5i; and (4) continuous PDE5i (either daily or every other day for 3 months). No significant difference in terms of average IIEF-EF domain score between patients who received on-demand versus continuous PDE5i was found at the 12-month postoperative FU. However, additional large randomized trials are needed to confirm the validity of these preliminary data.

Few objective data are available regarding the PDE5i discontinuation rate in patients after RP. Therefore, we analyzed real-life discontinuation data of 100 consecutive, age-comparable, preoperatively self-reported potent BNS RRP patients who received a PDE5i prescription at their discharge from the hospital *(64)*. Patients did not receive any specific counseling about the ED treatment aside from the standard instructions throughout the entire FU period, and they freely decided to use or not use any ED therapy. Thereafter, IIEF was compiled every 6 months postoperatively, and patients completed a semi-structured interview about the treatment adherence at the 18-month FU. Surprisingly, 49% of patients decided not to even begin any ED therapy. The remainder were subdivided into patients who preferred an on-demand PDE5i (36%) and men who decided to use a continuous PDE5i approach (15%). At the 18-month FU, the overall discontinuation rate from both treatment modalities was 73%. Treatment effect below expectations was the main reason for treatment dropout, followed by loss of interest in sex due to partners' causes. Results from this study show that roughly half of the patients preoperatively self-reporting to be fully potent and strongly motivated to maintain postoperative EF actually decided not to take any ED compound at the hospital discharge. Moreover, a significant proportion of inadequately counseled patients discontinued PDE5i treatment after BNS RRP. Thus, specific counseling on ED treatment modalities coupled with re-education of patients may represent key points in promoting reduction of the discontinuation rate *(63)*.

1.2 Tadalafil

Tadalafil is a potent orally active cGMP-specific PDE5i that acts as a peripheral conditioner treatment of ED of broad-spectrum etiology *(65,66)*.

1.2.1 Pharmacology and Pharmacokinetics

Tadalafil inhibits human recombinant PDE5 activity in vitro, with an IC_{50} of 1 nM *(67)*. With the exception of two PDE families (i.e., PDE6 and PDE11), tadalafil is at least 9000-fold selective for PDE5 inhibition over other PDEs *(65–68)*. Over a dose range of 2.5–20 mg, AUC increases proportionally with dose *(65,66)*. After oral administration of a 20-mg dose, tadalafil is readily absorbed with a median T_{max} of 2 h (range, 0.5–12.0) and mean peak plasma concentrations (C_{max}) of 378 ng/mL. Mean $T_{1/2}$ is 17.5 h *(66,67)*. A high-fat meal has no significant impact on tadalafil T_{max}, C_{max}, systemic exposure (AUC), or plasma half-life *(65,66)*. In daily dosing studies, steady-state plasma levels were achieved within 5 days, with AUC approximately 1.6 that of a single dose *(65,66)*.

Tadalafil is predominantly metabolized via CYP3A4. Lower doses of tadalafil should be considered when taken concomitantly with drugs that inhibit CYP3A4 activity. Tadalafil is well-tolerated with an efficacy profile that should provide effective treatment of ED in most men. Because tadalafil has an efficacy period longer than 36 h, together with its effectiveness and safety profile, this drug is an interesting adjunct to the armamentarium available to the physician taking care of ED patients. Tadalafil pharmacokinetics should guide the practicing physician in the best use of the drug.

1.2.2   Tadalafil as an On-Demand Treatment Option in Post-RP Patients

Based on the pathophysiological findings reported earlier in this chapter, PDE5i other than sildenafil should be considered for use in patients undergoing NS RP. The efficacy and safety of on-demand fixed-dose tadalafil (20 mg) were studied in 303 post-BNS RRP ED men from Europe and North America in a randomized, double-blind, placebo-controlled, multi-center study consisting of a 12-week treatment period (*69*). Patients were enrolled from 12 to 48 months following BNS RRP, to increase the possibility that the process of postoperative neuropraxia had subsided. Those patients who had evidence of postoperative penile tumescence (defined as the ability to achieve at least some erection in more than 50% of intercourse attempts) constituted a pre-specified subgroup for analysis, likely to have some residual cavernous nerve function and a higher chance to respond to tadalafil treatment. Previous experience with PDE5i was not considered as an exclusion criterion. Patients (mean age, 60 years) had a postoperative low-mean baseline IIEF-EF domain score (12.3–12.5); half of them (52%) had severe ED, while roughly 66% had evidence of postoperative drug-free penile tumescence. Of the randomized patients, 237 completed the study. Seventy-one percent of patients treated with tadalafil reported an improvement of their EF as compared with only 24% of those in the placebo group ($p < 0.001$). Overall, the IIEF-EF domain score was significantly ($p < 0.001$) higher after treatment with the active compound than with placebo (21 vs. 15, respectively). For all randomized patients mean $\pm$ SEM improvement in IIEF-EF domain score was 5 ± 0.5 versus 1 ± 0.6 with placebo ($p < 0.001$); this difference remained significant in patients with postoperative evidence of spontaneous penile erections ($p < 0.001$) but not in patients without such evidence ($p = 0.43$). In the post hoc analysis, significantly ($p < 0.001$) more tadalafil-treated patients attained normal scores on the IEEF-EF domain. A significantly larger group of tadalafil-treated patients also reported improved erections with successful intercourse attempts as compared with the placebo group (52% vs. 26%; $p < 0.001$). In addition, mean EDITS scores for patients treated with tadalafil were significantly greater than in placebo-treated patients (58 vs. 34; $p < 0.001$) and for the subgroup with post-RP drug-free tumescence (64 vs. 37; $p < 0.001$), indicating greater treatment satisfaction with the active compound.

Sixty-six patients dropped out of the trial; the most frequently reported reasons for early discontinuation were lack of effectiveness (tadalafil 8% vs. placebo 10%), AEs (tadalafil 5.5% vs. placebo 2%), and personal conflict or other personal decisions (tadalafil 2% vs. placebo 9%). To the best of our knowledge, there are no published long-term FU studies on the effectiveness and discontinuation rate in post-BNS RP ED patients treated with tadalafil.

1.2.3 Tadalafil as a Potentially Effective Prophylactic Approach in Post-RP Patients: Evidence from an Animal Model

Although no data supporting the usefulness of tadalafil as a prophylactic treatment in post-BNS RRP patients have been published, we believe that there is no reason not to expect results similar to those obtained with sildenafil and other PDE5i. For instance, Vignozzi et al. *(70)* reported the results of an animal study investigating whether chronic tadalafil may preserve bilateral cavernous neurotomy (BCN)-induced penile damage and hypo-oxygenation. The study evaluated the in vitro and ex vivo effects of 2 mg/kg/day tadalafil for 3 months in a rat model of BCN; they found that the BCN-induced massive hypoxia and decreased muscle/fiber ratio was completely restored by chronic tadalafil use. In their rat model, Vignozzi et al. also showed that hypoxic penis had an increased sensitivity to the relaxant effect of the NO donor sodium nitroprusside, whereas acute tadalafil (100 nM) did not amplify the effect. Similarly, PDE5 mRNA and protein were reduced in BCN penile tissues. By restoring PDE5, chronic tadalafil decreased sodium nitroprusside-induced relaxation and rescued sensitivity to acute tadalafil. In hypoxic penis, however, chronic tadalafil normalized neither acetylcholine hyporesponsiveness nor nNOS or eNOS expression. Based on these preliminary findings, the authors concluded that chronic tadalafil may restore some of the investigated BCN-induced alterations, including acute tadalafil efficacy *(70)*. Due to its unique pharmacokinetic properties, we feel that adequately designed randomized clinical trials are urgently needed to explore the potential application of tadalafil as a prophylactic approach in post-RP patients.

1.2.4 Safety of Tadalafil in Post-RP Patients

The safety and tolerability of tadalafil have been clearly demonstrated in multiple studies *(65,66)*, and the safety profile is high in post-RP patients as well. Patients enrolled in the above-mentioned Montorsi et al. trial reported significantly more headache (20.9% vs. 5.9%; $p < 0.001$), dyspepsia (13.4% vs. 5.9%; $p < 0.001$), and myalgia (6.5% vs. 0%; $p < 0.001$) in the tadalafil group as compared with the placebo group *(69)*. Non-serious AEs were reported in patients taking tadalafil, and the percentage of men reporting at least one severe AE with tadalafil was not statistically different from the rate reported by the placebo group (5% vs. 3%; $p = 0.55$). In addition, the dropout rate resulting from AEs was not statistically significant between groups (5.5% vs. 2.0%; $p = 0.231$).

1.3 Vardenafil

Vardenafil is the third highly selective, orally bioavailable, potent PDE5i *(71)*. Rapid onset and long-term reliability appear to be key features of vardenafil's clinical profile. These features may be a consequence of the high potency of vardenafil for PDE5 inhibition, and they provide patients with a high degree of convenience in the timing of dosing and sexual activity. Vardenafil provides reliable efficacy, with most men experiencing consistent improvement in EF during long-term use. Clinical studies have demonstrated that vardenafil is a well-tolerated and effective treatment for ED and represents a valuable therapy option for men with ED and their partners *(71–73)*.

1.3.1   Pharmacology and Pharmacokinetics

Vardenafil's chemical structure differs from those of sildenafil and tadalafil, reflecting its differing pharmacological properties. In vitro studies have shown that the potency of vardenafil in inhibiting PDE5 purified from human corpus cavernosum tissue was approximately 15–25-fold greater than that of sildenafil and 48-fold greater than that of tadalafil (IC_{50} values, 0.14, 3.5, and 6.74 nmol/L, respectively) *(68,71,74)*. Studies in men with ED showed that single doses of vardenafil (10–40 mg) were rapidly absorbed following oral administration, with C_{max} reached in some men within 15 min (median, 0.6–0.9 h) *(71,74)*. Mean C_{max} and AUC increased in a nearly dose-proportional manner. Vardenafil has a mean absolute bioavailability of 15%. The rate and extent of absorption were not altered when 20 mg of vardenafil was administered immediately after a typical meal (approximately 30% of calories as fat) compared with the fasting state. A high-fat meal (57% of calories as fat), however, reduced the rate of absorption (with an increase in T_{max} of 1 h) and reduced the C_{max} by 18%.

Based on our experience in the use of all three available PDE5i, it is wise to suggest to patients to initially use them on an empty stomach (at least 2 h after finishing a meal or pre-prandially) to maximize the therapeutic effect and optimize onset time. Responders are then routinely allowed to ingest these drugs irrespective of food or alcohol intake, with the possibility that the overall therapeutic effect may be reduced.

Because vardenafil is also predominantly metabolized by the hepatic enzyme CYP3A4, and to a lesser extent by CYP3A5 and CYP2C, inhibitors of these enzymes may reduce vardenafil clearance. Consequently, according to the product labeling concomitant use of vardenafil with potent CYP3A4 inhibitors is not recommended.

1.3.2   Vardenafil as an On-Demand Treatment Option in Post-RP Patients

In a multi-center, prospective, randomized, double-blind, placebo-controlled, parallel-group sponsored trial in the United States and Canada, the safety and efficacy of a 12-week regimen of fixed 10- and 20-mg doses of vardenafil were evaluated in 440 men with ED from 6 months to 5 years after NS RRP *(75)*. Overall, patients underwent surgery a mean of 1.7 years before entering the study, and most patients (73%) underwent BNS RRP. All enrolled patients had normal EF 6 months before surgery as objectively assessed with the IIEF-EF domain, but at immediately after surgery, mean EF domain score was roughly 9 and 70% of men had severe postoperative ED. Sildenafil failures were excluded from enrollment in the study. After 12 weeks, the IIEF-EF domain score, sexual encounter profile question 2 (SEP-2: Were you able to insert your penis into your partner's vagina?), SEP-3 (Did your erections last long enough to have successful intercourse?), and GAQ were significantly improved following vardenafil treatment relative to placebo. In men who had undergone BNS RRP, 71% experienced improved erections with 20 mg vardenafil, 60% with 10 mg vardenafil, and only 11% with placebo ($p < 0.0001$). Patients with residual post-RRP spontaneous EF experienced greater improvements in each of these efficacy parameters (75). A positive answer to the SEP-2 question was reported in 47 and 48% of patients using 10 and 20 mg vardenafil, respectively. A positive answer to the more challenging SEP-3 question was reported in 37 and 34% of patients using these doses, respectively (75). A post hoc analysis revealed that previous sildenafil use did not influence efficacy relative to sildenafil-naïve participants. More recently, Nehra et al. (76) demonstrated that both 10- and 20-mg doses of vardenafil were significantly ($p < 0.0009$) superior to placebo in improving the IIEF domains of intercourse satisfaction, orgasmic function, and overall satisfaction with sexual experience in the same group of patients who had previously undergone RRP (75). Moreover, significant improvements in the satisfaction rate with erection hardness were also demonstrated for each vardenafil dose as compared with placebo ($p < 0.0001$) (76).

1.3.3 Safety of Vardenafil in Post-RP Patients

Treatment with vardenafil is generally well-tolerated, although the incidence of treatment-emergent AEs increased with vardenafil dose. Similar to what has been observed for each PDE5-I, the most frequently reported drug-related AEs were headache (16 and 22% for vardenafil 10 and 20 mg, respectively, as compared with 4% in the placebo group), cutaneous flushing (19 and 20% vs. 0%), and rhinitis (16 and 20% vs. 6%). These AEs were generally mild or moderate in intensity. Overall, vardenafil induced a low incidence of serious AEs, with the highest incidence (2%), curiously, being reported in the 10-mg vardenafil group.

2 Conclusions

Radical prostatectomy of any form (i.e., open, laparoscopic, or robotic) is an increasingly and widely performed procedure for patients with clinically localized prostate cancer. This procedure may be associated with treatment-specific sequelae affecting health-related quality of life, mainly including ED. Formal use of on-demand PDE5i in patients undergoing RP has been shown to be effective and safe, with better results in younger patients, those preoperatively objectively fully potent and strongly motivated to maintain postoperative sexual activity, and those surgically treated with an anatomic procedure ensuring the preservation of at least one neurovascular bundle. Although recent evidence appears to suggest the presence of residual EF as early as the first night after catheter removal when an NS procedure has been performed, other data have also suggested that some time after surgery is needed to attain the best response to on-demand PDE5i. Pharmacological prophylaxis with PDE5i may have a significantly expanding role in future strategies aimed at preserving postoperative EF.

References

1. Walsh, P.C. (2000) Radical prostatectomy for localized prostate cancer provides durable cancer control with excellent quality of life: a structured debate. *J. Urol.* **163**, 1802–1807.
2. Palisaar, R.J., Noldus, J., Graefen, M., Erbersdobler, A., Haese, A., and Huland, H. (2005) Influence of nerve-sparing (NS) procedure during radical prostatectomy (RP) on margin status and biochemical failure. *Eur. Urol.* **47**, 176–184.
3. Oliver, S.E., Donovan, J.L., Peters, T.J., Frankel, S., Hamdy, F.C., and Neal, D.E. (2003) Recent trends in the use of radical prostatectomy in England: the epidemiology of diffusion. *BJU Int.* **91**, 331–336.
4. Cooperberg, M.R., Broering, J.M., Litwin, M.S., Lubeck, D.P., Mehta, S.S., Henning, J.M., Carroll, P.R., for CaPSURE. (2004) The contemporary management of prostate cancer in the United States: lessons from the cancer of the Prostate Strategic Urologic Research Endeavor (CaPSURE), a national disease registry. *J. Urol.* **171**, 1393–1401.
5. Salomon, L., Saint, F., Anastasiadis, A.G., Sebe, P., Chopin, D., and Abbou, C.C. (2003) Combined reporting of cancer control and functional results of radical prostatectomy. *Eur. Urol.* **44**, 656–660.
6. Roehl, K.A., Han, M., Ramos, C.G., Antenor, J.A.V., and Catalona, W.J. (2004) Cancer progression and survival rates following anatomical radical retropubic prostatectomy in 3478 consecutive patients: long-term results. *J. Urol.* **172**, 910–914.
7. Lubeck, D.P., Litwin, M.S., Henning, J.M., Stoddard, M.L., Flanders, S.C., and Carroll, P.R. (1999) Changes in health-related quality of life in the first year after treatment for prostate cancer: results from CaPSURE. *Urology* **53**, 180–186.
8. Madalinska, J.B., Essink-Bot, M.L., de Koning, H.J., Kirkels, W.J., van der Maas, P.J., and Schroder, F.H. (2001) Health-related quality of life effects of radical prostatectomy and primary radiotherapy for screen-detected or clinically diagnosed localized prostate cancer. *J. Clin. Oncol.* **19**, 1619–1628.
9. Matthew, A.G., Goldman, A., Trachtenberg, J., Robinson, J., Horsburgh, S., Currie, K., and Ritvo, P. (2005) Sexual dysfunction after radical prostatectomy: prevalence, treatments, restricted use of treatments and distress. *J. Urol.* **174**, 2105–2110.
10. Cooperberg, M.R., Koppie, T.M., Lubeck, D.P., Ye, J., Grossfeld, G.D., Mehta, S.S., Carroll, P.R., for CaPSURE. (2003) How potent is potent? Evaluation of sexual function and bother in men who report potency after treatment for prostate cancer: data from CaPSURE. *Urology* **61**, 190–196.
11. Hollenbeck, B.K., Dunn, R.L., Wei, J.T., Montie, J.E., and Sanda, M.G. (2003) Determinants of log-term sexual health outcome after radical prostatectomy measured by a validated instrument. *J. Urol.* **169**, 1453–1457.
12. Schover, L.R., Fouladi, R.T., Warneke, C.L., Neese, L., Klein, E.A., Zippe, C., and Kupelian, P.A. (2002) Defining sexual outcomes after treatment for localized prostate carcinoma. *Cancer* **95**, 1773–1785.
13. Mirone, V., Imbimbo, C., Palmieri, A., Longo, N., and Fusco, F. (2003) Erectile dysfunction after surgical treatment. *Int. J. Androl.* **26**, 137–140.

14. Briganti, A., Salonia, A., Gallina, A., Chun, F.K., Karakiewicz, P.I., Graefen, M., Huland, H., Rigatti, P., and Montorsi, F. (2007) Management of erectile dysfunction after radical prostatectomy in 2007. *World J. Urol.* **25**, 143–148.

15. Salonia, A., Zanni, G., Gallina, A., Saccà, A., Sangalli, M., Naspro, R., Briganti, A., Farina, E., Roscigno, M., DaPozzo, L.F., Rigatti, P., and Montorsi, F. (2006) Baseline potency in patients candidates to bilateral nerve sparing radical retropubic prostatectomy. *Eur. Urol.* **50**, 360–365.

16. Michl, U.H., Friedrich, M.G., Graefen, M., Haese, A., Heinzer, H., and Huland, H. (2006) Prediction of postoperative sexual function after nerve sparing radical retropubic prostatectomy. *J. Urol.* **176**, 227–231.

17. Dubbelman, Y.D., Dohle, G.R., and Schroder, F.H. (2006) Sexual function before and after radical retropubic prostatectomy: a systematic review of prognostic indicators for a successful outcome. *Eur. Urol.* **50**, 711–718.

18. Walsh, P.C., and Donker, P.J. (1982) Impotence following radical prostatectomy: insight into etiology and prevention. *J. Urol.* **128**, 492–497.

19. Rabbani, F., Stapleton, A.M., Kattan, M.W., Wheeler, T.M., and Scardino, P.T. (2000) Factors predicting recovery of erections after radical prostatectomy. *J. Urol.* **164**, 1929–1934.

20. Montorsi, F., Salonia, A., Suardi, N., Gallina, A., Zanni, G., Briganti, A., Dehò, F., Naspro, R., Farina, E., and Rigatti, P. (2005) Improving the preservation of the urethral sphincter and neurovascular bundles during open radical retropubic prostatectomy. *Eur. Urol.* **48**, 938–945.

21. Graefen, M., Walz, J., and Huland, H. (2006) Open retropubic nerve-sparing radical prostatectomy. *Eur. Urol.* **49**, 38–48.

22. Kessler, T.M., Burkhard, F.C., and Studer, U.E. (2007) Nerve-sparing open radical retropubic prostatectomy. *Eur. Urol.* **51**, 90–97.

23. Touijer, K., and Guillonneau, B. (2006) Laparoscopic radical prostatectomy: a critical analysis of surgical quality. *Eur. Urol.* **49**, 625–632.

24. Menon, M., Shrivastava, A., Kaul, S., Badani, K.K., Fumo, M., Bhandari, M., and Peabody, J.O. (2007) Vattikuti Institute prostatectomy: contemporary technique and analysis of results. *Eur. Urol.* **51**, 648–657.

25. Neese, L.E., Schover, L.R., Klein, E.A., Zippe, C., and Kupelian, P.A. (2003) Finding help for sexual problems after prostate cancer treatment: a phone survey of men's and women's perspectives. *Psychooncology* **12**, 463–473.

26. Heaton, J.P.W., Adams, M.A., and Morales, A. (1997) A therapeutic taxonomy of treatments for erectile dysfunction: an evolutionary imperative. *Int. J. Impot. Res.* **9**, 115–121.

27. Salonia, A., Rigatti, P., and Montorsi, F. (2003) Sildenafil in erectile dysfunction: a critical review. *Curr. Med. Res. Opin.* **19**, 241–262.

28. Montorsi, F., Briganti, A., Salonia, A., Rigatti, P., and Burnett, A.L. (2004) Current and future strategies for preventing and managing erectile dysfunction following radical prostatectomy. *Eur. Urol.* **45**, 123–133.

29. Moreland, R.B. (1998) Is there a role of hypoxemia in penile fibrosis: a viewpoint presented to the Society for the Study of Impotence. *Int. J. Impot. Res.* **10**, 113–120.

30. User, H.M., Hairston, J.H., Zelner, D.J., McKenna, K.E., and McVary, K.T. (2003) Penile weight and cell subtype specific changes in a post–radical prostatectomy model of erectile dysfunction. *J. Urol.* **169**, 1175–1179.

31. Mulhall, J.P., and Graydon, R.J. (1996) The hemodynamics of erectile dysfunction following nerve-sparing radical retropubic prostatectomy. *Int. J. Impot. Res.* **8**, 91–94.

32. Marshall, F.F., Chan, D., Partin, A.W., Gurganus, R., and Hortopan, S.C. (1998) Minilaparotomy radical retropubic prostatectomy: technique and results. *J. Urol.* **160**, 2440–2445.

33. Stanford, J.L., Feng, Z., Hamilton, A.S., Gilliland, F.D., Stephenson, R.A., Eley, J.W., Albertsen, P.C., Harlan, L.C., and Potosky, A.L. (2000) Urinary and sexual function after radical prostatectomy for clinically localized prostate cancer: the Prostate Cancer Outcomes Study. *JAMA* **283**, 354–360.

34. Mulhall, J.P., Slovick, R., Hotaling, J., Aviv, N., Valenzuela, R., Waters, W.B., and Flanigan, R.C. (2002) Erectile dysfunction after radical prostatectomy: hemodynamic profiles and their correlation with the recovery of erectile function. *J. Urol.* **167**, 1371–1375.

35. McCullough, A., Woo, K., Telegrafi, S., and Lepor, H. (2002) Is sildenafil failure in men after radical retropubic prostatectomy (RRP) due to arterial disease? Penile duplex Doppler findings in 174 men after RRP. *Int. J. Impot. Res.* **14**, 462–465.

36. Rogers, C.G., Trock, B.P., and Walsh, P.C. (2004) Preservation of accessory pudendal arteries during radical retropubic prostatectomy: surgical technique and results. *Urology* **64**, 148–151.

37. Zippe, C.D., Kedia, A.W., Kedia, K., Nelson, D.R., and Agarwal, A. (1998) Treatment of erectile dysfunction after radical prostatectomy with sildenafil citrate (Viagra). *Urology* **52**, 963–966.

38. Marks, L.S., Duda, C., Dorey, F.J., Macairan, M.L., and Santos, P.B. (1999) Treatment of erectile dysfunction with sildenafil. *Urology* **53**, 19–24.

39. Lowentritt, B.H., Scardino, P.T., Miles, B.J., Orejuela, F.J., Schatte, E.C., Slawin, K.M., Elliott, S.P., and Kim, E.D. (1999) Sildenafil citrate after radical retropubic prostatectomy. *J. Urol.* **162**, 1614–1617.

40. Hong, E.K., Lepor, H., and McCullough, A.R. (1999) Time dependent patient satisfaction with sildenafil for erectile dysfunction (ED) after nerve-sparing radical retropubic prostatectomy. *Int. J. Impot. Res.* **11**(Suppl 11), S15–S22.

41. Zagaja, G.P., Mhoon, D.A., Aikens, J.E., and Brendler, C.B. (2000) Sildenafil in the treatment of erectile dysfunction after radical prostatectomy. *Urology* **56**, 631–634.

42. Blander, D.S., Sanchez-Ortiz, R.F., Wein, A.J., and Broderick, G.A. (2000) Efficacy of sildenafil in erectile dysfunction after radical prostatectomy. *Int. J. Impot. Res.* **12**, 165–168.

43. Baniel, J., Israilov, S., Segenreich, E., and Livne, P.M. (2001) Comparative evaluation of treatments for erectile dysfunction in patients with prostate cancer after radical retropubic prostatectomy. *BJU Int.* **88**, 58–62.

44. Zippe, C.D., Jhaveri, F.M., Klein, E.A., Kedia, S., Pasqualotto, F.F., Kedia, A.W., Agarwal, A., Montague, D.K., and Lakin, M.M. (2000) Role of Viagra after radical prostatectomy. *Urology* **55**, 241–245.

45. Raina, R., Lakin, M.M., Agarwal, A., Sharma, R., Goyal, K.K., and Montague, D.K. (2003) Long-term effect of sildenafil citrate on erectile dysfunction after radical prostatectomy: 3-year follow-up. *Urology* **62**, 110–115.

46. Raina, R., Lakin, M.M., Agarwal, A., Mascha, E., Montagne, D.K., Klein, E., and Zippe, C.D. (2004) Efficacy and factors associated with successful outcome of sildenafil citrate use for erectile dysfunction after radical prostatectomy. *Urology* **63**, 960–966.

47. Wille, S., Heidenreich, A., Hofmann, R., and Engelmann, U. (2007) Preoperative erectile function is one predictor for post prostatectomy incontinence. *Neurourol. Urodyn.* **26**, 140–143.

48. Althof, S.E., Corty, E.W., Levine, S.B., Levine, F., Burnett, A.L., McVary, K., Stecher, V., and Seftel, A.D. (1999) EDITS: development of questionnaires for evaluating satisfaction with treatments for erectile dysfunction. *Urology* **53**, 793–799.

49. Shimizu, T., Hisasue, S., Sato, Y., Kato, R., Kobayashi, K., and Tsukamoto, T. (2005) Erectile dysfunction following nerve-sparing radical retropubic prostatectomy and its treatment with sildenafil. *Int. J. Urol.* **12**, 552–557.

50. Cappelleri, J.C., Rosen, R.C., Smith, M.D., Mishra, A., and Osterloh, I.H. (1999) Diagnostic evaluation of the erectile function domain of the International Index of Erectile Function. *Urology* **54**, 346–351.

51. Zanni, G., Salonia, A., Briganti, A., Gallina, A., Barbieri, L., Suardi, N., Fabbri, F., Dehò, F., Rigatti, P., and Montorsi, F. (2004) Efficacy of sildenafil 100 mg on demand in selected young patients after bilateral nerve sparing radical prostatectomy. *J. Sex. Med.* **2**(Suppl 1):A094.

52. Lowentritt, B.H. (2000) Sildenafil citrate after radical retropubic prostatectomy. *Urology* **55**, 241–245.
53. McMahon, C.G. (2002) High dose sildenafil citrate as a salvage therapy for severe erectile dysfunction. *Int. J. Impot. Res.* **14**, 533–538.
54. Montorsi, F., and McCullough, A. (2005) Efficacy of sildenafil citrate in men with erectile dysfunction following radical prostatectomy: a systematic review of clinical data. *J. Sex. Med.* **2**, 658–667.
55. Moreira, S.G., Brannigan, R.E., Spitz, A., Orejuela, F.J., Lipshultz, L.I., and Kim, E.D. (2000) Side-effect profile of sildenafil citrate (Viagra) in clinical practice. *Urology* **56**, 474–476.
56. Montorsi, F., Guazzoni, G., Strambi, L.F., Da Pozzo, L.F., Nava, L., Barbieri, L., Rigatti, P., Pizzini, G., and Miani, A. (1997) Recovery of spontaneous erectile function after nerve-sparing radical retropubic prostatectomy with and without early intracavernous injections of alprostadil: results of a prospective, randomized trial. *J. Urol.* **158**, 1408–1410.
57. Bannowsky, A., Schulze, H., van der Horst, C., Seif, C., Braun, P.M., and Junemann, K.P. (2006) Nocturnal tumescence: a parameter for postoperative erectile integrity after nerve sparing radical prostatectomy. *J. Urol.* **175**, 2214–2217.
58. Schwartz, E.J., Wong, P., and Graydon, J. (2004) Sildenafil preserves intracorporeal smooth muscle after radical retropubic prostatectomy. *J. Urol.* **171**, 771–774.
59. Behr-Roussel, D., Gorny, D., Mevel, K., Ciasey, S., Bernabè, J., Burgess, G., Wayman, C., Alexandre, L., and Giuliano, F. (2005) Chronic sildenafil improves erectile function and endothelium-dependent cavernosal relaxations in rats: lack of tachyphylaxis. *Eur. Urol.* **47**, 87–91.
60. Montorsi, F., Maga, T., Strambi, L.F., Salonia, A., Barbieri, L., Scattoni, V., Guazzoni, G., Losa, A., Rigatti, P., and Pizzini, G. (2000) Sildenafil taken at bedtime significantly increases nocturnal erections: results of a placebo-controlled study. *Urology* **56**, 906–911.
61. Padma-Nathan, H., McCullough, A.R., Giuliano, F., Toler, S.M., Wohlhuter, C., and Shpilsky, A. (2003) Postoperative nightly administration of sildenafil citrate significantly improves the return of normal spontaneous erectile function after bilateral nerve-sparing radical prostatectomy. *J. Urol.* **4**(Suppl), 375.
62. Mulhall, J., Land, S., Parker, M., Waters, W.B., and Flanigan, R.C. (2005) The use of an erectogenic pharmacotherapy regimen following radical prostatectomy improves recovery of spontaneous erectile function. *J. Sex. Med.* **2**, 532–540.
63. Montorsi, M., Salonia, A., Gallina, A., Zanni, G., Saccà, A., Dehò, F., Briganti, A., Ghezzi, M., Barbieri, L., Farina, E., Schuit, J.S., and Rigatti, P. (2006) There is no significant difference between on-demand PDE5-I vs. PDE5-I as rehabilitative treatment in patients treated by bilateral nerve-sparing radical retropubic prostatectomy. *Eur. Urol.* **5**(Suppl 2), A472.
64. Salonia, A., Gallina, A., Zanni, G., Saccà, A., Schuit, J.S., Barbieri, L., Briganti, A., Farina, E.P., Rigatti, P., and Montorsi, F. (2006) Severe dropout rate from the treatment for erectile dysfunction in non-counselled patients who underwent bilateral nerve sparing radical retropubic prostatectomy. *Eur. Urol.* **5**(Suppl 2), A474.
65. Curran, M., Keating, G., and Tadalafil. (2003) *Drugs* **63**, 2203–2212.
66. Lilly ICOS LLC. (Nov 2003) Cialis summary of product characteristics. Available via www.emea.eu.int/humandocs/Humans/EPAR/cialis/cialis
67. Francis, S.H., Turko, I.V., and Corbin, J.D. (2001) Cyclic nucleotide phosphodiesterases: relating structure and function. *Prog. Nucleic Acid Res. Mol. Bio.***65**, 1–52.
68. Saenz de Tejada, I., Spain, J., and Angulo Frutos, M. (2002) Comparative selectivity profiles of tadalafil, sildenafil and vardenafil using an in vitro phosphodiesterase activity assay. *Int. J. Impot. Res.* **14**(Suppl 4), S20.
69. Montorsi, F., Padma-Nathan, H., McCullough, A., Brock, G.B., Broderick, G., Ahuja, S., Whitaker, S., Hoover, A., Novack, D., Murphy, A., and Varanese, L. (2004) Tadalafil in the treatment of erectile dysfunction following bilateral nerve sparing radical retropubic prostatectomy: a randomized, double-blind, placebo controlled trial. *J. Urol.* **172**, 1036–1041.

70. Vignozzi, L., Filippi, S., Morelli, A., Ambrosini, S., Luconi, M., Vannelli, G.B., Donati, S., Crescioli, C., Zhang, X.H., Mirone, V., Forti, G., and Maggi, M. (2006) Effect of chronic tadalafil administration on penile hypoxia induced by cavernous neurotomy in the rat. *J. Sex. Med.* **3**, 419–431.

71. Montorsi, F., Salonia, A., Briganti, A., Barbieri, L., Zanni, G., Suardi, N., Cestari, A., Montorsi, P., and Rigatti, P. (2005) Vardenafil for the treatment of erectile dysfunction: a critical review of the literature based on personal clinical experience. *Eur. Urol.* **47**, 612–621.

72. Padma-Nathan, H., Montorsi, F., Giuliano, F., Meuleman, E., Auerbach, S., Eardley, I., McCullough, A., Homering, M., Segerson, T., for the North American and European Vardenafil Study Group. (2007) Vardenafil restores erectile function to normal range in men with erectile dysfunction. *J. Sex. Med.* **4**, 152–161.

73. Goldstein, I., Fisher, W.A., Sand, M., Rosen, R.C., Mollen, M., Brock, G., Karlin, G., Pommerville, P., Bangerter, K., Bandel, T.J., Derogatis, L.R., for the Vardenafil Study Group. (2005) Women's sexual function improves when partners are administered vardenafil for erectile dysfunction: a prospective, randomized, double-blind, placebo-controlled trial. *J. Sex. Med.* **2**, 819–832.

74. Gbekor, E., Bethell, S., Fawcett, L., Mount, N., and Phillips, S. (2002) Selectivity of sildenafil and other phosphodiesterase type 5 (PDE5) inhibitors against all human phosphodiesterase families. *Eur Urol.* **1**(Suppl 1), 63.

75. Brock, G., Nehra, A., Lipshultz, L.I., Karlin, G.S., Gleave, M., Seger, M., and Padma-Nathan, H. (2003) Safety and efficacy of vardenafil for the treatment of men with erectile dysfunction after radical retropubic prostatectomy. *J. Urol.* **170**, 1278–1283.

76. Nehra, A., Grantmyre, J., Nadel, A., Thibonnier, M., and Brock, G. (2005) Vardenafil improved patient satisfaction with erectile hardness, orgasmic function and sexual experience in men with erectile dysfunction following nerve sparing radical prostatectomy. *J. Urol.* **173**, 2067–2071.

Chapter 13
Injectable Therapies After Prostate Cancer Therapy

Andrew McCullough

Abstract Erectile dysfunction (ED) is a common sequela of the treatment of prostate cancer that negatively impacts quality of life. Though the phosphodiesterase inhibitors (PDE5i) are popular for the treatment of ED because of their ease in administration, they are frequently ineffective after surgery and radiation therapy for prostate cancer.

Intracavernosal therapy (ICT) was the first effective medical therapy for erectile dysfunction and is the most effective therapy for post-treatment ED. Patient and physician resistance contributes to its low acceptance despite its clear superior efficacy. The rationale for the use of ICT in the treatment and possible prevention of ED after prostate cancer therapy is presented along with strategies for facilitating its implementation.

Keywords Erectile dysfunction; prostate cancer; erectile dysfunction; injection therapy.

From: *Current Clinical Urology* Series, *Sexual Function in the Prostate Cancer Patient* 197
Edited by John P. Mulhall, DOI 10.1007/978-1-60327-555-2_13,
© Humana Press, a part of Springer Science+Business Media, LLC 2009

1   Introduction

Men with prostate cancer are being treated more aggressively, earlier and are living longer. In 1983, approximately 10% of new cases of prostate cancer underwent radical prostatectomy, 25% had radiation therapy, 15% had hormonal therapy, and 50% had no therapy. Sixty percent of men had disease outside of the prostate at the time of diagnosis. In 1986, the prostate-specific antigen test was approved by the FDA. Soon thereafter the relatively non-invasive transrectal ultrasound biopsy was introduced facilitating the diagnosis of prostate cancer. These two technological advances led to a downward stage and age migration at the time of diagnosis. Ninety percent of men are currently diagnosed with clinically localized disease. In 1995, 35% of men underwent radical prostatectomy, 30% had radiation therapy, less than 10% had hormonal therapy, and slightly less than 30% had no therapy. Despite advances in surgical and radiation treatment, many men will experience a treatment-related decline in their erectile function that inexorably progresses with time, age, and increasing ED co-morbidities, regardless of their chosen treatment. Substantial decreases in erectile function as high as 61% and 79% at 2 years in patients treated with RT and RP, respectively, have been reported (1–3). Erectile dysfunction is a substantial problem following treatment for localized prostate cancer and is associated with a self-perceived decrease in overall quality of life (4). Yet, despite the high incidence of erectile dysfunction after treatment and its negative impact on quality of life only 50% of patients use treatments for ED (5). Of the ED treatments, oral PDE5i are the most popular. Of those using only PDE5i, only 12% felt that

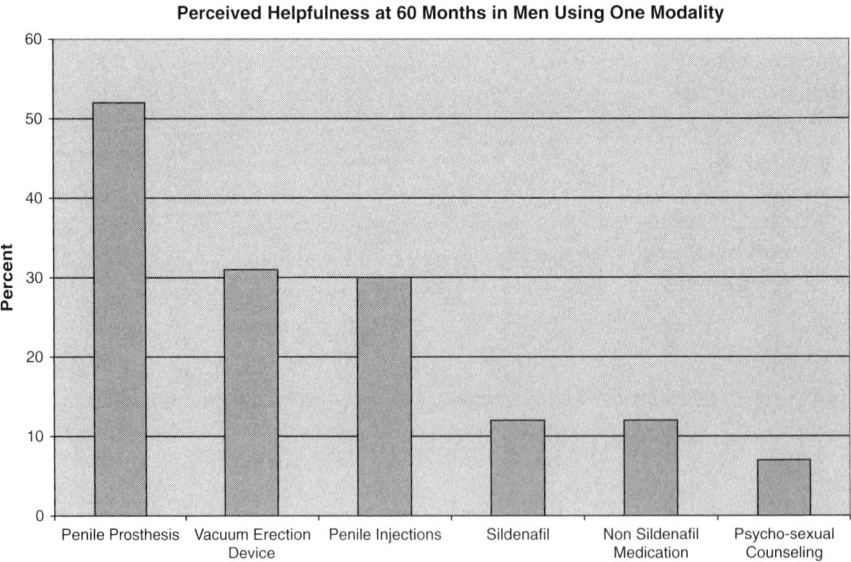

Fig. 1 Perceived helpfulness of ED therapies (5)

it helped a lot. The penile implant was perceived as the most helpful followed by the vacuum device and penile injections (Fig. 1). Despite their superior effectiveness at 60 months the prosthesis, vacuum device, and penile injections were used in only 1.6, 5, and 2% of patients, whereas the PDE5i alone or in combination were used in over 37% of patients. In this group of patients that respond so poorly to the PDE5 inhibitors why is injection therapy so infrequently used? The purpose of this chapter is to review the use of penile injection therapy in the treatment and possible prevention of erectile dysfunction after prostate cancer treatment.

2   Penile Intracorporal Therapy (ICT)

ICT was introduced dramatically in the USA at the 1983 American Urological Association Meeting by Giles Brindley *(6)*. This represented the first effective medical treatment for Erectile Dysfunction (ED). Prior to 1983 the only effective treatment was the penile implant (1972), or the vacuum erection device (1986). ED had long been associated with vascular disease *(7)* and initially ICT was used most often for vascular ED. Between 1983 and 1994, ICT evolved using either monotherapy or combination therapy of generic papaverine, phentolamine, prostaglandin E_1 or atropine (Table 1). The most common form of ICT currently used by urologists is

Table 1 Common ICT Treatments

Drug	Cost/dose	Dose range	Advantages	Disadvantages
Papaverine	$6–$60	7.5–60 mg	Low cost (Generic) Stable at room temp	Penile induration Priapism Elevation of liver enzymes Not FDA approved
Phentolamine	$6–$60	0.5–2 mg	Low cost (Generic) Stable at room temp No priapism	Low efficacy as monotherapy Not FDA approved
Alprostadil	$33–$38	1–40 µg	Commercially available FDA approved Priapism rare Room temp storage	Requires refrigeration after reconstitution Expensive Complicated reconstitution High volume of injection Penile pain
Papaverine/ Phentolamine	$2–$20	0.1–60 mg/ 0.2–2 mg	low cost (Generic)	Priapism Penile indurations
Papaverine/ Phentolamine/ Alprostadil	$2–$20	0.1–60 mg/ 0.1–2 mg/ 0.2 µg	Low cost (Generic) Low volume injection Highly effective Stock vial can be frozen	Priapism Penile induration Requires refrigeration

alprostadil (Caverjet® Pfizer, Ny, and Edex®, Schwarz Pharma) though combinations of generic formulations of the generic vasodilators papaverine, alprostadil and phentolamine are also popular.

In 1995, intracorporal alprostadil (Caverjet®) was approved by the FDA. Efficacy in the pivotal trials with alprostadil was over 90%, with patient and partner satisfaction of over 85% *(8)*. Despite the overall effectiveness of ICT, fewer than 6% of men suffering from ED sought treatment before the advent of oral therapy. In 1995 *(9)*, a goal-directed approach was adopted by most physicians as ED was considered a "functional disease and not life-threatening." Patients were encouraged, with counseling, to choose their form of treatment. Not surprisingly, patients chose medical therapy over surgery, yet as many as 25% failed to start ICT therapy and only 40–50% continued therapy, despite its high degree of effectiveness *(10,11)*. Mulhall et al. catalogued the reasons for dropout of injection therapy, with expense and dislike of injections being the two most common reasons (Table 2) *(12)*. Confounding the patient resistance issues, is a general reluctance of physicians, including urologists, to promote ED treatments largely because of lack of time and a belief that the patient will initiate the conversation if ED is an issue *(13)*. In addition, the urologist or radiation therapist may be concerned that a discussion about post-treatment erectile dysfunction may underscore unrealistic pretreatment claims of post-treatment erectile function recovery.

The etiology of ED in men after prostate cancer treatment is multifactorial as well as treatment dependent. Clearly, epidemiologic studies such as the Massachusetts Male Aging Study (MMAS) established the incidence of pretreatment ED in the age group of men diagnosed with prostate cancer as high as 60%. Psychogenic, vascular, neurogenic, myogenic, and endocrine etiologies have all been implicated after treatment (Table 3).

Table 2 Reasons for Dropping Out of Self-Injection Program *(12)*

	% Patients.
Therapy too expensive	28.3
Did not like the idea of injecting penis	27.6
Partner did not like injections	19.3
Partner not available	17.0
Erections improved spontaneously	15.3
Injections were not effective	14.2
Development of penile curvature	11.2
Development of other medical problems	10.6
Lost interest in sex	8.1
Undertook alternative treatment	7.6
Lost interest in partner	7.2
Development of penile lump	5.8
Injections thought to be unnatural	6.1
Erections lasted too long	4.9
Injections painful	4.9
Fear of needles	4.5

Table 3 Etiologies of ED After Prostate Cancer Treatment

Observation	Psychogenic, natural progression
Radiation	Arteriogenic, neurogenic, myogenic
Radical prostatectomy	Neurogenic, myogenic, arteriogenic
Cryosurgery	Vascular
Androgen ablation	Endocrine deficiency

Regardless of the etiology or mode of treatment ICT has been shown to be effective.

3 Mechanism of Action of ICT

3.1 Alprostadil

Unlike oral therapy, the mechanism of action for ICT is independent of nerve function. The ability of ICT to work independent of the nerves is particularly appealing for post-prostatectomy men, where there is an obligate early (first 12 months after RP) neuropraxia that occurs after surgery and makes oral therapy ineffective. The responsiveness to oral therapy follows the time course of resolution of the neuropraxia *(14)*. Alprostadil is the exogenous synthetic form of a naturally occurring fatty acid, PGE_1. It causes smooth muscle relaxation, vasodilatation, and inhibition of platelet aggregation through elevation of intracellular cAMP. Alprostadil is then metabolized in the corpora cavernosa by the enzyme prostaglandin 15-hydroxy-dehydrogenase. After ICI, 96% of alprostadil is locally metabolized within 60 min and peripheral blood levels return to baseline. In patients with veno-occlusive dysfunction, serum alprostadil levels may rise to tenfold, but up to 90% is metabolized on the first-pass through the lungs.

3.2 Papaverine

The molecular mechanism of papaverine action is through its non-specific inhibitory effect on phosphodiesterase (PDE), leading to increased cAMP and cGMP in penile erectile tissue. It also blocks voltage-dependent calcium channels, thus impairing calcium influx, and it may also impair calcium-activated potassium and chloride currents. The end result is relaxation of cavernous smooth muscle and penile vessels. The plasma half-life is 1–2 h as papaverine is metabolized in the liver. The increased half-life and requisite systemic metabolism are believed to contribute to the suggested higher rate of priapism with papaverine. The suggested increase in corporal fibrosis with papaverine may possibly be secondary to the high degree of acidity of the papaverine solution (pH of 3 or 4) *(15)*.

3.3 Phentolamine

Phentolamine is a non-specific α-adrenergic antagonist with equal affinity for blocking both α-1 and α-2 adrenoreceptors as adrenergic agents are anti-erectile. Endogenous norepinephrine (NE) contracts corporal smooth muscle primarily through its effects on post-junctional α-1 receptors and is the principal neurotransmitter of detumescence. ICT monotherapy with phentolamine results in penile tumescence but not rigidity. Combination therapy results in synergy between different agents as the local mechanisms of action are different. This synergy allows the use of very small doses of injected dose in men with no preexisting ED prior to radical prostatectomy. Excellent response to doses as low as 0.3 mg papaverine, 0.1 μg of alprostadil, and 0.01 mg of phentolamine is not uncommon, requiring dilution of the stock solution to allow the patient to work with measurable quantities of the injectate. At these low concentrations and volumes corporal fibrosis is highly unlikely.

4 Complications with ICT

4.1 Priapism

The most feared complication by urologists from ICT is priapism (Table 4). Priapism occurs in men with an intact veno-occlusive mechanism. A man suffering from pretreatment ED secondary to veno-occlusive disease (VOD) is likely to require larger doses of injectate and is unlikely to encounter priapism. A pretreatment history of PDE5i refractory or dependent ED, or the presence of multiple endothelial disease risk factors (diabetes, hypertension, dyslipidemia, age>65, obesity) or exposure to a prior priapism episode or pelvic radiation therapy is likely to result in VOD and a high-dose ICT requirement to achieve an erection. The initial etiology for ED after RRP is neuropathic and secondarily myogenic. The contribution of arterial insufficiency to the development of post-RP is discussed in Chapter 5. Dosage requirements for ICT in the neuropathic patients have long been documented to be much lower than men with ED secondary to vascular disease *(16)*. Approximately 50% of preoperatively potent men without arterial disease on penile duplex Doppler after RRP will not demonstrate VOD by Doppler criteria *(17)*. In a

Table 4 Complications of Injection Therapy

Complications of injection therapy	%
Temporary ecchymosis/hematoma	25
Induration/subcutaneous nodules	6
Priapism	0.1–5

cross-sectional study, VOD after prostatectomy appeared to worsen with time and to be associated with a poorer long-term prognosis with respect to eventual return of natural function (18). VOD progression is most likely related to progressive corporal smooth muscle fibrosis but may improve with time with treatment within the first 2 years after surgery (19).

Because of the increased risk of priapism in the post-RRP patient without preoperative ED, gradual dose titration is very important. My typical testing initial dose in the office is 0.1 ml of trimix (30 mg/ml papaverine/20 μg/ml alprostadil, 0.2 mg/ml phentolamine) containing 3 mg of papaverine, 2 mg of alprostadil, and 0.2 mg of phentolamine, although other dose combinations are used. The patient is observed for approximately 45 min and reversed with phenylephrine if necessary. If a reversal dose is needed, the patient is started on 0.05 ml of a half-strength solution of trimix. If no reversal dose is used and a strong erection was obtained, the dose is reduced to 0.05 ml of full-strength solution. If the erection was not sufficient for penetration, the patient is started on the 0.15 ml of full-strength solution. The latter scenario is uncommon and is a very poor prognostic sign. Men frequently report subsequent better efficacy in their home environment than in the office. Using this regimen I have minimized priapism in the early postoperative period. A recent review describes an excellent titration schedule (20).

A confounding variable with priapism in the post-RRP man is the recovery of function that occurs in the first 2 years. Whereas men with vasculogenic ED can be stable on the same dose of ICT for years, men after RRP are experiencing a gradual return of their natural function in the first 2 postoperative years and their dosage requirements may actually decrease. Though it is frightening to the patient that his erections may be lasting longer on an established dose, the man should be heartened that the decreased dose requirement is a sign of recovery of natural function.

Unlike after RRP where the PDE5 refractory ED is immediate, after radiation therapy ED is typically manifest years after treatment and is most likely the result of radiation damage to the proximal corpora with the resulting nerve, muscle, and vascular damage (19). Priapism is therefore unlikely to result in men after RT. A systematic slow titration of ICT is the best way to prevent priapism. The use of liberal communication between the patient and the urologist's office can go a long way to achieve the correct dose without priapism.

Current AUA guidelines on priapism recommend a stepwise approach to the treatment of priapism (21) (Table 5). It should be assumed that the priapism after

Table 5 AUA Guidelines for Ischemic Priapism

1. Therapeutic aspiration (with or without irrigation)
2. Intracavernous injection of sympathomimetics (e.g., phenylephrine, epinephrine, norepinephrine, metaraminol)
3. Systemic treatment of underlying disease (e.g., sickle-cell disease) plus intracavernous treatment for patients with underlying disorders or hematologic pathology
4. Surgical shunts, including distal shunts; the caverno spongious shunt; and caverno saphenous shunt

ICT is ischemic or low flow as it carries the poorest prognosis. Priapism in the post-ICT may be mechanistically different from idiopathic priapism where the erection should be reversed within 6 h to prevent irreversible corporal fibrosis. Kulmala found that men treated for less than 36 h after an ICT induced-priapic episode reversed without a long-term impact on there subsequent ICT responsiveness. If a delay greater than 36 h occurs corporal fibrosis ensues *(22)*. Caution is advised, as the impact of an early priapic episode on the eventual return of function has not been evaluated. In over 20 years of experience with ICT, I have never had to perform a shunt in a post-ICT priapism. The priapism either resolves spontaneously, with aspiration or injection of sympathomimetics. Though phenylephrine, epinephrine, norepinephrine, metaraminol have all been used, the preferred reversal agent is phenylephrine because it minimizes the risk of cardiovascular side effects that are more common for other sympathomimetic medications. An initial dose of 500 μg of intracorporal phenylephrine is prescribed with monitoring of blood pressure and pulse followed with repeat injection 15–20 min later. As many as six such consecutive injections have been used although no maximum dose has been defined, and as long as the patient does not develop hypertension and reflex bradycardia repeat dosing can continue *(23)*.

4.2   Penile Pain

Intracorporal pain in the penis is one of the most common complaints with ICT, being reported in as many as 80% of men. The pain is usually tolerable and severe in less than 20%. It is not associated with the injection process but appears to be activation of intrapenile pain receptors and is seen more often after RRP (early or late), with increasing doses and concentrations of PGE_1; sometimes lasting after detumescence has occurred. The exact mechanism has not been elucidated. Trimix has been associated with a decreased incidence of pain compared to alprostadil alone *(24)*. If the pain persists with trimix, a formulation of papaverine and phentolamine, without alprostadil, can be used though higher doses of the injectate will be necessary with less efficacy. Attempts to alkalinize or add lidocaine to the injectate have been successful in decreasing but not eliminating the penile pain *(25–27)*.

4.3   Penile Fibrosis

Ever since the introduction of ICT, penile fibrosis and Peyronie's disease have always been a concern. Loss of penile length and circumference has been described after radiation therapy, prostatectomy, and androgen ablation and is independent of the use of erectogenic aids. Fibrotic penile changes have been described in 11% of men after RRP *(28)*. Fibrotic nodules from ICT do not appear to lead to Peyronie's disease, do not worsen, and sometimes resolve despite continued use of ICT *(29)*. The presence of fibrotic nodules or Peyronie's disease does not significantly complicate penile prosthesis implantation should it subsequently be required. The occurrence of fibrotic nodules should not be used as a reason to cease ICT.

5   Benefit of ICT in Penile Rehabilitation

Anecdotally the use of ICT has been reported to improve spontaneous erectile function in men with ED *(29–31)*. In 1997 Montorsi in a small randomized series reported that the introduction of ICT in the early postoperative period resulted in the earlier and more complete return of natural erectile function *(32)*. The study has never been replicated though it is generally believed that the introduction of ICT in the postoperative period is beneficial in increasing corporal oxygenation *(33)*. The use of ICT has been shown to increase corporal oxygenation *(34)*. In men who have failed oral therapy after RP the use of ICT can result in improved PDE5i responsiveness *(35,36)*. Because of patient resistance and the expense of commercial alprostadil, postoperative ICT has not been adopted by most urologists or patients.

6   Conclusions

ICT is underutilized but still plays an important role in the treatment of the man with erectile dysfunction after treatment for prostate cancer. Though the PDE5i have been beneficial, the ED after prostatectomy is frequently refractory to oral therapy. Urologists should encourage their patients to explore ICT at all stages of their recovery. In the early postoperative period ICT has been shown to not only improve quality of life but also enhance the return of natural erectile function. In the late convalescence it has been shown to enhance responsiveness to PDE5i. In both phases it will allow the patient to resume penetrative sexual function. As men suffer the long-term effects of prostate radiation and the PDE5i fail, ICT remains the best medical alternative. The complications of ICT (priapism, penile pain, and penile fibrosis) can be managed easily with good patient education and follow up.

References

1. Stanford, J.L., Feng, Z., Hamilton, A.S., et al. (2000) Urinary and sexual function after radical prostatectomy for clinically localized prostate cancer: the Prostate Cancer Outcomes Study. *JAMA* **283(3),** 354–360.
2. Litwin, M.S., Flanders, S.C., Pasta, D.J., Stoddard, M.L., Lubeck, D.P., and Henning, J.M. (1999) Sexual function and bother after radical prostatectomy or radiation for prostate cancer: multivariate quality-of-life analysis from CaPSURE. Cancer of the Prostate Strategic Urologic Research Endeavor. *Urology* **54**(3), 503–508.
3. Lilleby, W., Fossa, S.D., Waehre, H.R., and Olsen, D.R. (1999) Long-term morbidity and quality of life in patients with localized prostate cancer undergoing definitive radiotherapy or radical prostatectomy. *Int. J. Radiat. Oncol. Biol. Phys.* **43**(4), 735–743.

4. Penson, D.F., Feng, Z., Kuniyuki, A., et al. (2003) General quality of life 2 years following treatment for prostate cancer: what influences outcomes? Results from the prostate cancer outcomes study. *J. Clin. Oncol.* **21**(6), 1147–1154.

5. Stephenson, R.A., Mori, M., and Hsieh, Y.C., et al. (2005) Treatment of erectile dysfunction following therapy for clinically localized prostate cancer: patient reported use and outcomes from the Surveillance, Epidemiology, and End Results Prostate Cancer Outcomes Study. *J. Urol.* **174**(2), 646–650; discussion 50.

6. Brindley, G.S. (1983) Cavernosal alpha-blockade: a new technique for investigating and treating erectile impotence. *Br. J. Psychiatry* **143**, 332–337.

7. O'Conor, V.J., Jr. (1958) Impotence and the Leriche syndrome: an early diagnostic sign; consideration of the mechanism; relief by endarterectomy. *J. Urol.* **80**(3), 195–198.

8. Linet, O.I., and Ogrinc, F.G. (1996) Efficacy and safety of intracavernosal alprostadil in men with erectile dysfunction. The Alprostadil Study Group. *N. Engl. J. Med.* **334**(14), 873–877.

9. Lue, T.F. (1995) A patient's goal-directed approach to erectile dysfunction and Peyronie's disease. *Can. J. Urol.* **2**(Suppl 1), 13–17.

10. Jarow, J.P., Nana-Sinkam, P., Sabbagh, M., and Eskew, A. (1996) Outcome analysis of goal directed therapy for impotence. *J. Urol.* **155**(5), 1609–1612.

11. Derouet, H., Caspari, D., Munch, M., and Ziegler, M. (1991) [Acceptance of corpus cavernosum auto-injection therapy in long-term treatment of erectile dysfunction]. *Urologe A* **30**(6), 423–427.

12. Mulhall, J.P., Jahoda, A.E., Cairney, M., et al. (1999) The causes of patient dropout from penile self-injection therapy for impotence. *J. Urol.* **162**(4), 1291–1294.

13. Perttula, E. (1999) Physician attitudes and behaviour regarding erectile dysfunction in at- risk patients from a rural community. *Postgrad. Med. J.* **75**(880), 83–85.

14. Hong, E.K., Lepor, H., and McCullough, A.R. (1999) Time dependent patient satisfaction with sildenafil for erectile dysfunction (ED) after nerve-sparing radical retropubic prostatectomy (RRP). *Int. J. Impot. Res.* **11**(Suppl 1), S15–S22.

15. van Ahlen, H., Peskar, B.A., Sticht, G., and Hertfelder, H.J. (1994) Pharmacokinetics of vasoactive substances administered into the human corpus cavernosum. *J. Urol.* **151**(5), 1227–1230.

16. Hirsch, I.H., Smith, R.L., Chancellor, M.B., Bagley, D.H., Carsello, J., and Staas, W.E., Jr. (1994) Use of intracavernous injection of prostaglandin E1 for neuropathic erectile dysfunction. *Paraplegia* **32**(10), 661–664.

17. McCullough, A., Woo, K., Telegrafi, S., and Lepor, H. (2002) Is sildenafil failure in men after radical retropubic prostatectomy (RRP) due to arterial disease? Penile duplex Doppler findings in 174 men after RRP. *Int. J. Impot. Res.* **14**(6), 462–465.

18. Mulhall, J.P., Slovick, R., Hotaling, J., et al. (2002) Erectile dysfunction after radical prostatectomy: hemodynamic profiles and their correlation with the recovery of erectile function. *J. Urol.* **167**(3), 1371–1375.

19. Mulhall, J.P., Yonover, P., Sethi, A., Yasuda, G., and Mohideen, N. (2002) Radiation exposure to the corporeal bodies during 3-dimensional conformal radiation therapy for prostate cancer. *J. Urol.* **167**(2 Pt 1), 539–542.

20. Albaugh, J.A. (2006) Intracavernosal injection algorithm. *Urol. Nurs.* **26**(6), 449–453.

21. Berger, R., Billups, K., Brock, G., et al. (2001) Report of the American Foundation for Urologic Disease (AFUD) Thought Leader Panel for evaluation and treatment of priapism. *Int. J. Impot. Res.* **13**(Suppl 5), S39–S43.

22. Kulmala, R.V., and Tamella, T.L. (1995) Effects of priapism lasting 24 hours or longer caused by intracavernosal injection of vasoactive drugs. *Int. J. Impot. Res.* **7**(2), 131–136.

23. Muruve, N., and Hosking, D.H. (1996) Intracorporeal phenylephrine in the treatment of priapism. *J. Urol.* **155**(1), 141–143.

24. Baniel, J., Israilov, S., Engelstein, D., Shmueli, J., Segenreich, E., and Livne, P.M. (2000) Three-year outcome of a progressive treatment program for erectile dysfunction with intracavernous injections of vasoactive drugs. *Urology* **56**(4), 647–652.

25. Godschalk, M., Gheorghiu, D., Katz, P.G., and Mulligan, T. (1996) Alkalization does not alleviate penile pain induced by intracavernous injection of prostaglandin E1. *J. Urol.* **156**(3), 999–1000.

26. Schouman, M., Lacroix, P., and Amer, M. (1992) Suppression of prostaglandin E1-induced pain by dilution of the drug with lidocaine before intracavernous injection. *J. Urol.* **148**(4), 1266.

27. Kattan, S. (1995) Double-blind randomized crossover study comparing intracorporeal prostaglandin E1 with combination of prostaglandin E1 and lidocaine in the treatment of organic impotence. *Urology* **45**(6), 1032–1036.

28. Ciancio, S.J., and Kim, E.D. (2000) Penile fibrotic changes after radical retropubic prostatectomy. *BJU Int.* **85**(1), 101–106.

29. Canale, D., Giorgi, P.M., Lencioni, R., Morelli, G., Gasperi, M., and Macchia, E. (1996) Long-term intracavernous self-injection with prostaglandin E1 for the treatment of erectile dysfunction. *Int. J. Androl.* **19**(1), 28–32.

30. Rowland, D.L., Boedhoe, H.S., Dohle, G., and Slob, A.K. (1999) Intracavernosal self-injection therapy in men with erectile dysfunction: satisfaction and attrition in 119 patients. *Int. J. Impot. Res.* **11**(3), 145–151.

31. Imagawa, A., Kawanishi, Y., and Tamura, M. (1989) Intracavernous injection therapy in recovery of spontaneous erection (not for self-injection) – its mechanism and indications. *Hinyokika Kiyo* **35**(7), 1145–1148.

32. Montorsi, F., Guazzoni, G., Strambi, L.F., et al. (1997) Recovery of spontaneous erectile function after nerve-sparing radical retropubic prostatectomy with and without early intracavernous injections of alprostadil: results of a prospective, randomized trial. *J. Urol.* **158**(4), 1408–1410.

33. van der Horst, C., Martinez-Portillo, F.J., and Junemann, K.P. (2005) [Pathophysiology and rehabilitation of erectile dysfunction after nerve-sparing radical prostatectomy]. *Urologe A* **44**(6), 667–673.

34. Knispel, H.H., and Andresen, R. (1993) Evaluation of vasculogenic impotence by monitoring of cavernous oxygen tension. *J. Urol.* **149**(5 Pt 2), 1276–1279.

35. Mydlo, J.H., Viterbo, R., and Crispen, P. (2005) Use of combined intracorporal injection and a phosphodiesterase-5 inhibitor therapy for men with a suboptimal response to sildenafil and/or vardenafil monotherapy after radical retropubic prostatectomy. *BJU Int.* **95**(6), 843–846.

36. Gutierrez, P., Hernandez, P., and Mas, M. (2005) Combining programmed intracavernous PGE1 injections and sildenafil on demand to salvage sildenafil nonresponders. *Int. J. Impot. Res.* **17**(4), 354–358.

Chapter 14
Non-pharmacologic Erectile Dysfunction Treatments After Prostate Cancer Therapy

Brian R. Lane and Drogo K. Montague

Abstract Erectile dysfunction (ED) after treatment for prostate cancer (radical prostatectomy, radiotherapy, or androgen deprivation therapy) is common. Systemic therapy with the PDE5 inhibitors is successful in a lower percentage of these patients than it is in men with ED of other etiologies. Penile injection therapy often results in usable erections in these men but its acceptability may be limited because of pain which is more common in this subset of patients. Vacuum erection device therapy and penile prosthesis implantation are non-pharmacologic options available for the treatment of ED after prostate cancer therapy.

The literature is surveyed for penile prosthesis implantation in men treated for prostate cancer and an overview of the results is presented. Special considerations for penile prosthesis implantation before, after, and during radical prostatectomy are discussed. Some surgeons prefer two-piece inflatable penile prosthesis implantation after radical prostatectomy because of concerns regarding scarring of the lower abdominal fascia and the retropubic space which might complicate reservoir placement. Evidence is presented that three-piece inflatable penile prosthesis implantation can safely be accomplished in these patients.

Penile prosthesis implantation before and after radiation therapy for prostate cancer is reviewed as is penile prosthesis placement after androgen ablation therapy. Vacuum constriction devices remain an option for prostate cancer patients in whom

From: *Current Clinical Urology* Series, *Sexual Function in the Prostate Cancer Patient*
Edited by John P. Mulhall, DOI 10.1007/978-1-60327-555-2_14,
© Humana Press, a part of Springer Science+Business Media, LLC 2009

pharmacologic agents are ineffective or contraindicated and who are not interested in or are poor operative candidates for penile prosthesis implantation.

Keywords Penile prosthesis; vacuum constriction device; prostatic neoplasms; prostatectomy; radiotherapy.

Abbreviations Prostate cancer; erectile dysfunction; radical prostatectomy; radiation therapy; phosphodiesterase-5; inflatable penile prosthesis; vacuum constriction device.

1 Introduction

Sexual dysfunction of various etiologies is common in older men in the presence *or absence* of prostate cancer (PC), and erectile function is commonly negatively affected by treatment for prostate cancer. A recent investigation of sexual function outcomes in men with localized PC revealed that more than half of these men used some form of treatment for ED within 5 years of treatment *(1)*. While approximately 75% were sexually active prior to treatment for PC, only about one in eight men retained adequate sexual function without assistance after treatment *(1)*. The use of any ED treatment increased after the introduction of oral PDE5 inhibitors, and these agents were the most frequently used treatment (38% of all patients at 5 years) *(1)*. Although penile prosthesis was the least commonly used treatment (<2%), it was associated with the highest rates of patient satisfaction, full erections, sexual frequency, and maintenance of erection *(1)*.

Prior to 1983 almost all men who received treatment for prostate cancer were rendered sexually non-functional. Men treated with systemic hormonal therapy for PC experience a reduction in circulating and intraprostatic levels of testosterone. Clinical (or subclinical) hypogonadism reduces libido, impairs sexual arousal, and can reduce the quality of erections *(2,3)*. Treatment for localized PC in previous decades almost uniformly resulted in erectile dysfunction (ED), because radical prostatectomy (RP) for prostate cancer, as originally described, involved wide resection of the tissue lateral to the prostate that contains the parasympathetic nerve fibers that are responsible for normal erectile function. Therefore, the likely etiology of post-prostatectomy ED is disruption of the neurovascular bundle that courses alongside the posterolateral aspects of the prostate, although thermal or stretch injury and vascular compromise may also contribute. In the mid-1980s, the nerve-sparing, or anatomic, RP, in which the lateral dissection along the prostate preserves one or both neurovascular bundles, was developed by Walsh and colleagues *(4–6)*. Nerve-sparing RP often preserves satisfactory erections after an oncologically sound surgery for localized PC. Several studies during the last 20 years have demonstrated that the percentages of patients with ED after RP are highest following a non-nerve-sparing operation and lowest when both nerves can be preserved *(7–13)*.

Despite undergoing a nerve-sparing RP, almost all patients will experience ED immediately after surgery, but the length of time to recovery and the rigidity of erections after RP are variable *(8–10,14)*. The percentage of patients experiencing adequate erections continues to rise over the first 12–24 months after surgery, when ED rates stabilize or increase gradually as expected due to advancing age *(8–10,12,14)*. In one single surgeon series, 76% of the 1,770 men who were potent prior to bilateral nerve-sparing RP had erections sufficient for intercourse at a mean of 18 months after surgery *(11)*. In another large series, 63 and 70% of previously potent men ($n = 785$) were capable of achieving erections (with or without pharmacologic treatment) at 18 and 24 months after bilateral nerve-sparing RP, respectively *(13)*. Erectile function retention 5 years after RP in the Prostate Cancer Outcomes Study was lower overall (bilateral 41%, unilateral 23%, non-nerve-sparing 23%), but showed the same trend with nerve-sparing status *(12)*. Younger patients and those with excellent preoperative sexual function often have higher objective measures of erectile function after RP *(10–12)*, but it is not always possible to predict which patients will regain satisfactory erectile function.

Similarly, ED is common after radiation therapy (RT) for localized prostate cancer. The etiology of post-radiation ED is thought to be vascular, resulting from radiation damage to small vessels leading to ischemic injury. In contrast to post-prostatectomy ED, which occurs immediately and improves without treatment during the first 12–24 months after surgery and plateaus thereafter, sexual function is not negatively affected immediately after RT, but decreases over time in a manner that is not accounted for solely by advancing age *(14–17)*. In one large series, "impotence" was reported in 50 and 64% of patients 2 and 5 years after RT *(14)*, In another series, at a median of 2.6 and 6.2 years, 69 and 82% of those receiving three-dimensional conformal RT and 75 and 89% of those receiving brachytherapy reported erections not firm enough for intercourse, respectively *(17)*. The likelihood and severity of ED vary with the type, technique, and radioisotope used during RT *(14–16)*. The extent of sexual dysfunction after RT may decrease as technological refinements improve the targeting of radiation within the pelvis. After three-dimensional computer-optimized high-dose-rate prostate brachytherapy in conjunction with highly conformal external beam RT, 80% were able to achieve erections satisfactory for intercourse *(18)*. However, 43% of these patients required sildenafil citrate for adequate erections, and the 5-year actuarial likelihood of potency was only 53% in the 47 patients who were potent prior to treatment *(18)*. While sexual function immediately after treatment may be higher in patients receiving RT when compared with those receiving RP, the negative effects on sexual function are comparable or worse at a longer duration of follow-up *(14–17)*.

ED is defined as the consistent inability to attain or maintain penile erections of sufficient quality to allow satisfactory sexual performance *(19)*. Clinical judgment best helps determine that an individual is consistently not able to obtain sufficient erections after pelvic surgery, and long-term treatment recommendations may be best made once the severity of ED is assessed at an adequate period of follow-up. Oral phosphodiesterase-5 (PDE5) inhibitors must be considered as first-line therapy for all patients with ED, although in some patients they are poorly tolerated or contraindicated. In the major studies of oral PDE5 inhibitors, PC patients consistently respond more poorly than other men *(20,21)*. This may be a reflection of etiology and/or severity of ED in these patients. Other options, including intraurethral prostaglandin, intracavernosal injection of prostaglandin or combination therapy, vacuum-constriction devices, and penile prostheses, must be discussed with the patient. While these therapies are considered second-line therapies in the average ED patient, they must be considered and discussed for all PC patients with ED.

The purview of this chapter is to discuss the indications, techniques, and outcomes of non-pharmacologic therapies for ED in the patient with PC. A systematic review of articles available on MEDLINE® as of March 2006 using the MeSH terms "penile prosthesis" or "penile implantation" revealed 679 articles. The titles and abstracts of all 95 English-language references listing cancer as a subheading were reviewed and the complete text of 23 of these manuscripts were examined further. In addition, review of the titles of all 101 non-English-language references revealed 1 manuscript regarding penile prostheses in PC patients. Finally, 18 references were identified by a search using "penile prosthesis" or "penile implantation" and "prostatic neoplasms" and 4 additional references by combining "radiotherapy" and these 2 terms. Each of these relevant manuscripts were reviewed and included.

2   Implantation of Inflatable Penile Prostheses

Penile prostheses can be classified as inflatable and non-inflatable. The benefits of non-inflatable, or semi-rigid, prostheses include lower cost and low mechanical failure rate, but disadvantages include continuous penile rigidity and increased risk of erosion *(22)*. Most specialists recommend malleable prostheses in a minority of patients, given the excellent outcomes observed with the inflatable penile prosthesis (IPP) *(23–30)*. These devices are composed of two or three parts: paired inflatable cylinders, a pump that regulates fluid transit from the reservoir to the cylinders, and a fluid-filled reservoir. In three-piece IPP the reservoir is typically placed in the perivesical space, while in two-piece devices, it is an integrated part of the cylinders. Since the initial prototypes were developed in 1973, IPP have undergone major modifications that have resulted in lower rates of infection and technical failure *(28,30,31)*. These include design modifications to all components and the addition of an antibiotic-containing or hydrophilic coating to reduce infections, each of which has been described in detail elsewhere *(28,30)*.

Several articles have detailed the surgical technique for placement of these devices *(32,33)*. Our preferred approach involves placement of a three-piece device under either spinal or general anesthesia. In the operating room, skin shaving is performed followed by a 10 min skin prep and isolation of the surgical field with paper drapes. A transverse incision is made about 1 cm below the penoscrotal junction and directed toward the urethra and corpora cavernosa, rather than the scrotum. Dartos fascia is dissected off the urethra and proximal corpora (crura) and a ring retractor is placed to maintain exposure using a combination of hook stays and retractor blades. Paired 2 cm corporotomies are made and two horizontal mattress

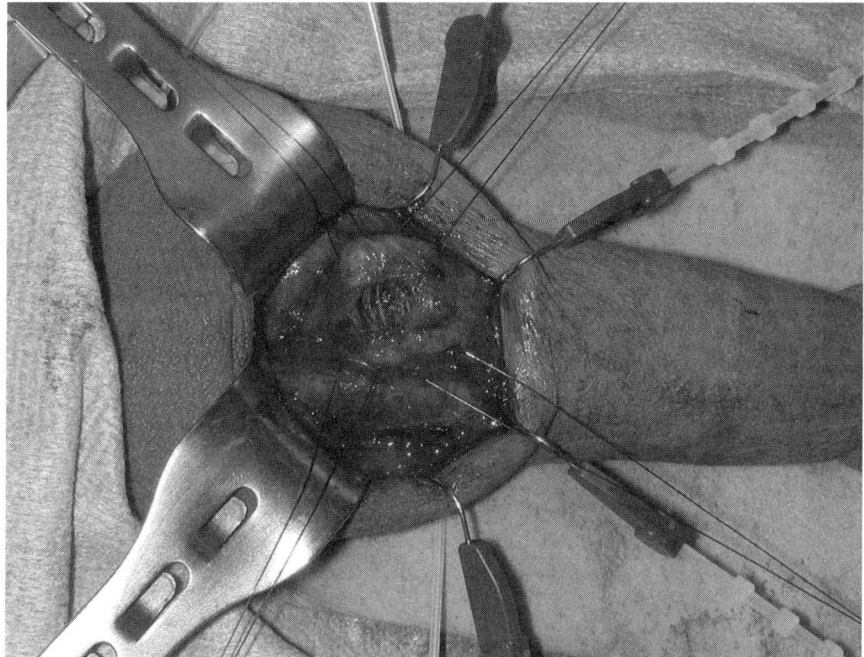

Fig. 1 After making a transverse incision 1 cm below the penoscrotal junction, and dissecting toward the urethra and corpora cavernosa, a ring retractor has been placed to maintain exposure using a combination of hook stays and retractor blades. Dartos fascia has been dissected off the urethra and proximal corpora, and a 2 cm right corporotomy has been made. Two horizontal mattress sutures of 2-O PDS II serve as guide sutures during dilation and measurement of the corpora, and are later used to close the corporotomies after cylinder placement

sutures of 2-O PDS II (polydioxanone, Ethicon, Inc., Somerville, NJ) are placed on each side of each corporotomy (Fig. 1). These sutures serve as guide sutures during dilation and measurement of the corpora, and are later used to close the corporotomies after cylinder placement *(34)*. Dilation and calibration begins with an 8 mm Hegar dilator and proceeds to 14 mm distally (Fig. 2) and to 16 mm proximally. The larger size proximally allows for both the device and device tubing. If the corpora cannot be dilated without force, rounded-tip Metzenbaum scissors can be used with or without special cutting dilators, and in some cases, extension of the corporotomies is necessary *(33,35,36)*. Where dilation to 14 mm and 16 mm cannot be achieved, we recommend that smaller diameter cylinders be used *(33)*.

The proximal and distal corporal lengths are measured internally from the respective ends of the corporotomies. The appropriate cylinder size is selected by summing these measurements without including the 2 cm corporotomy *(37)*. All device components are filled with normal saline to displace air and, for placement, the reservoir is emptied and the cylinders are left rounded, but not inflated. Irrigation containing antibiotics (typically, bacitracin) is used immediately prior to placement of all

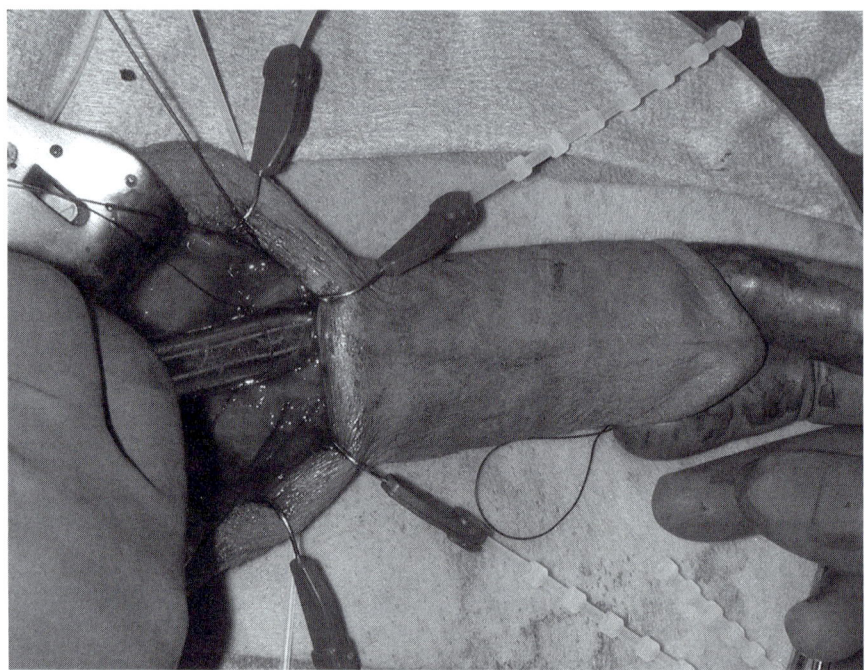

Fig. 2 Dilation and calibration of the right distal corpus cavernosum is performed using a 14-mm Hegar dilator. Dilation of the proximal erectile body to 16 mm allows for both the cylinder and tubing of the IPP

components and tubing connections. A Furlow cylinder inserter aids distal cylinder placement, delivering the needle and guide sutures through the tip of the corpus cavernosum and out through the glans (Fig. 3). Rear tip extenders are added (if needed), and the proximal tip is inserted, ensuring that the rounded visible portion of the cylinder lies flatly within the open corporotomy (Fig. 4). The corporotomies are closed using the preplaced horizontal mattress sutures *(34)*.

A second incision through dartos fascia in the scrotal septum is used to place the pump, which is oriented at the base of the scrotum in the midline with the reservoir tubing in front and the two cylinder tubings behind (Fig. 5). All three tubes are routed separately into the first incision through the back wall of the pouch (Fig. 6), which is then irrigated with antibiotic solution and closed with running 3-O Dexon II (polyglycolic acid suture, United States Surgical, Tyco Healthcare Group, Norwalk, CT). The redundant tubing between the pump and cylinders is cut prior to making straight, sutureless connections (Fig. 7). A 50-ml syringe filled with normal saline serves as a temporary reservoir, while the device is cycled to ensure adequate rigidity and straightening and proper fit (Figs. 8 and 9).

A urethral catheter is inserted and the bladder is drained until completely empty with suprapubic pressure to ensure safe reservoir insertion into the retropubic space.

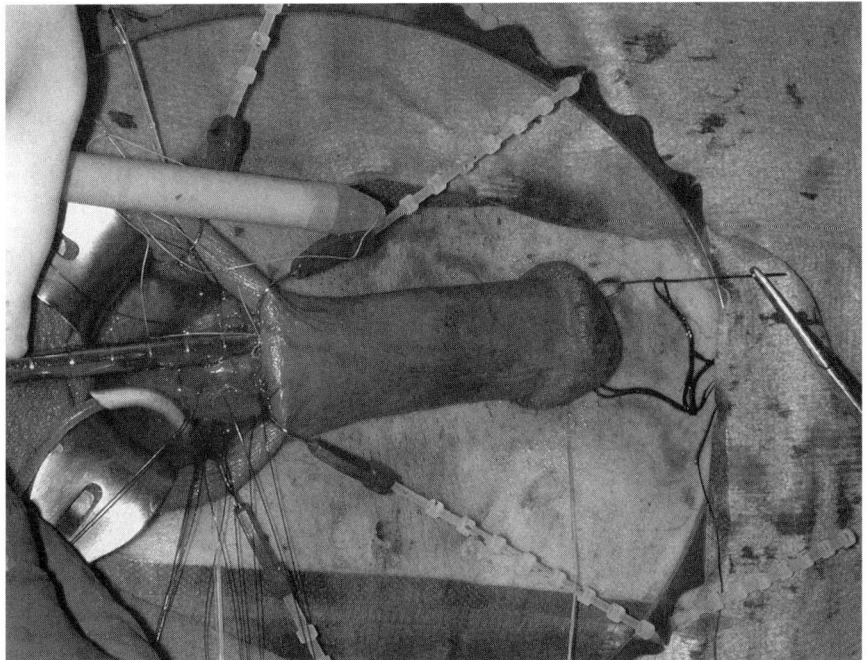

Fig. 3 The Furlow cylinder inserter has been placed within the corpus cavernosum, and the Ultrex cylinder is shown beside the penis. A needle and guide sutures will be passed out through the tip of the glans to guide distal placement of the cylinder

The surgeon's index finger identifies the external inguinal ring, or if not palpable, a point just above the pubic tubercle. The transversalis fascia is perforated using Metzenbaum scissors or a Kelly clamp medial to the finger. If all fascial layers are perforated, the surgeon's index finger will enter the retropubic space without a "trampoline" effect and the back of the symphysis pubis and balloon within the empty bladder will be palpated. In post-prostatectomy patients, scarring of the fascia may make perforation somewhat more difficult; however, this maneuver can still be made safely. A nasal speculum with long blades guides placement of the empty reservoir into the retropubic space and the device is filled with normal saline. If properly situated, only the tubing hub of the reservoir should be palpable protruding through the fascia (Fig. 10). The fluid pressure in the reservoir is zeroed by applying manual suprapubic pressure and allowing fluid to escape from the reservoir into an empty 50-ml syringe held at bladder level. The reservoir tubing is then brought into the incision in the upper scrotum and the third straight, sutureless connection is made. A closed suction drain is introduced through a separate stab inguinal incision and laid along the tubes and connectors at the base of the penis. Dartos fascia is closed transversely with running 3-O Dexon and the skin is closed with running subcuticular 4-O Vicryl suture.

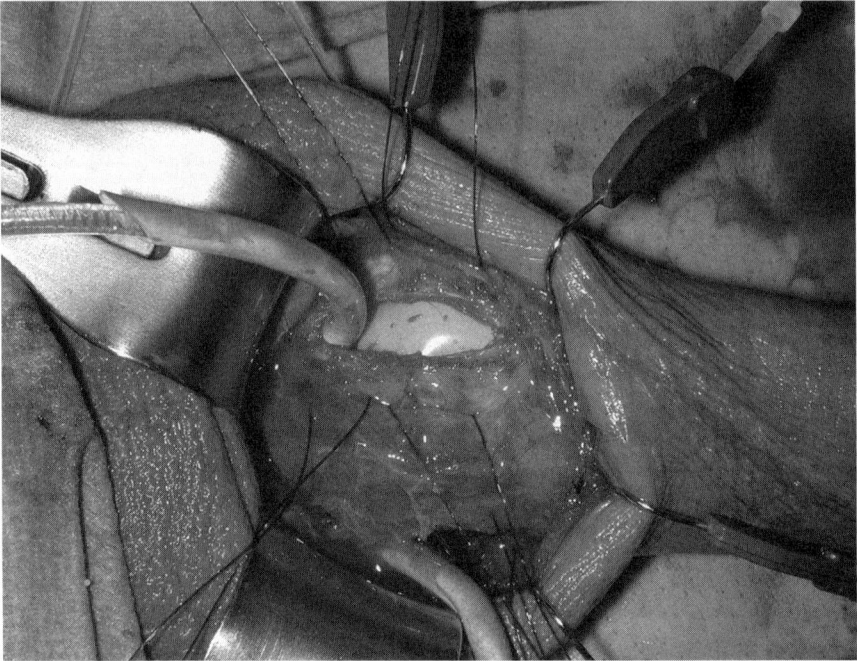

Fig. 4 After inserting the proximal tip of the cylinder, the rounded visible portion of the cylinder lies flatly within the open corporotomy. The preplaced horizontal mattress sutures are then used to close the corporotomies

After an overnight stay in the ambulatory surgery center, the closed suction drain and urethral catheter are removed. Patients are instructed to take an oral cephalosporin for 1 week after surgery, and typically require oral narcotics for this duration as well. After this, non-steroidal anti-inflammatory agents usually suffice. The patient is instructed to restrict lifting and other activities that might displace the reservoir and to keep his penis up on the lower abdomen to prevent ventral curvature for 1 month. Most men are ready for instructions on device cycling 1 month after surgery, and coitus can begin when inflation can be accomplished without discomfort *(33)*.

3 Outcomes of Penile Prosthesis Placement

The Cleveland Clinic experience with IPP placement prior to and after the 1993 modification of the American Medical Systems Ultrex device has previously been reported, and our experience with re-operation for failed prostheses and in post-prostatectomy patients has been recently updated *(28,38,39)*. Since the 1993 modification of the Ultrex, an estimated 94% of devices are free of mechanical

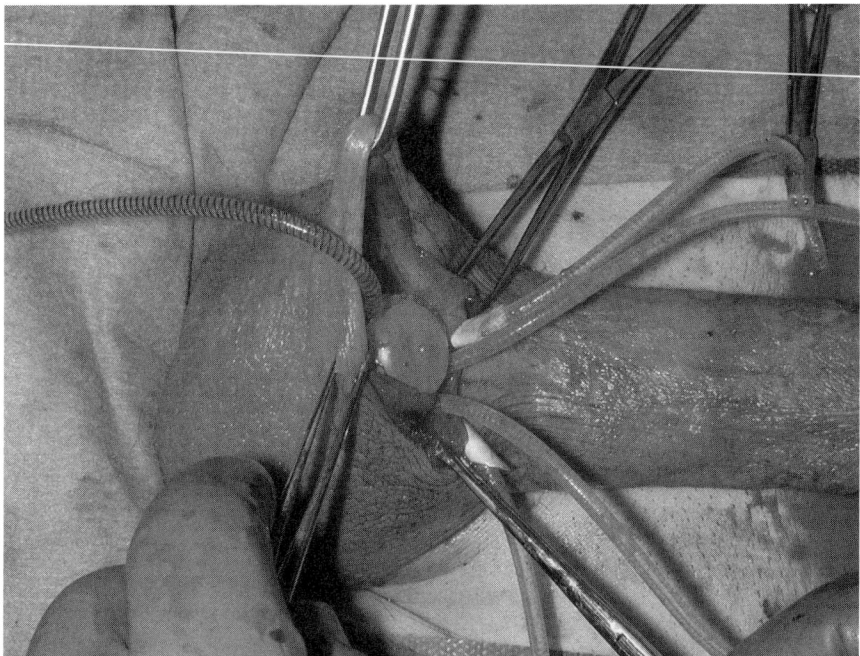

Fig. 5 After incising dartos fascia in the scrotal septum, space for the pump is developed using a ring forceps. The pump is then oriented at the base of the scrotum in the midline with the reservoir tubing in front and the tubing to the two cylinders behind

failure at 5 years after placement *(28)*. Kaplan–Meier projections of survival free of mechanical failure at 5 years range from 80 to 96% in various published series of three-piece IPP *(23–30)*. Infection of the periprosthetic space usually requires removal of all components of the prosthesis, although salvage in a single operation is sometimes possible *(40)*. Device manufacturers have introduced surface treatments combining rifampin and minocycline (InhibiZone™) or polyvinylpyrrolidone in an attempt to reduce infections. Large studies comparing coated devices to controls have shown reductions in early rates of infection from 1.6 to 0.7% with InhibiZone™, and from 2 to 1% with polyvinylpyrrolidone *(41,42)*. Although previous reports indicate a higher infection rate (up to 16%) during replacement of failed devices, our recent experience demonstrates an acceptable rate of infections (1.8%) using antibiotic-coated devices *(38)*. Management of complications and other special situations is discussed in more detail elsewhere *(33)*.

After IPP placement, 83–85% of men and 70–76% of their partners are satisfied with the use of the device *(43,44)*. Satisfaction continues to improve between 3 and 12 months after surgery, with highest patient satisfaction at 1 year after surgery *(45,46)*. Comparative studies indicate that ED patients managed with IPP have the highest levels of satisfaction when compared with patients receiving other forms of therapy *(1,47,48)*.

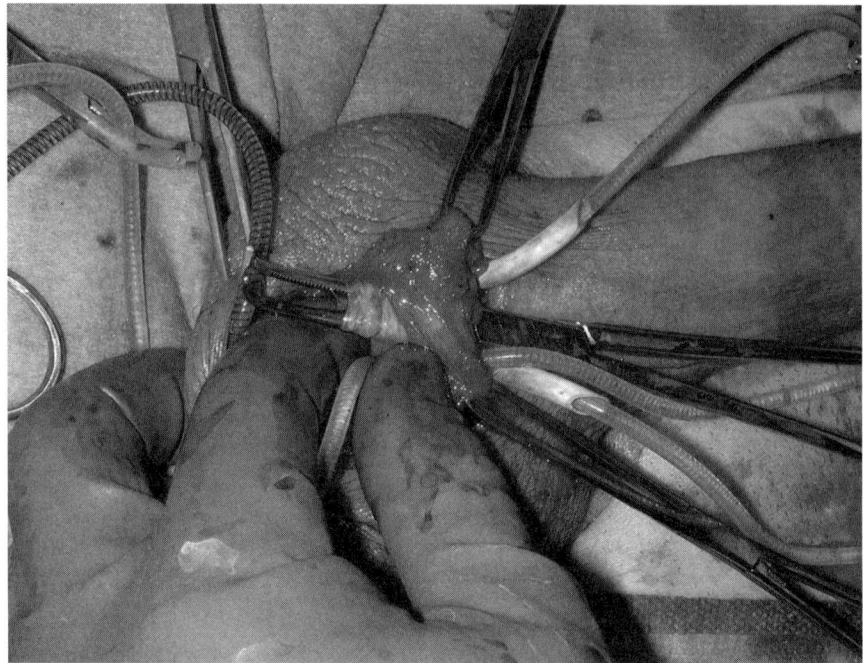

Fig. 6 The tubing to each cylinder and the reservoir (three in total) is routed separately into the first incision through the back wall of the scrotal pouch

4 Penile Prosthesis Placement Before Radical Prostatectomy

Multiple small series have reported RP in patients who had previously undergone IPP placement *(49–53)*. In 1992, the technique used to perform retropubic RP in eight patients with preexisting IPP cases was first reported *(49)*. In two patients in whom the reservoir was in the perivesical space, RP was completed without modification *(49)*. Reservoir removal was required in order to complete the RP in six patients, three of whom had the reservoir replaced between 3 and 6 months after RP and three others who never had the reservoir replaced *(49)*. Prosthesis infection occurred in one of the two patients in whom the reservoir was left in place *(49)*. The authors conclude that prior IPP should not preclude RP, but the reservoir may need to be temporarily removed in order to complete the procedure. A different technique was reported in 1997, in which the reservoir of a three-piece IPP was dissected out of the pseudocapsule and placed above the pubis during RP and replaced in the perivesical space at the end of the case *(50)*. No intraoperative or post-operative complications were observed in either of the two patients *(50)*. The group at Wayne State subsequently reported a similar technique during RP in eight men with prior IPP *(51)*. The cylinders were fully inflated to remove fluid from the reservoir, which was then dissected free of its pseudocapsule using only cutting cautery *(51)*. The

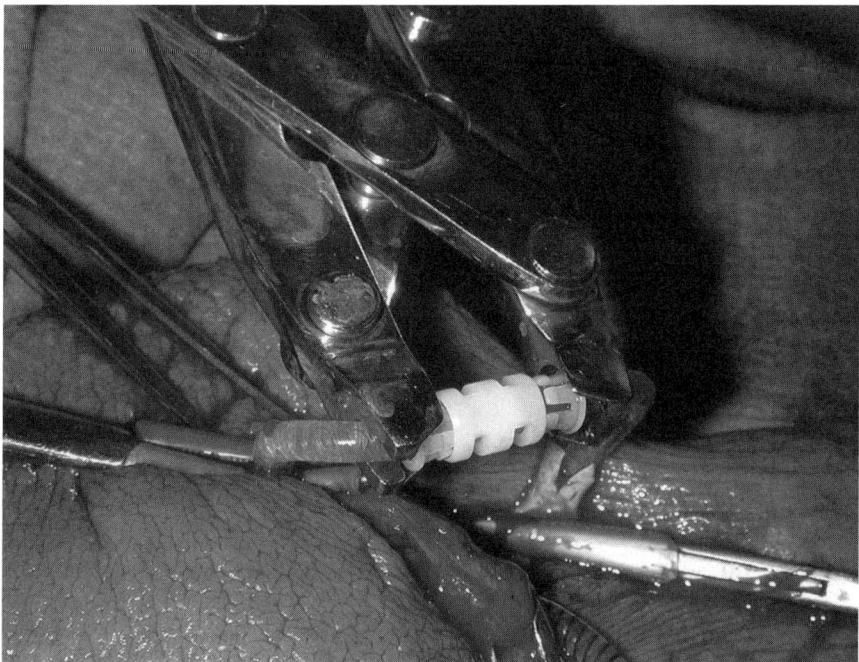

Fig. 7 The tubing between the pump and each cylinder is cut to eliminate redundant length prior to making straight, sutureless connections

reservoir was placed out of the field in an antibiotic-soaked sponge until completion of the RP. At that point, the device was cycled to ensure proper function, and the reservoir was re-placed in the perivesical space along with two closed-suction drains *(51)*. In one case, the reservoir tubing was punctured during closure of the abdominal fascia wall and immediately repaired *(51)*. All eight patients had a functioning penile prosthesis after RP and the authors concluded that patients with a preexisting penile prosthesis should not be denied RP *(51)*. Schanne et al. reported three cases in which the IPP reservoir was relocated within the extraperitoneal space without disrupting the tubing in order to facilitate dissection *(52)*. They reported no complications or injuries to the IPP, and reactivation was successful 6 weeks after surgery *(52)*. Mireku et al. reported that RP was accomplished without complication in 6 patients with previously placed IPPs without injury to the device or other pelvic organs *(53)*. The prosthesis was inflated to reduce the volume of fluid in the reservoir and otherwise left intact *(53)*. We were unable to identify any reports in which perineal RP was performed in a patient with a preexisting IPP, although this approach might be feasible without injury to the device or need to relocate the reservoir. Similarly, no reports of laparoscopic or robotic RP in patients with previously placed prostheses were identified. In summary, the most commonly used technique involves relocation of the reservoir above the pubis during retropubic RP and

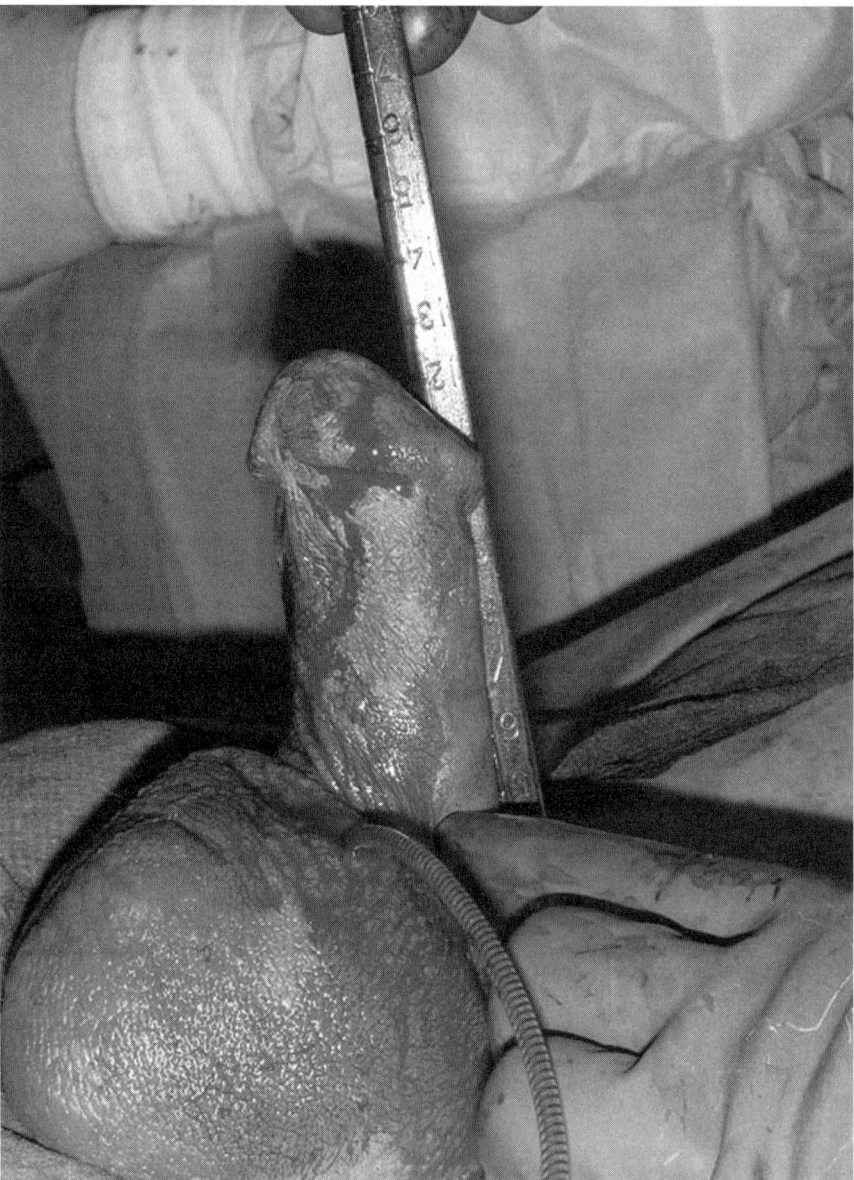

Fig. 8 After both cylinders have been connected to the pump, a syringe filled with 50 ml of normal saline serves as a temporary reservoir. In this patient, the length of the flaccid penis with both cylinders in place is between 12 and 13 cm

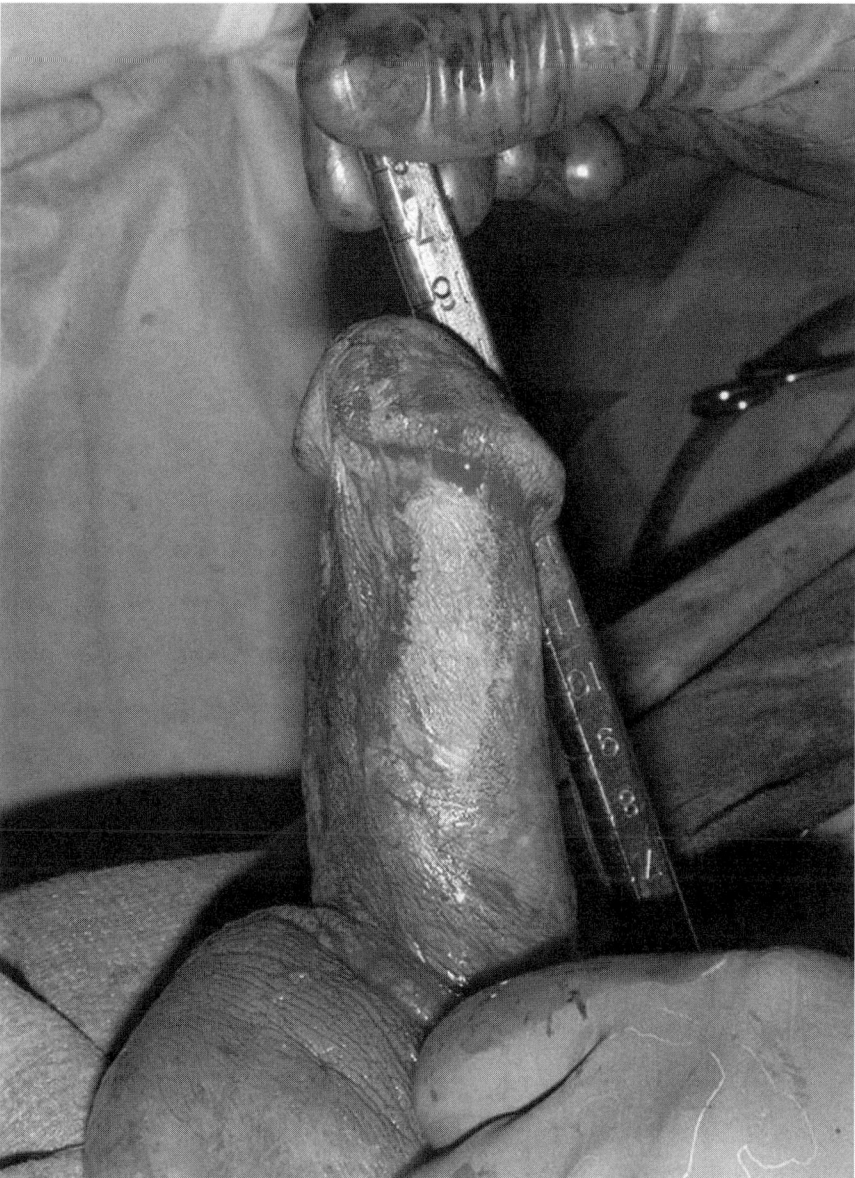

Fig. 9 Using the syringe as a temporary reservoir, the device can be cycled to evaluate the length and quality of erection with the prosthesis in place. The erect penis in this patient has a gentle dorsal curve and measures 16 cm

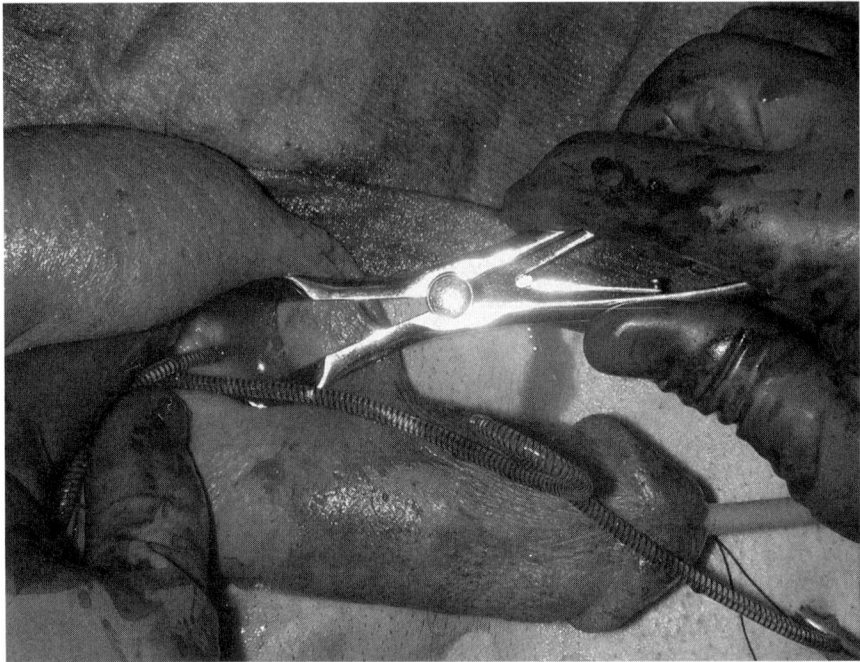

Fig. 10 After the bladder has been drained completely using a urethral catheter, the transversalis fascia is perforated medial to the surgeon's index finger in the external inguinal ring. The empty reservoir is then placed in the perivesical space guided by a nasal speculum with long blades. When properly situated, only the tubing hub of the reservoir is palpable protruding through the fascia

replacement within the perivesical space after the completion of the vesicourethral anastomosis. This technique was utilized in 13 patients, with only 1 minor complication (5%). An alternative technique involves inflation of the prosthesis to reduce the reservoir volume, without relocating the reservoir, although the single prosthesis infection (4%) among the 27 reported cases occurred in 1 of the 8 patients treated in this manner *(49)*.

5   Penile Prosthesis Placement Simultaneously with Radical Prostatectomy

Several surgeons have advocated concurrent placement of IPP following completion of RP in certain patients. Candidates would include those in whom RP has been completed without undue length of anesthesia or blood loss in whom a significant amount of ED is expected after surgery based on preoperative sexual function and intraoperative results (non-nerve-sparing RP). In the initial report of concurrent non-nerve-sparing RP and IPP placement, 50 patients were treated successfully with an additional operative time of 82 min *(54)*. No intraoperative complications related to placement of the prosthesis were reported and during the mean follow-up of 1.7 years, no prosthesis infections occurred and 4 revisions were performed *(54)*. In comparison with 72 patients who underwent RP alone, the additional procedure did not increase blood loss, hospital stay, or analgesic requirements, and the patients resumed intercourse 13 weeks after surgery *(54)*. This group later reported quality of life data in 51/120 men (43%) that had undergone simultaneous procedures (RP/IPP) between 1993 and 2000 *(55)*. Outcomes in these patients were compared with 47 men who had undergone RP alone and the subgroup of 15 patients who had undergone nerve-sparing RP *(55)*. In this study, one RP/IPP patient underwent removal of IPP for device failure and five patients underwent IPP placement after RP alone *(55)*. The majority of patients in the RP alone group used sexual aids, including injections (60%), oral PDE5 inhibitors (55%), and/or vacuum constriction device (45%). Erectile function, as assessed by the Erectile Dysfunction Inventory of Treatment Satisfaction score, was highest in the RP/IPP group, and these patients reported a greater frequency of sexual contacts (mean 2.4 per month) than either of the RP or nerve-sparing RP groups (mean 1.0 and 1.1 per month). Overall quality of life was assessed using the total score of a 30-question instrument, the prostate cancer-specific European Organization for the Research and Treatment of Cancer QOL questionnaire. Total score and sexual function subscale were highest in the RP/IPP group, reflecting a potential advantage of this approach, although the study methodology was somewhat flawed and the sample size is small *(55)*. The authors conclude that simultaneous RP and IPP placement is well-tolerated and may be desirable in patients in whom post-operative ED is likely, including those in whom a nerve-sparing RP is not performed.

Some have reported anecdotal placement of the reservoir at the time of retropubic RP in order to facilitate placement of an IPP at a later date. As we have not encountered significant difficulty in placing a reservoir in patients who had previously undergone RP, we do not feel that this maneuver will benefit a given patient significantly. In our opinion, simultaneous RP and IPP placement is a reasonable option and could be offered to a greater number of patients than currently undergo concurrent procedures. The risks of any combined procedure, however, are theoretically higher than either procedure alone and planned IPP placement should be aborted if non-nerve-sparing RP does not proceed smoothly, within the expected operative time, and with no more than the expected amount of blood loss.

6 Penile Prosthesis Placement After Radical Prostatectomy

There are a few published surgical series regarding IPP placement in RP patients *(39,56)*. Nevertheless, post-prostatectomy ED patients represent between 9 and 25% of the patients who have undergone IPP placement in most surgical series. Some reports specifically identify factors contributing to ED, including surgical or radiation therapy for prostate cancer, and in these, between 9 and 13% of patients had undergone prior prostatectomy *(23,44,46)*. The majority of reports group patients undergoing RP into various categories, such as "pelvic trauma," "iatrogenic surgery," or "pelvic trauma/surgery," which represent 10–25% of patients *(24,26,28)*, or "other," which represents 16–20% of patients *(29,30)*. Some series do not report potential etiologies of ED *(25,47,57)*. The results of IPP in each of these reports are analyzed for patients with ED of all etiologies, without specific mention of prostate cancer patients who had undergone RP or other forms of treatment. We feel that conclusions drawn from these reports can, in general, be applied to this subgroup of ED patients.

However, two points deserve further mention in regards to patients with post-prostatectomy ED. First, optimal timing of surgical intervention depends upon the severity and progression of ED in an individual patient. Erectile function continues to improve until between 12 and 24 months after surgery *(8–10,12–14)*, so conservative management of ED in patients with some return of erectile function during this time is reasonable. On the other hand, management with IPP should be discussed with and strongly considered for patients with more significant ED, ED that is refractory to other treatment modalities, or profound ED 12 months after RP. Secondly, some surgeons do not offer three-piece devices to patients who have undergone previous retropubic or inguinal surgery because of a perceived increased intraoperative risk. In our experience, while the fascia is scarred and may be more difficult to perforate, implantation of a retropubic reservoir is safe in these patients. We have not observed any intraoperative complications during three-piece IPP placement in 115 patients who had undergone RP previously *(39)*. We, therefore, do not feel that prostatectomy should be a contraindication for placement of a retropubic reservoir, and these patients should be offered the same prostheses as other patients.

7 Penile Prosthesis Placement Before Radiation Therapy for Prostate Cancer

When considering radiotherapy for prostate cancer, a history of prior pelvic or abdominal surgery may increase the likelihood of complications and radiation treatment planning should be tailored accordingly. In patients who have undergone placement of an IPP or artificial urinary sphincter, state-of-the-art conformal techniques should be employed to limit the radiation dose that will be administered in the region of the device, but portions of the device will inevitably receive some degree of radiation. Limited in vitro testing has revealed that certain prosthetic devices can withstand 40–100 Gy given using a 6 MV photon beam without malfunction *(58)*. The worldwide reported clinical experience is limited to a single patient who received external beam radiotherapy and five patients who received brachytherapy with coexistent penile prostheses *(58,59)*. A man with clinically localized Gleason 9 PC received 60 Gy to a field encompassing the prostate and proximal ends of an IPP, with the other components of the device receiving no more than an exit dose *(58)*.

Although the patient developed radiation proctitis, the device continued to function normally until his demise 18 months after treatment *(58)*.

Li et al. reported successfully administering transperineal interstitial brachytherapy to five patients with a previously placed and functioning penile prosthesis, including four patients with semi-rigid implants and one patient with a three-piece IPP *(59)*. Unfortunately, transrectal ultrasound was unable to reliably visualize the cylinders during needle placement *(59)*. Therefore, CT of the pelvis obtained prior to treatment in order to exclude that the needle path would traverse either the pubic arch or the cylinders *(59)*. Brachytherapy was performed according to standard protocol in all five cases, without suspected injury or infection to the prosthesis. No patient experienced prosthesis-related pain, infection, or malfunction during the first year after brachytherapy. The patient with the three-piece IPP developed a fluid leak from the reservoir tubing 8 years after device placement and 13 months after brachytherapy, making it unclear whether the malfunction was related to the radiotherapy *(59)*. The authors propose that prosthesis malfunction and infection should be unlikely if brachytherapy is performed after an adequate pseudocapsule has formed, given that the majority of infections occur shortly after IPP placement *(59)*. To reduce the chance of prosthetic infection, they advocate delaying brachytherapy until at least 6 months after IPP placement, full bowel preparation prior to brachytherapy, and administration of intravenous broad-spectrum antibiotics before and after brachytherapy *(59)*.

We feel that when considering RT for a patient with a preexisting prosthesis, options include removal of the device prior to conformal radiotherapy, delivering a reduced dose or using a modified template, or giving standard treatment despite the poorly understood effects of radiation on various prosthetic devices. The likelihood of prosthetic infection or failure after radiotherapy is unclear, but does not appear to be unreasonable. Therefore, alternative treatments should be considered strongly and patients should be adequately informed of the paucity of available data and potential risks inherent with such treatment.

8   Penile Prosthesis Placement After Radiation Therapy

As with post-prostatectomy ED, few of the major series mention RT specifically as a causative factor prior to IPP placement *(24–26,28–30,46,47,57)*. In one series of 145 patients, 1 patient each had received brachytherapy or external beam RT prior to IPP placement *(44)*. In another series, 5 of 371 patients (1.3%) had a history of "pelvic irradiation" *(23)*. In none of these reports is there mention of technique modification or outcomes in patients with prior radiotherapy *(23–26,28–30,44,46,47,57)*.

A single series reported outcomes in 43 patients who underwent penile implant after radiation therapy for prostate cancer *(60)*. Multi-component IPP, single component IPP, and semi-rigid rods were implanted in 76, 13, and 11% of patients, respectively *(60)*. The reported surgical technique in these patients was identical to that performed in other patients, which included use of an "infection minimization protocol" *(60)*. No patient in their surgical series experienced device infection or erosion, although one patient had undergone three prior prosthesis surgeries elsewhere, including placement, removal of an infected device, and subsequent failed re-implantation. At median follow-up of 24 months (range 8–145 months), three patients (7%) had required repeat surgical procedures due to fluid leak *(60)*. Of note, two of the three mechanical failures occurred in devices no longer on the market *(60)*. Of the 34 monitored patients, 32 (94%) stated they would undergo the surgery again and recommend the same surgery to others; including 24 patients (71%) who use the device at least once weekly. The two dissatisfied individuals included one patient who could not learn to cycle the device and one patient who was placed on a luteinizing hormone-releasing hormone analogue for advanced prostate cancer but attributes loss of libido to the implant *(60)*.

In this series, 35 patients (81%) underwent definitive RT to the prostate and seminal vesicles with total photon equivalent dose of 67–0 Gy, 9 of whom also received a neutron dose of 9–5 nGy 67 to the prostatic bed after RP. Contemporary radiation dosages for prostate cancer are somewhat higher (78–81 Gy), but provide less of a dose to off-target tissue *(61)*. We do not feel that pelvic irradiation as treatment for prostate cancer or otherwise should alter management options for patients in whom penile prosthesis surgery is being considered; three-piece IPPs are likely to provide the best results in these patients.

9 Penile Prosthesis Placement After Hormonal or Other Systemic Therapy for Prostate Cancer

Placement of a device in patients who have undergone pharmacologic castration or other systemic therapy is the same as for any other patient. There are no studies that specifically address technical outcomes or patient satisfaction in patients treated with hormones for PC or other hypogonadal patients who have undergone IPP placement. However, these patients in particular should be reminded that IPP will only correct ED, and will not increase libido or alter penile sensation or ejaculatory function. Outcomes would be expected to be no different than for other patients with ED.

10 Vacuum Erection Device Therapy

Vacuum constriction devices (VCD) are a non-pharmacologic, non-invasive, mechanical means to achieve a functional erection in motivated patients *(62,63)*. Most devices work by drawing blood into the penis using negative pressure and then affixing a ring around the base of the engorged penis. Widespread use of VCD has been limited by low acceptability to both patients and their sexual partners.

Although early reports estimated overall satisfaction rates greater than 80% *(62)*, more recent studies have demonstrated relatively high rates of dissatisfaction with and discontinuation of VCD *(12,64,65)*. In a review of sexual function outcomes in 1,288 men with prostate cancer who had undergone RP, 25% reported that they had used a vacuum erection device. Of these men, 35% reported that the VED helped "a lot" and 25% reported that erections were firm enough for intercourse *(12)*. In one study of 129 ED patients, the attrition rate was 65%, with discontinuation occurring at a median of 1 month after initiation of treatment *(65)*. The 2005 AUA ED guideline update panel recommended using only VCD containing a vacuum limiter (pop-off valve), in order to avoid injury to the penis at high negative pressure *(66)*. VCD remains a reasonable alternative for prostate cancer patients in whom pharmacologic agents are ineffective or contraindicated and are not interested in or poor operative candidates for IPP.

Other external erectile aids are an intriguing alternative for ED treatment in highly motivated patients, but other than a single case report *(67)* scientific data on this strategy are lacking.

11 Conclusions

ED is common in patients with prostate cancer and can be the result of neural injury from pelvic surgery or radiation or any of the other etiologies responsible for ED in other patients. Pharmacologic interventions can be attempted in most patients without detriment, but ED patients who have received treatment for PC respond less well to PDE5 inhibitors than other ED patients. Penile prostheses consistently provide the greatest patient (and partner) satisfaction and should be considered in patients who wish to maintain sexual activity despite poor erectile function after PC treatment. IPP can be considered prior to or shortly after RP in patients unlikely to retain sufficient erectile function. Placement of IPP after RP is safe and effective as a second-line therapy in those who have ED refractory to oral pharmacologic agents. Other non-pharmacologic interventions are used by a minority of men, but can be an effective alternative in the motivated patient.

References

1. Stephenson, R.A., Mori, M., Hsieh, Y.C., Beer, T.M., Stanford, J.L., Gilliland, F.D., et al. (2005 Aug) Treatment of erectile dysfunction following therapy for clinically localized prostate cancer: patient reported use and outcomes from the Surveillance, Epidemiology, and End Results Prostate Cancer Outcomes Study. *J. Urol.* **174**(2), 646–650; discussion 650.
2. Fowler, F.J., Jr., McNaughton C.M., Walker C.E., Elliott, D.B., and Barry, M.J. (2002 Jul 15) The impact of androgen deprivation on quality of life after radical prostatectomy for prostate carcinoma. *Cancer* **95**(2), 287–295.
3. Sharifi, N., Gulley, J.L., and Dahut, W.L. (2005 Jul 13) Androgen deprivation therapy for prostate cancer. *JAMA* **294**(2), 238–244.

4. Walsh, P.C., and Donker, P.J. (1982 Sep) Impotence following radical prostatectomy: insight into etiology and prevention. *J. Urol.* **128**(3), 492–497.
5. Walsh, P.C. (1998 Dec) Anatomic radical prostatectomy: evolution of the surgical technique. *J. Urol.* **160**(6 Pt 2), 2418–2424.
6. Walsh, P.C. (2007) Anatomic radical retropubic prostatectomy. In: Wein, A.J., Kavoussi, L.R., Novick, A.C., Partin, A.W., and Peters, C.A., eds. *Campbell-Walsh Urology*, 9th edn. New York: W.B. Saunders.
7. Quinlan, D.M., Epstein, J.I., Carter, B.S., and Walsh, P.C. () Sexual function following radical prostatectomy: influence of preservation of neurovascular bundles. *J. Urol.* 1991 May;145(5):998–1002.
8. Stanford, J.L., Feng, Z., Hamilton, A.S., Gilliland, F.D., Stephenson, R.A., and Eley, J.W., et al. (2000 Jan 19) Urinary and sexual function after radical prostatectomy for clinically localized prostate cancer: the Prostate Cancer Outcomes Study. *JAMA* **283**(3), 354–360.
9. Walsh, P.C., Marschke, P., Ricker, D., and Burnett, A.L. (2000 Jan) Patient-reported urinary continence and sexual function after anatomic radical prostatectomy. *Urology* **55**(1), 58–61.
10. Rabbani, F., Stapleton, A.M., Kattan, M.W., Wheeler, T.M., and Scardino, P.T. (2000 Dec) Factors predicting recovery of erections after radical prostatectomy. *J. Urol.* **164**(6), 1929–1934.
11. Kundu, S.D., Roehl, K.A., Eggener, S.E., Antenor, J.A., Han, M., and Catalona, W.J. (2004 Dec) Potency, continence and complications in 3,477 consecutive radical retropubic prostatectomies. *J. Urol.* **172**(6 Pt 1), 2227–2231.
12. Penson, D.F., McLerran, D., Feng, Z., Li, L., Albertsen, P.C., Gilliland, F.D., et al. (2005 May) 5-year urinary and sexual outcomes after radical prostatectomy: results from the prostate cancer outcomes study. *J. Urol.* **173**(5), 1701–1705.
13. Bianco, F.J., Jr., Scardino, P.T., and Eastham, J.A. (2005 Nov) Radical prostatectomy: long-term cancer control and recovery of sexual and urinary function ("trifecta"). *Urology* **66**(5 Suppl), 83–94.
14. Potosky, A.L., Davis, W.W., Hoffman, R.M., Stanford, J.L., Stephenson, R.A., Penson, D.F., et al. (2004 Sep 15) Five-year outcomes after prostatectomy or radiotherapy for prostate cancer: the prostate cancer outcomes study. *J. Natl. Cancer Inst.* **96**(18), 1358–1367.
15. Talcott, J.A., Rieker, P., Clark, J.A., Propert, K.J., Weeks, J.C., Beard, C.J., et al. (1998 Jan) Patient-reported symptoms after primary therapy for early prostate cancer: results of a prospective cohort study. *J. Clin. Oncol.* **16**(1), 275–283.
16. Litwin, M.S., Flanders, S.C., Pasta, D.J., Stoddard, M.L., Lubeck, D.P., and Henning, J.M. (1999 Sep) Sexual function and bother after radical prostatectomy or radiation for prostate cancer: multivariate quality-of-life analysis from CaPSURE. Cancer of the Prostate Strategic Urologic Research Endeavor. *Urology* **54**(3), 503–508.
17. Miller, D.C., Sanda, M.G., Dunn, R.L., Montie, J.E., Pimentel, H., Sandler, H.M., et al. (2005 Apr 20) Long-term outcomes among localized prostate cancer survivors: health-related quality-of-life changes after radical prostatectomy, external radiation, and brachytherapy. *J. Clin. Oncol.* **23**(12), 2772–2780.
18. Yamada, Y., Bhatia, S., Zaider, M., Cohen, G., Donat, M., Eastham, J., et al. (2006 Jul–Sep) Favorable clinical outcomes of three-dimensional computer-optimized high-dose-rate prostate brachytherapy in the management of localized prostate cancer. *Brachytherapy* **5**(3), 157–164.
19. NIH Consensus Conference. (1993 Jul 7) Impotence. NIH Consensus development panel on impotence. *JAMA* **270**(1), 83–90.
20. Martinez-Jabaloyas, J.M., Gil-Salom, M., Villamon-Fort, R., Pastor-Hernandez, F., Martinez-Garcia, R., and Garcia-Sisamon, F. (2001 Dec) Prognostic factors for response to sildenafil in patients with erectile dysfunction. *Eur. Urol.* **40**(6), 641–646; discussion 647.
21. Gontero, P., Fontana, F., Zitella, A., Montorsi, F., and Frea, B. (2005 Feb) A prospective evaluation of efficacy and compliance with a multistep treatment approach for erectile dysfunction in patients after non-nerve sparing radical prostatectomy. *BJU Int.* **95**(3), 359–365.

22. Steidle, C.P., and Mulcahy, J.J. (1989 Sep) Erosion of penile prostheses: a complication of urethral catheterization. *J. Urol.* **142**(3), 736–739.
23. Carson, C.C., Mulcahy, J.J., and Govier, F.E. (2000 Aug) Efficacy, safety and patient satisfaction outcomes of the AMS 700CX inflatable penile prosthesis: results of a long-term multicenter study. AMS 700CX Study Group. *J. Urol.* **164**(2), 376–380.
24. Deuk Choi, Y., Jin Choi, Y., Hwan Kim, J., and Ki Choi, H. (2001 Mar) Mechanical reliability of the AMS 700CXM inflatable penile prosthesis for the treatment of male erectile dysfunction. *J. Urol.* **165**(3), 822–824.
25. Dubocq, F., Tefilli, M.V., Gheiler, E.L., Li, H., and Dhabuwala, C.B. (1998 Aug) Long-term mechanical reliability of multicomponent inflatable penile prosthesis: comparison of device survival. *Urology* **52**(2), 277–281.
26. Daitch, J.A., Angermeier, K.W., Lakin, M.M., Ingleright, B.J., and Montague, D.K. (1997 Oct) Long-term mechanical reliability of AMS 700 series inflatable penile prostheses: comparison of CX/CXM and Ultrex cylinders. *J. Urol.* 158(4), 1400–1402.
27. Montorsi, F., Rigatti, P., Carmignani, G., Corbu, C., Campo, B., Ordesi, G., et al. (2000 Jan) AMS three-piece inflatable implants for erectile dysfunction: a long-term multi-institutional study in 200 consecutive patients. *Eur. Urol.* **37**(1), 50–55.
28. Milbank, A.J., Montague, D.K., Angermeier, K.W., Lakin, M.M., and Worley, S.E. (2002 Jun) Mechanical failure of the American Medical Systems Ultrex inflatable penile prosthesis: before and after 1993 structural modification. *J. Urol.* **167**(6), 2502–2506.
29. Goldstein, I., Newman, L., Baum, N., Brooks, M., Chaikin, L., Goldberg, K., et al. (1997 Mar) Safety and efficacy outcome of mentor alpha-1 inflatable penile prosthesis implantation for impotence treatment. *J. Urol.* **157**(3), 833–839.
30. Wilson, S.K., Cleves, M.A., and Delk, J.R., II. (1999 Sep) Comparison of mechanical reliability of original and enhanced Mentor Alpha I penile prosthesis. *J. Urol.* **162**(3 Pt 1), 715–718.
31. Scott, F.B., Bradley, W.E., and Timm, G.W. (1973 Jul) Management of erectile impotence. Use of implantable inflatable prosthesis. *Urology* **2**(1), 80–82.
32. Carson, C.C. (2005 Nov) Penile prosthesis implantation: surgical implants in the era of oral medication. *Urol. Clin. North Am.* **32**(4), 503–509, vii.
33. Montague, D.K. (2007) Prosthetic surgery for erectile dysfunction. In: Wein, A.J., Kavoussi, L.R., Novick, A.C., Partin, A.W., and Peters, C.A., eds. *Campbell-Walsh Urology*, 9th edn. New York: W.B. Saunders.
34. Montague, D.K. (1993 Sep) Penile prosthesis corporotomy closure: a new technique. *J. Urol.* **150**(3), 924–925.
35. Mooreville, M., Adrian, S., Delk, J.R., II, and Wilson, S.K. (1999 Dec) Implantation of inflatable penile prosthesis in patients with severe corporeal fibrosis: introduction of a new penile cavernotome. *J. Urol.* **162**(6), 2054–2057.
36. Montague, D.K., and Angermeier, K.W. (2006 May) Corporeal excavation: new technique for penile prosthesis implantation in men with severe corporeal fibrosis. *Urology* **67**(5), 1072–1075.
37. Montague, D.K., and Angermeier, K.W. (2003 Oct) Cylinder sizing: less is more. *Int. J. Impot. Res.* **15**(Suppl 5), S132–S133.
38. Abouassaly, R.A., Angermeier, K.W., and Montague, D.K. (2006) Risk of infection with an antibiotic coated penile prosthesis at device replacement for mechanical failure. *J. Urol.* **176**(12), x–y.
39. Lane, B.R., Abouassaly, R.A., Angermeier, K.W., and Montague, D.K. (2007) Three-piece inflatable penile prostheses can be safely implanted following radical prostatectomy. *Urol.* **70**(3), 539–542.
40. Mulcahy, J.J. (2000 Feb) Long-term experience with salvage of infected penile implants. *J. Urol.* **163**(2), 481–482.
41. Carson, C.C., III. (2004 Apr) Efficacy of antibiotic impregnation of inflatable penile prostheses in decreasing infection in original implants. *J. Urol.* **171**(4), 1611–1614.

42. Wolter, C.E., and Hellstrom, W.J. (2004 Sep) The hydrophilic-coated inflatable penile prosthesis: 1-year experience. *J. Sex. Med.* **1**(2), 221–224.

43. McLaren, R.H., and Barrett, D.M. (1992 Jan) Patient and partner satisfaction with the AMS 700 penile prosthesis. *J. Urol.* **147**(1), 62–65.

44. Holloway, F.B., and Farah, R.N. (1997 May) Intermediate term assessment of the reliability, function and patient satisfaction with the AMS700 Ultrex penile prosthesis. *J. Urol.* **157**(5), 1687–1691.

45. Tefilli, M.V., Dubocq, F., Rajpurkar, A., Gheiler, E.L., Tiguert, R., Barton, C., et al. (1998 Dec) Assessment of psychosexual adjustment after insertion of inflatable penile prosthesis. *Urology* **52**(6), 1106–1112.

46. Mulhall, J.P., Ahmed, A., Branch, J., and Parker, M. (2003 Apr) Serial assessment of efficacy and satisfaction profiles following penile prosthesis surgery. *J. Urol.* **169**(4), 1429–1433.

47. Sexton, W.J., Benedict, J.F., and Jarow, J.P. (1998 Mar) Comparison of long-term outcomes of penile prostheses and intracavernosal injection therapy. *J. Urol.* **159**(3), 811–815.

48. Rajpurkar, A., and Dhabuwala, C.B. (2003 Jul) Comparison of satisfaction rates and erectile function in patients treated with sildenafil, intracavernous prostaglandin E1 and penile implant surgery for erectile dysfunction in urology practice. *J. Urol.* **170**(1), 159–163.

49. Davis, B.E., DeBrock, B.J., Lierz, M.F., and Weigel, J.W. (1992 Oct) Management of pre-existing inflatable penile prosthesis during radical retropubic prostatectomy. *J. Urol.* **148**(4), 1198–1200.

50. Dunsmuir, W.D., and Kirby, R.S. (1997 Feb) Conservation of inflatable penile prosthesis during radical retropubic prostatectomy. *Br. J. Urol.* **79**(2), 283–284.

51. Tiguert, R., Hurley, P.M., Gheiler, E.L., Tefilli, M.V., Gudziak, M.R., Dhabuwala, C.B., et al. (1998 Dec) Treatment outcome after radical prostatectomy is not adversely affected by a pre-existing penile prosthesis. *Urology* **52**(6), 1030–1033.

52. Schanne, F.J., Carpiniello, V., and Chaikin, D. (1998 Oct) Radical prostatectomy in patients with indwelling inflatable penile prosthesis. *Urology* **52**(4), 715–716.

53. Mireku-Boateng, A.O., and Oben, F. (2005) Surgical outcome of radical retropubic prostatectomy is not adversely affected by preexisting three-piece inflatable penile implant. *Urol. Int.* **74**(3), 221–223.

54. Khoudary, K.P., DeWolf, W.C., Bruning, C.O., III, Morgentaler, A. (1997 Sep) Immediate sexual rehabilitation by simultaneous placement of penile prosthesis in patients undergoing radical prostatectomy: initial results in 50 patients. *Urology* **50**(3), 395–399.

55. Ramsawh, H.J., Morgentaler, A., Covino, N., Barlow, D.H., and DeWolf, W.C. (2005 Oct) Quality of life following simultaneous placement of penile prosthesis with radical prostatectomy. *J. Urol.* **174**(4 Pt 1), 1395–1398.

56. Telang, D.J., and Farah, R.N. (1992) Management of impotence after treatment of carcinoma of the prostate. *Henry Ford Hosp Med. J.* **40**(1–2), 111–113.

57. Brinkman, M.J., Henry, G.D., Wilson, S.K., Delk, J.R., II, Denny, G.A., Young, M., et al. (2005 Jul) A survey of patients with inflatable penile prostheses for satisfaction. *J. Urol.* **174**(1), 253–257.

58. Christie, D.R., Hulbert, P., and Christiansen, P. (2001 Nov) Prosthetic devices within radiotherapy fields: planning implications and results. *Australas. Radiol.* **45**(4), 528–530.

59. Li, P., Wallner, K., Ellis, W., Blasko, J., and Corman, J.M. (2001 May) Prostate brachytherapy in patients with a penile prosthesis. *BJU Int.* **87**(7), 712–713.

60. Dubocq, F.M., Bianco, F.J., Jr., Maralani, S.J., Forman, J.D., and Dhabuwala, C.B. (1997 Nov) Outcome analysis of penile implant surgery after external beam radiation for prostate cancer. *J. Urol.* **158**(5), 1787–1790.

61. Speight, J.L., and Roach, M., III. (2006 Apr) Radiotherapy in the management of common genitourinary malignancies. *Hematol. Oncol. Clin. North Am.* **20**(2), 321–346.

62. Nadig, P.W., Ware, J.C., and Blumoff, R. (1986 Feb) Noninvasive device to produce and maintain an erection-like state. *Urology* **27**(2), 126–131.

63. Lewis, R.W., and Witherington, R. (1997) External vacuum therapy for erectile dysfunction: use and results. *World J. Urol.* **15**(1), 78–82.
64. Earle, C.M., Seah, M., Coulden, S.E., Stuckey, B.G., and Keogh, E.J. (1996 Dec) The use of the vacuum erection device in the management of erectile impotence. *Int. J. Impot. Res.* **8**(4), 237–240.
65. Dutta, T.C., and Eid, J.F. (1999 Nov) Vacuum constriction devices for erectile dysfunction: a long-term, prospective study of patients with mild, moderate, and severe dysfunction. *Urology* **54**(5), 891–893.
66. Montague, D.K., Jarow, J.P., Broderick, G.A., Dmochowski, R.R., Heaton, J.P., Lue, T.F., et al. (2005 Jul) Chapter 1: The management of erectile dysfunction: an AUA update. *J. Urol.* **174**(1), 230–239.
67. Gray, R.E., and Klotz, L.H. (2004 Jun) Restoring sexual function in prostate cancer patients: an innovative approach. *Can. J. Urol.* **11**(3), 2285–2289.

Chapter 15
Androgen Supplementation in the Prostate Cancer Patient

Abraham Morgentaler

Contents

Abstract Testosterone (T) deficiency, also termed hypogonadism, affects a substantial proportion of older men, and causes a variety of symptoms and signs, such as erectile dysfunction, diminished libido, fatigue, depression, and diminished bone mineral density. Testosterone replacement therapy (TRT) can be an effective therapy, but there has been a long-standing and widely held fear of offering TRT in the prostate cancer (PCa) patient due to the concern that higher T levels may "awaken" dormant PCa cells, and cause a recurrence or progression of the cancer. Indeed, product information packaging for testosterone products includes FDA-mandated language stating that TRT is contraindicated in men with a history of, or suspicion of prostate cancer.

From: *Current Clinical Urology* Series, *Sexual Function in the Prostate Cancer Patient*
Edited by John P. Mulhall, DOI 10.1007/978-1-60327-555-2_15,
© Humana Press, a part of Springer Science+Business Media, LLC 2009

However, scientific literature fails to provide support for this concept. The origin of the concern stems from the landmark work by Huggins and co-workers, who reported in 1941 that severe reductions in serum T by castration or estrogen therapy caused regression of prostate cancer (PCa), and also that administration of T caused "enhanced growth" of PCa. Remarkably, the assertion by Huggins regarding the "enhanced growth" of PCa was based on a single patient. A number of reports prior to 1982 described the use of daily T injections in men with advanced PCa, with some men experiencing subjective benefits, and without any indication of unexpected disease progression. Although there is little modern experience with administration of T in men with known history of PCa, there is a varied and extensive literature indicating that higher T does not pose any increased risk of PCa growth, in men with or without prior treatment. For instance, the cancer rate in TRT trials is only approximately 1%, similar to detection rates in screening programs, yet biopsy detectable PCa is found in one of seven hypogonadal men. Moreover, PCa is almost never seen in the peak T years of the early twenties despite autopsy evidence that men in this age group already harbor microfoci of PCa in substantial numbers. Finally, a recent report showed that concentrations of T and DHT within the prostate were unchanged after 6 months of TRT, thus providing an explanation why TRT may not cause increased PCa growth.

The growing number of PCa survivors who happen to be hypogonadal and requesting treatment has spurred a change in attitude toward this topic, with increasing numbers of physicians now offering TRT to men who appear cured of their disease. Publications have now reported no PSA recurrence with TRT in small numbers of men who had undetectable PSA values following radical prostatectomy. Although still controversial, there appears little justification to withhold TRT from men with favorable outcomes after definitive treatment for PCa.

Keywords Testosterone; androgen; prostate cancer; hypogonadism; testosterone replacement therapy; libido; erectile dysfunction.

1 Introduction

1.1 Testosterone Deficiency and the Prostate Cancer Patient

Testosterone deficiency, also termed hypogonadism, can cause a variety of symptoms and signs, such as erectile dysfunction, diminished libido, increased fatigue, depression, and decreased bone mineral density *(1)*. Testosterone replacement therapy (TRT) is often effective in treating these symptoms and signs *(2)*; however, there has been a long-standing and widely held taboo against offering TRT to men with a history of prostate cancer (PCa), regardless of disease status. This taboo arose from the concern that higher serum T levels would "awaken" dormant PCa cells, thus causing disease progression or recurrence. The prohibition against TRT has particular poignancy for PCa survivors, who often have already experienced significant compromise of their sexual function from their cancer treatments, and also because their cancer treatment may have directly caused the reduction in serum T that has contributed to their symptoms.

1.2 The Origin of the Prohibition Against TRT in Prostate Cancer Patients

The origin of the prohibition against TRT in prostate cancer patients a rose from the work of Huggins and co-workers in 1941, who reported that castration or lowering of T by estrogen administration caused PCa to regress *(3)*, and that T administration caused "enhanced growth" of PCa. This prohibition against TRT in men with a history of PCa reaches to the highest levels of medicine. Product labeling for T formulations includes a contraindication against using T in men with "a history of, or suspicion of, prostate cancer" *(4)*. Several years ago, the NIH temporarily halted T-related research, in part due to prostate safety concerns, until the Institute of Medicine could make recommendations regarding effective and ethical T trials. It has even been suggested that men who only have a family history of PCa should not be offered TRT *(5)*.

However, with the increased interest in TRT over the last decade, the relationship of T to PCa has come under greater scrutiny. Surprisingly, multiple reviews have failed to find any compelling evidence supporting the decades-old assumption that higher T causes PCa growth *(6–10)*. And there is now a growing population of otherwise healthy men who have survived definitive treatment for PCa and who happen to have symptomatic hypogonadism, and are requesting treatment. These events have conspired to create a new environment regarding the use of TRT in men with PCa or at risk for it.

The change in attitudes regarding this issue is manifest by the appearance of publications questioning the relationship of T to PCa *(6,9,10)*, by several small publications reporting no ill-effects of TRT in men who appear cured of PCa *(11,12)*, and by substantial interest in the topic at medical meetings with lectures addressing this issue.

2 Historical Experience with Testosterone and Prostate Cancer

2.1 The Original Report: Huggins

In 1941 Huggins and co-workers reported that men with metastatic PCa demonstrated significant reductions in serum acid phosphatase when T was severely reduced by castration or with estrogen treatment *(3)*. In the same publication, Huggins and co-workers also administered T for short duration in several of these men,

Table 1 Long-Standing Arguments Versus Facts Regarding the Relationship Between Testosterone and Prostate Cancer

---

Lowering testosterone to castrate levels causes PCa to regress, so raising T is likely to increase growth
  – Data support a saturation curve, in which cancer growth follows T levels only with changes at very low levels
Huggins reported that T supplementation caused enhanced growth of PCa
  – Data presented for only a single patient who had not been previously manipulated hormonally
Fowler and Whitmore reported that 45 of 52 men with metastatic PCa treated with T had an "unfavorable response"
  – Only 4 men in their study population had not been castrated or treated with estrogen to lower testosterone, and those 4 men had a fairly unremarkable clinical course. The authors concluded that endogenous levels of testosterone may be enough to provide "near-maximal stimulation" of prostate cancer growth.
Men castrated early in life never develop PCa
  – First asserted in 1948. Widely repeated, but incorrect, and without scientific support.
The transient rise in testosterone with LHRH agonists, termed testosterone flare, is associated with poor clinical outcomes due to PCa progression.
  – In two studies that reported PSA values during the course of the testosterone flare, no increase in PSA was noted during or after the observed increase in testosterone levels.

---

and reported that acid phosphatase levels rose, leading them to conclude that T administration caused "enhanced growth" of PCa. This paper established the hormonal dependence of prostate cancer, and forms the basis for current treatment with the use of LHRH agonists in men with advanced PCa. Huggins eventually was awarded the Nobel Prize for this landmark work (Tables 1 and 2).

However, the portion of the paper that addressed the effects of T administration fails to stand up to scientific scrutiny, at least by today's standards. Whereas three men were reported to have received T injections, results were provided for only two men, and one of these men had been previously castrated. Thus, the original assertion that T administration in previously untreated men would cause "enhanced growth" of PCa was based on short-term blood test results in only a single patient!

Table 2 Inconsistencies in Current Approach to Testosterone and Prostate Cancer

---

  – If testosterone were truly a major stimulus for PCa growth, why is it that we rarely see clinical PCa in the peak testosterone years of 20–39, despite the presence of PCa in substantial numbers of men in this age group, as shown by autopsy studies?
  – Why does the prevalence of PCa rise dramatically with advancing age, when testosterone levels are low, and is almost never seen in young men, when testosterone levels are high?
  – We deny testosterone supplementation to men who appear to have been cured of PCa after definitive treatment, with the rationale that higher testosterone levels might "awaken" dormant malignant cells, yet we make no attempt to reduce testosterone in men with normal endogenous levels.
  – If the concern is that testosterone causes progression of PCa after a delay of 20–30 years, then why do we have any hesitation in offering testosterone treatment to men in their sixties and seventies?

2.2 Historical Experience with T Administration in Men with PCa

Other investigators of that era failed to find worrisome progression of PCa in men receiving T administration. Prout et al. *(13)* administered daily injections of T propionate to 26 men, of whom 20 had not been castrated. Although no regression of PCa was noted in any of these men, some did experience beneficial subjective responses, such as increased appetite, decreased bone pain, and an improved sense of well-being. The improvement in bone pain reported by these investigators is in contrast to the conventional modern wisdom that higher T routinely causes worse bone pain among men with bone metastases. No obvious or precipitous progression of PCa with T administration was reported in these men.

2.3 The Memorial Sloan-Kettering Experience

Fowler and Whitmore reported on the experience of T administration in men with a history of bone metastases from PCa treated at the Memorial Sloan-Kettering Cancer Center over a period of 18 years *(14)*. Of 52 men, 45 were reported to have experienced an "unfavorable response," a broad category that included clinical progression, worse bone pain, or an increase in acid phosphatase. This report is often cited as proof that T administration is dangerous for men with PCa.

However, a close reading provides a different conclusion. Of these 52 men, only four had not previously undergone castration or estrogen treatment. Since we know that PCa will recur if T deprivation is reversed, there should be no surprise that most of these previously treated men experienced negative outcomes with restoration of T levels. The group of greater interest is the men who had not been previously treated. Of these four, one had an early "unfavorable" response, not otherwise specified, one had a beneficial subjective response, and the remaining two had "unfavorable" responses at 56 and 310 days of T administration. The authors concluded from this experience that endogenous levels of T may be enough to provide "near-maximal stimulation" of PCa growth *(14)*.

3 Modern Evidence Regarding Testosterone and the Risk of PCa

3.1 Natural History

The concept that higher T represents a risk for PCa growth or subsequent development has been a touchstone of uro-oncology, but the evidence to support this belief has been elusive, and the logic has always been strained. Reviews have failed to find compelling evidence demonstrating a link between higher T and PCa. And the concept defies the epidemiology of PCa, rarely occurring during the peak T years of the twenties and thirties, but becoming highly prevalent when men are older and T levels have declined substantially. Moreover, it is known from autopsy studies that a significant percentage of men in their twenties already harbor microfoci of PCa *(15)*. If high T caused enhanced PCa growth, one would expect to find a much greater number of PCa cases in young men.

3.2 Longitudinal Studies of Serum Testosterone and Subsequent Risk of Prostate Cancer

3.2.1 Overview

There are at least 16 sizable longitudinal studies investigating the relationship of endogenous levels of multiple hormones and the subsequent risk of PCa *(16–22)*. In these studies, blood is obtained at baseline, men are followed for periods of up to 20 years or longer, and a group of men is identified who has developed PCa in the interim. A control group of an equal or greater number of age-matched individuals who did not develop PCa is then identified. Samples frozen from study entry are then thawed and tested for various hormone levels. Not one has shown an association between total testosterone and subsequent risk of PCa. A few have shown weak associations with minor androgens or ratios of T to other hormones, but those findings have not been reproducible. The largest of these studies, from Scandinavia, actually reported an association between PCa and *low* serum testosterone *(18)*.

3.2.2 Reported Associations Between PCa and T in Longitudinal Studies

Three of these longitudinal studies have suggested a relationship with androgens. One of these reported an association with the weak androgen androstenedione *(22)*, and another reported an association with calculated free testosterone *(17)*. Neither of these results has stood up to subsequent investigation. Another study reported a relationship between PCa and ratios of T to sex hormone binding globulin, as well as a relationship to T when adjusted simultaneously for four other hormones *(21)*.

This latter study was derived from the Physician's Health Study, published in 1996 *(20)*. It can be instructive to examine the details of such studies, in particular what relationships proved *not* to be significant, and the ways in which positive associations were identified. In this study, 222 men developed PCa between 1982 and 1992. An age-matched group of 390 men who did not develop PCa served as a control population. The primary findings were that no significant differences were seen in test results between the PCa and non-PCa groups with regard to any of the hormones studied, including total testosterone, estradiol, SHBG, and DHT. There was also no increased risk found for increasing levels of T, or for any other hormone. Among the many additional analyses, a significant association was found for a rising ratio of T/SHBG, and also for increasing T levels, but only with simultaneous adjustment for four other hormones. Subsequent studies have failed to confirm any relationship between T/SHBG ratios and PCa *(16)*. In addition, the validity of adjusting for four other variables simultaneously has dubious clinical merit.

3.2.3 The Baltimore Longitudinal Aging Study

More recently, an analysis of data from the Baltimore Longitudinal Aging Study reported that higher levels of calculated free T were associated with an increased risk of PCa, based on quartile analysis *(17)*. However, there was no association noted for total T, or for any other hormone. This relationship is suspect for two primary reasons. First, men in the PCa group were significantly older than men without PCa, and age represents the strongest known risk factor for PCa. Second, mean levels of calculated free T were actually numerically lower in the cancer group than in the group without PCa, raising concerns regarding the validity of quartile analysis. Subsequent studies in larger populations using the same methodology for calculated free T have failed to support this finding *(18)*.

In summary, these longitudinal studies involving several hundred thousand men, have consistently and uniformly found no association whatsoever between PCa and total T levels, and occasional reports of associations with other androgen measures have failed to be confirmed with subsequent investigations. If higher T truly caused significant PCa growth, why would it be so difficult to demonstrate a relationship between T and PCa in these sophisticated large studies, particularly since occult PCa is present in as many as 15% of older men *(23)*?

3.3 Clinical TRT Trials

No large-scale, long-term TRT trials have yet been performed, although planning for such a trial is currently in progress, sponsored by the NIH. No definitive assurances of safety and efficacy may be possible until such a trial is completed, yet there have been a modest number of smaller trials to review. In TRT trials of 6–36 month duration, the cancer detection rate was approximately 1% *(1)*. These studies have included regular PSA tests and DREs, with biopsy triggered by development of abnormalities. This rate of cancer is similar to that found in prostate screening studies *(1)*.

3.4 TRT in Men with Prostatic Intraepithelial Neoplasia

A group of 20 hypogonadal men with high-grade PIN and 55 hypogonadal men with benign prostate biopsies underwent 12 months of TRT *(24)*. One of the men in the PIN group was found to have cancer, with biopsy triggered by development of an abnormal DRE. This represents a 5% cancer rate in this population, and a 1.3% cancer rate for the group as a whole. Since development of frank cancer has been reported to occur within several years in 25% or more of men with PIN *(25)*, these data suggest that TRT did not cause any precipitous progression of cancer in these men.

3.5   Prostate Biopsy in Men with Low Testosterone

The notion that higher T causes increased PCa growth should also mean that men with lower T should be relatively protected against the growth of PCa. However, this also appears to not be the case. Sextant prostate biopsy in untreated hypogonadal men with PSA of 4.0 or less revealed cancer in 11 of 77 men, or 14% *(26)*. This rate is not dissimilar to the cancer rate of 15% in men with PSA of 4.0 or less noted by Thompson et al. in the placebo arm of the Prostate Cancer Prevention Trial (PCPT) *(23)*. The mean age of men in the hypogonadal series was approximately 10 years younger than men in the PCPT trial. In a recent report of 345 men with low T and PSA ≤4.0 ng/ml, men with more severe reductions in T had a significantly greater risk of cancer than men with milder reduction in T *(27)*. This again suggests the possibility of an important association between low T and PCa.

3.6   Testosterone Flare and PSA

Testosterone flare refers to the transient rise in T that occurs within 7–10 days of administration of LHRH agonists, before T levels drop to castrate levels. Several publications have reported that the T flare is associated with increased bone pain, cancer progression, urinary retention, or vertebral collapse with spinal cord compression *(28)*. However, only two studies appear to have measured PSA acutely, during the flare interval, and in neither instance did mean PSA levels increase during the T flare *(29,30)*. Since PSA is the best available indicator of PCa progression and volume, these results fail to support the concept that a rise in T causes growth of PCa. Reports of negative effects seen in association with the T flare were uncontrolled, and occurred in men with advanced disease. One must consider the possibility that the reported negative clinical effects seen during the period of testosterone flare may have been due to the natural history of the disease itself, or possibly, via direct effects of T on bone.

4   Testosterone Treatment in Men with Prostate Cancer

4.1   Rationale

Treatment of PCa with LHRH agonists or radiation treatment may cause testosterone deficiency, and cause symptoms of erectile dysfunction, diminished libido, difficulty achieving orgasm, and fatigue. With severely depressed T levels, men may also experience hot flushes. Even when LHRH therapy is discontinued, there may be long-lasting suppressive effects on serum T, and in some cases T levels never return to normal. Men who are symptomatic from testosterone deficiency, particularly if they appear stable with regard to PCa, may request treatment for their hypogonadal symptoms. If there is little evidence that higher T causes PCa growth, then why withhold treatment that may be symptomatically beneficial?

4.2 Testosterone Following Radical Prostatectomy

The "cleanest" population in whom to consider TRT following treatment of PCa is the group of men with undetectable PSA several years following radical prostatectomy. If no cancer cells are evident, as suggested by undetectable PSA, then there should be no concern that T administration would cause them to grow. If the concern is that dormant cells might "awaken" with higher T, causing cancer progression, then why do we not act to reduce T levels in men with high endogenous T levels?

Two small studies *(11,12)*, in seven and ten men, have been published reporting the use of TRT in men following radical prostatectomy and with undetectable PSA. No PSA recurrence was noted in any of the men, with the longest follow-up being 12 years.

4.3 Testosterone Following Other Treatments for PCa

In men following PCa treatment with external beam radiation, brachytherapy, or cryotherapy, there is usually a measurable PSA value, and this value can fluctuate over time, raising anxieties for clinician and patient alike. There has thus been greater reluctance to initiate TRT in these men. However, the theoretical arguments remain the same. If no cancer is present, then there should be no concern regarding growth. And even if cancer is present in small volumes, the existing evidence fails to indicate that higher T values cause cancer growth or progression. To date, no publications have confirmed this concept, however, an abstract presented at the meeting of the American Urological Association in 2006 indicated a lack of PSA progression in men treated with TRT following brachytherapy.

5 TRT in Men with Untreated or Recurrent PCa

There is little modern experience of administering TRT to men with known PCa who have not otherwise undergone treatment, or with recurrent PCa. Historical papers, described above, were uncontrolled and accurate measures of progression, i.e., PSA, were unavailable. It is therefore impossible to state with any certainty what the effect of TRT might be in men with active PCa.

Nevertheless, available evidence suggests that once a testosterone threshold, or saturation point, has been reached, higher levels of T are unlikely to cause any further increase in PCa growth *(6)*. A recent report provides support for this concept. In a prospective study *(31)*, 40 hypogonadal men were randomized to 6 months of placebo or T injections. Prostate biopsies were obtained at the beginning and end of the trial, and assayed also for hormone levels and gene markers of interest. Although serum T and DHT increased significantly in men receiving TRT, prostate tissue levels demonstrated no change in T or DHT, and tumor markers were also unchanged. Prostate hormone levels thus do not appear to reflect the increases in hormone values seen in serum with TRT.

6   Conclusions

Over the last several years there has been a gradual reassessment of the relationship of T and PCa. Although traditionally, it has been considered taboo to offer TRT to any man with a history of PCa, regardless of disease status, many clinicians have begun to offer treatment to selected patients. The most common clinical scenario is for the symptomatically hypogonadal man with undetectable PSA following radical prostatectomy. The near future is likely to provide additional evidence regarding safety and degree of risk regarding TRT and PCa.

It is difficult to discard old ideas, particularly when they conjure up concerns regarding progression or recurrence of cancer. However, in this age of evidence-based medicine, it is imperative that we examine the basis for risk-related concerns as carefully as we do other parameters of health care. With regard to TRT and PCa, it is important to acknowledge that the putative risk of TRT causing PCa progression does not stand up to scientific scrutiny. Until such time as we have more definitive data, it may be reasonable to offer TRT to selected PCa patients, taking care to disclose that there is an unknown degree of risk with regard to PCa recurrence or progression. In partnership with our patients, it may then be possible to strike a proper balance between risk and benefit, allowing for the best possible quality of life while still acknowledging the limits of scientific knowledge.

References

1. Rhoden, E.L., and Morgentaler, A. (2004) Risks of testosterone-replacement therapy and recommendations for monitoring. *N. Engl. J. Med.* **350,** 482–492.
2. Morgentaler, A. (2004) Clinical crossroads: a 66-year-old man with sexual dysfunction. *JAMA* **291,** 2994–3003.
3. Huggins, C., and Hodges, C.V. (1941) Studies on prostatic cancer I. the effect of castration, of estrogen and of androgen injection on serum phosphatases in metastatic carcinoma of the prostate. *Cancer Res.* **1,** 293–7.

4. *Physician's, Desk Reference.* (2005) Montvale, NJ: Thomson, PDR, p. 3245.
5. Vaughan, D., Gaylis, F.D., et al. (2005) Re: Prostate cancer in men using testosterone supplementation. *J. Urol.* **174**, 534–538.
6. Morgentaler, A. (2006) Testosterone and prostate cancer: an historical perspective on a modern myth. *Eur. Urol.* **50**, 935–939.
7. Gould, D.C., and Kirby, R.S. (2006) Testosterone replacement therapy for late onset hypogonadism: what is the risk of inducing prostate cancer? *Prostate Cancer Prostatic Dis.* **9**, 14–18.
8. Bhasin, S., Singh, A.B., Mac, R.P., Carter, B., Lee, M.I., and Cunningham, G.R. (2003) Managing the risks of prostate disease during testosterone replacement therapy in older men: recommendations for a standardized monitoring plan. *J. Androl.* **24**, 299–311.
9. Morgentaler, A. (2006) Testosterone replacement therapy and prostate risks: where's the beef? *Can. J. Urol.* **13**, S40–S43.
10. Barqawi, A.B., and Crawford, E.D. (2005) Testosterone replacement therapy and the risk of prostate cancer: a perspective view. *Int. J. Impot. Res.* **17**, 462–463.
11. Kaufman, J.M., and Graydon, R.J. (2004) Androgen replacement after curative radical prostatectomy for prostate cancer in hypogonadal men. *J. Urol.* **172**, 920–922.
12. Agarwal, P.K., and Oefelein, M.G. (2005) Testosterone replacement therapy after primary treatment for prostate cancer. *J. Urol.* **173**, 533–536.
13. Prout, G.R., and Brewer, W.R. (1967) Response of men with advanced prostatic carcinoma to exogenous administration of testosterone. *Cancer* **20**, 1871–1878.
14. Fowler, J.E., and Whitmore, W.F., Jr. (1981) The response of metastatic adenocarcinoma of the prostate to exogenous testosterone. *J. Urol.* **126**, 372–375.
15. Sakr, W.A., Grignon, D.J., Crissman, J.D., Heilbrun, L.K., Cassin, B.J., Pontes, J.J., and Haas, G.P. (1994) High grade prostatic intraepithelial neoplasia (HGPIN) and prostatic adenocarcinoma between the ages of 20–69: an autopsy study of 249 cases. *In Vivo* **8**, 439–443.
16. Hsing, A.W. (2001) Hormones and prostate cancer: what's next? *Epidemiol. Rev.* **23**, 42–58.
17. Parsons, J.K., Carter, H.B., Platz, E.A., Wright, E.J., Landis, P., and Metter, E.J. (2005) Serum testosterone and the risk of prostate cancer: potential implications for testosterone therapy. *Cancer Epidemiol. Biomarkers Prev.* **14**, 2257–2260.
18. Stattin, P., Lumme, S., Tenkanen, L., et al. (2004) High levels of circulating testosterone are not associated with increased prostate cancer risk: a pooled prospective study. *Int. J. Cancer* **108**, 418–424.
19. Chen, C., Weiss, N.S., Stanczyk, F.Z., et al. (2003) Endogenous sex hormones and prostate cancer risk: a case-control study nested within the carotene and retinol efficacy trial. *Cancer Epidemiol Biomarkers Prev.* **12**, 1410–1416.
20. Platz, E.A., Leitzmann, M.F., Rifai, N., et al. (2005) Sex steroid hormones and the androgen receptor gene CAG repeat and subsequent risk of prostate cancer in the prostate-specific antigen era. *Cancer Epidemiol Biomarkers Prev.* **14**, 1262–1269.
21. Gann, P.H., Hennekens, C.H., Ma, J., et al. (1996) Prospective study of Sex hormone levels and risk of prostate cancer. *J. Natl. Cancer Inst.* **88**, 1118–1126.
22. Barrett-Connor, E., Garland, C., McPhillips, J.B., Khaw, K.T., and Wingard, D.L. (1990) A prospective, population-based study of androstenedione, estrogens, and prostatic cancer. *Cancer Res.* 50, 169–173.
23. Thompson, I.M., Pauler, D.K., Goodman, P.J., et al. (2004), Prevalence of prostate cancer among men with a prostate-specific antigen level £4 ng per milliliter. *N. Eng. J. Med.* **350**, 2239–2246.
24. Rhoden, E.L., and Morgentaler, A. (2003) Testosterone replacement therapy in hypogonadal men at high risk for prostate cancer: results of 1 year of treatment in men with prostatic intraepithelial neoplasia. *J. Urol.* **170**, 2348–2351.
25. Lefkowitz, G.K., Taneja, S.S., Brown, J., Melamed, J., and Lepor, H. (2002) Follow up interval prostate biopsy 3 years after diagnosis of high grade prostatic intraepithelial neoplasia is associated with high likelihood of prostate cancer, independent of change in prostate specific antigen levels. *J. Urol.* **168**, 1415–1418.

26. Morgentaler, A., Bruning, C.O., III, and DeWolf, W.C. (1996) Incidence of occult prostate cancer among men with low total or free serum testosterone. *JAMA* **276,** 1904–1906.

27. Morgentaler, A., and Rhoden, E.L. (2006) Prevalence of prostate cancer among hypogonadal men with prostate-specific antigen of 4.0 ng/ml or less. *Urology* **68,** 1263–1267.

28. Bubley, G.J. (2001) Is the flare phenomenon clinically significant? *Urology* **58** (Suppl 2A), 5–9.

29. Kuhn, J.M., Billebaud, T., Navratil, H., et al. (1989) Prevention of the transient adverse effects of a gonadotropin-releasing hormone analogue (Buserelin) in metastatic prostatic carcinoma by administration of an antiandrogen (Nilutamide). *NEJM* **321,** 413–418.

30. Tomera, K., Gleason, D., Gittelman, M., et al. (2001) The gonadotropin-releasing hormone antagonist Abarelix depot versus luteinizing hormone releasing hormone agonists leuprolide or goserelin: initial results of endocrinological and biochemical efficacies in patients with prostate cancer. *J. Urol.* **16,** 1585–1589.

31. Marks, L.S., Mazer, N.A., Mostaghel, E., Hess, D.L., Dorey, F.J., Epstein, J.I., Veltri, R.W., Makarov, D.V., Partin, A.W., Bostwick, D.G., Macairan, M.L., and Nelson, P.S. (2006) Effect of testosterone replacement therapy on prostate tissue in men with late-onset hypogonadism: a randomized controlled trial. *JAMA* **296,** 2351–2361.

Chapter 16
Future Therapies Applicable to Post-radical Pelvic Surgery Patients

Anthony J. Bella, William O. Brant, and Tom F. Lue

Abstract Despite advances in operative technique and pharmacotherapy, erectile function is compromised in a significant proportion of men undergoing radical pelvic surgery for prostate, bladder, and colorectal malignancies. Strategies to decrease the incidence or severity of post-operative erectile dysfunction may include pre-operative optimization of erectile function, risk factors, and/or other protective maneuvers, elimination or modulation of neural, vascular and corporal smooth muscle injury, and the use of novel pharmacotherapies. In this chapter, future strategies to optimize the recovery of erectile function, and ultimately increase patient quality of life, are outlined.

Keywords Prostate cancer; erectile dysfunction; neuroprotection; nerve regeneration; stem cells; quality of life; gene therapy.

From: *Current Clinical Urology* Series, *Sexual Function in the Prostate Cancer Patient*
Edited by John P. Mulhall, DOI 10.1007/978-1-60327-555-2_16,
© Humana Press, a part of Springer Science+Business Media, LLC 2009

1 Introduction

A paradigm shift in the management of prostate cancer occurred as a result of the introduction of cavernous nerve-sparing radical prostatectomy by Walsh and Donker, and the widespread availability of effective, safe, and well-tolerated pharmacotherapies for erectile dysfunction (ED) *(1,2)*. Although cancer-control is the primary and most important outcome measure for any surgical intervention for malignancy, a growing emphasis on health-related quality of life (QoL) has thrust sexual function into the forefront of post-operative clinical concerns. Mainstream media exposure for ED following the introduction of the oral phosphodiesterase-5 (PDE-5) inhibitors sildenafil, tadalafil and vardenafil, coupled with an enhanced understanding of the physiology and pathophysiology of erectile function and dysfunction, have contributed to a growing awareness by physicians and their patients of the possibility of maintaining satisfactory sexual function following cancer treatments.

Unfortunately, most men report some degree of compromised erectile function or complete loss of potency even with bilateral nerve-sparing modifications to open, laparoscopic, and robot-assisted approaches to curative prostatectomy, indicating that the cavernous nerves are inadvertently damaged by surgical manipulation *(3,5)*. The risk of ED is ever-present, even under optimal circumstances for men with normal pre-operative erectile function, and is influenced by several other factors, including advancing age and resection of the neurovascular bundles, which are discussed in detail elsewhere.

Here, we review future approaches and therapies, which may be used to optimize erectile function following radical pelvic surgeries for malignancy of the prostate, as well as muscle-invasive bladder or colorectal cancers. It is possible that future treatments will encompass a combination of strategies such as neuroprotection to counteract secondary injury, provision of scaffolds to replace lost tissue, and methods to enhance axonal regrowth, inhibition of apoptosis, and synaptic plasticity. Strategies include pre-operative protective measures, modulation of neural, vascular (including arterial insufficiency and veno-occlusive dysfunction), and corporal smooth muscle injury, further refinement of operative techniques such as the introduction of nerve "bridges" or "scaffolds," and novel monotherapy or combination drug therapies for ED induced by pelvic cancer treatments.

2 Pre-operative Optimization of Erectile Function

One of the most powerful predictors for satisfactory post-radical prostatectomy (RP) erectile recovery is sexual function prior to surgery *(6)*. To date, pharmacologic preconditioning, pre-operative modification of co-morbidities, and changes to patient lifestyle, have been underutilized as an adjunctive strategy for improving post-operative erectile function (EF).

2.1 Pharmacological Preconditioning

The concept of optimizing or enhancing recovery and minimizing post-operative tissue changes is intriguing. Cavernous nerve injury is known to induce cavernous smooth muscle apoptosis, denervation coupled with hypoxia increases scar tissue formation, and decreased arterial circulation can lead to increased production of TGF-β and corporal fibrosis. End-results of these changes include cavernosal insufficiency and veno-occlusive dysfunction (7).

Early animal and pilot human studies with pre-treatment regimens using various agents, including phosphodiesterase-5 inhibitors, have produced some encouraging results (8). Whether these findings prove translatable into a treatment advantage for men undergoing radical pelvic surgery remains to be seen. As well, more pathophysiology-specific approaches may prove feasible in the near future as the molecular understanding of neural, smooth muscle, and supportive tissue response to injury is further elucidated. For example, targeting signaling pathways for the initial inflammatory reaction or downstream prior to activation of putative factors such as TGF-β, halting the smooth muscle apoptotic cascade, or minimizing effects of vascular compromise by optimizing the cellular microenvironment prior to surgery may result in improved preservation of EF. After confirming oncologic safety, pre-treatment with novel, pathway-specific pharmacotherapeutic agents may prove to be an effective therapeutic strategy of the future (e.g., small interfering RNA, activation of the neuroregenerative pathways, or reduction of oxidative or nitrosative stress) (9,11).

2.2 Modification of Co-morbidities and Patient Lifestyle

Although most guidelines recommend definitive treatment within 2–4 weeks of the diagnosis of prostate cancer, surgical wait times approach 90 days or more in many instances due to patient concerns or preference (delay in decision-making, arranging for a second opinion), an imbalance between surgical demand and the number of procedures a center is able to offer, initial "treatment" with active surveillance for prostate cancer with favorable parameters, or other factors (12,13). Without well-designed, prospective studies to evaluate this concept, it is difficult to conclude that using this time-period to address co-morbidities or lifestyle factors will translate into a more rapid and/or robust return to potency. However, control of diabetes, hypertension, dyslipidemia, misuse of drugs and alcohol, depression, etc., are essential for maintaining satisfactory erectile function, as well as facilitating a less complicated anesthetic and in-hospital course, post-operative wound healing, and return to pre-operative levels of global function.

It is well established that ED is intimately related to atherosclerotic coronary and peripheral vascular diseases, as well as the metabolic syndrome, which is characterized by central obesity, abnormal lipids, insulin dysregulation, and borderline hypertension. In addition to optimizing pharmacotherapy for hypertension, dyslipidemia, and other medical co-morbidities, simple changes in day-to-day lifestyle may confer an advantage for EF recovery. For example, recent evidence suggests that a Mediterranean-style diet improves endothelial function scores and inflammatory markers (C-reactive protein) when compared to men on a control diet *(14)*. Smoking and obesity have also been prospectively identified as risk factors, while physical activity is inversely associated with the development of ED *(15)*. The beneficial effect of lifestyle change (total weight loss of 10% or more by reduction of caloric intake and increased physical activity) was demonstrated in a randomized, single-blind trial. Mean IIEF scores improved in the intervention group (from 14 ± 4 to 17 ± 5; $p < 0.001$), but remained stable in the control group who were given only general information about healthy food choices and exercise *(16)*.

In conclusion, the potential to reduce the risk of ED following RP may serve as a concrete motivation for men to engage in a variety of health promoting behaviors, including cessation of smoking, weight loss, dietary improvements, and/or pharmacotherapy, and translate into an overall improvement in patient health *(17)*.

3   Peri-operative Strategies

Refinements in anatomic surgical technique, specifically an improved understanding of penile autonomic innervation, and the implementation of innovative technological advances in laparoscopic and robot-assisted surgery, has led to significant improvements in post-operative erectile function. However, even with the advantages gained by using these approaches, ED remains a significant problem for at least 15–40% men treated with radical prostatectomy, and approaches 80–90% for men who are not candidates for nerve-sparing surgery *(4,5,18,19)*.

3.1   Modifying Surgical Approach

Advances using optical magnification to allow for precise visualization and localization of the neurovascular bundles, trials of intraoperative nerve stimulation, decreased use of electrocautery during dissection, sparing of accessory pudendal artery branches, and other refinements to surgical technique have allowed for a slow, but steady improvement in the understanding of factors placing a patient at risk of ED post-operatively and at times, modest gains in overall potency rates *(2,20)*. Although preservation of the cavernous nerves during radical prostatectomy is the most important factor for maintaining post-operative EF and downstream events, including apoptosis of smooth muscle, cavernosal fibrosis, and venous leak are thought to result from CN injury, strategies such as those outlined above are not likely to have a future meaningful impact for men in whom nerve-sparing is not feasible. Therefore, adjunctive peri-operative strategies, including nerve recovery conduit "bridges" or "scaffolds" and modulation of the local environment at the time of surgery, are future possibilities.

3.2 Nerve-Replacement Strategies and Optimization of Cavernous Nerve Regrowth

For men who are not candidates for nerve-sparing procedures, or those in whom sparing is deemed sub-optimal, intraoperative nerve grafting to supplement or replace cavernous nerve function has been attempted by multiple investigators and is discussed in detail elsewhere in this text. Although early enthusiasm for this approach has dampened somewhat, tissue engineering techniques may lead to a resurgence of this approach or variations using tissue engineered or biomaterial scaffolds and or novel drug delivery systems.

Biomaterials hold promise for the future as they have the major advantage over traditional autologous grafts: an ability to impart structural and chemical versatility into this treatment approach *(21)*. To date, several biomaterial polymers have been tested as delivery systems for cellular and non-cellular neuroprotective or neuroregenerative agents or as guidance channels for regenerating axons in experimental models. For example, seeded Schwann cells that had been expanded in tissue culture and placed in silicone tubes were subsequently placed into surgically created cavernous nerve defects in the rat. In comparison to animals treated with nerve reconstruction, genitofemoral nerve interposition, or interposition of empty silicone tubes, the group with the seeded tubes had better functional outcomes *(22)*. There is optimism that as the molecular understanding of nerve recovery expands, technology utilizing treatment strategies on a cellular level, including signaling pathway modulators, neurotrophic factors, or stem cells, can modulate the microenvironment and promote repair of the injury *(23)*. An optimal approach has yet to be determined; variables include device design, the use of degradable versus non-degradable biomaterials, development of new drug agents or novel application of currently available therapeutics, and combination strategies with conduit "bridges" of "scaffolds" used to maintain CN continuity after planned segmental excision (non-nerve-sparing) or functional compromise (laceration, stretch, thermal injury, ischemia, inflammation, or inadvertent resection) *(24)*.

3.3 Electrical Stimulation

For many men, erectile recovery may take 24 months or more after surgery even as recent reports demonstrate that most patients with good pre-operative erectile function (IIEF>18) maintain nocturnal penile tumescence during the acute phase after surgery *(25)*. However, not all of these men will maintain their erections, or demonstrate time-dependent improvement. In potent men undergoing bilateral nerve-sparing RP, the incidence of venous leakage was 14, 21, 35, and 50% at less than 4 months, 4–8 months, 8–12 months, and more than 12 months following surgery, respectively. In these patients, arterial insufficiency (approximately 60%) did not change over time *(26)*. For potent men treated with bilateral non-nerve-sparing surgery, complete tumescence and full rigidity after intracavernous injection of 20 µg prostaglandin E1 was 80% within the first 30 days of surgery, but declined to 37% at 7–12 months post-operatively *(27)*. Clearly, elements of smooth muscle degeneration following even partial nerve injury can have a meaningful clinical impact, compromising recovery of erectile function and translating into decreased penile rigidity, difficulties in maintaining an erection, and other sequelae of cavernous smooth muscle dysfunction or veno-occlusive disease.

A novel approach of some promise is the use of an implantable electrical neurostimulator (ENS) adjacent to the cavernous nerves at the time of radical prostatectomy. Previous animal and human studies have demonstrated improved EF following partial denervation, for patients with chronic ED, and at time of surgery for veno-occlusive disease. Although the precise mechanism of action is not known, preliminary findings are encouraging. A current clinical trial evaluating this approach (Advanced Bionics, Valencia, California) for men undergoing radical prostatectomy is ongoing and results are eagerly anticipated, as ENS may be identified as a new adjunctive treatment for enhanced recovery of erectile function in this population *(23)*.

4   Post-operative Strategies

Erectile dysfunction after radical prostatectomy may persist, despite surgical advances, neuroprotective strategies, and pre-operative treatment or optimization of erectile function and risk factors. Currently available medications, as well as novel ED therapies, may be used aiming to alleviate patient symptoms or stimulate recovery as monotherapies or in combination with other treatments. With profound end-organ damage and dysfunction, however, other strategies might be employed to create new, healthy tissue. Components of future therapy for patients following pelvic surgery are likely to focus upon regeneration or creation of functional erectile tissue, whether done on a tissue, cellular, or gene level and may include tissue engineering and stem-cell or gene-based approaches.

4.1   Post-operative Penile Rehabilitation

Although there is no unifying pathophysiological theory for the cause of post-operative ED to date, most investigators would agree that therapeutic inactivity in the motivated patient is counter-productive to a potential return to potency *(3,28)*. Rehabilitation strategies are varied, but literature suggests that early therapy using intracavernous injection of vasoactive agents (prostaglandin E-1 or combinations with papaverine or phentolamine, or all three), oral therapy with phosphodiesterase-5 inhibitors, or a combination of both may confer a recovery advantage to the patient as damage secondary to tissue hypoxia and subsequent atrophy of cavernosal smooth muscle is decreased *(25)*. These concepts are discussed in detail in Chapter 12, "Pharmacologic Penile Preservation and Rehabilitation."

The ability to deliver drugs directly into the corpora cavernosa via injection is a distinct advantage for treating the smooth muscle and neural (through retrograde transmission) components of the erectile tissues; novel growth factors such as the bone-morphogenic protein GDF-5 (growth-differentiation factor-5), PARP-1 (poly[adenosine diphosphate ribose] polymerase-1) inhibitors, and glial cell line derivatives such as neurturin, may represent the next generation of smooth-muscle protectants or neuromodulators *(23,29)*. Recent reports support continued investigation of the potential mechanisms by which PDE-5 inhibitors enhance tissue protection or regeneration as chronic administration of tadalafil reduced some effects of hypoxia following cavernous nerve neurotomy in the rat *(30)*. The development of these, and other promising therapies such as the immunophilin ligands, gene therapy, and stem cells (discussed below), represent some of the many potential postoperative approaches translated from the lab bench to clinical use. Although future forms of post-operative rehabilitation will likely share some characteristics with current regimens, the combination of novel therapies specifically tailored to apoptotic, neuroprotective, and neuroregenerative targets, at optimal doses and timing (therapeutic "windows of opportunity"), and adjunctive use of pre- and peri-operative strategies is most likely to yield a demonstrable improvement in post-operative EF.

4.2 *Tissue Engineering*

Total phallic reconstruction or replacement is not likely to be necessary, even in the face of severe endothelial dysfunction and/or loss of functional smooth muscle cells. More realistic approaches are cell or tissue (combination)-based therapies, and involve the injection of "functional" cells into the corpus cavernosum or regeneration of damaged tissues.

One of the first barriers to overcome in tissue engineering is to isolate the crucial cell populations without excessive contamination by other cell types. Pilatz et al. evaluated a wide variety of published and novel techniques for separation and culture of both endothelial and stromal cell populations *(31)*. Using a combination of elastase-treatment of tissue blocks and mechanical squeezing of the tissues with a metal spatula yielded an impressive 98% purity as confirmed by immunohistochemistry (IHC) and Western blotting. Their conclusion was that endothelial cell cultures derived from human corpora cavernosa are reproducible and reliable to serve for cell culture-based investigations of the endothelial dysfunction and may develop into a future therapy. Isolating pure cavernosal smooth muscle cells using current techniques is not as successful. The discrepancy in the purity of smooth muscle cell cultures might reflect laboratory and tissue source factors, lacking an exclusion of fibroblasts in other studies or changes in stromal phenotype under culture conditions. Further research is necessary to clarify a possible plasticity between smooth muscle cells and (myo)fibroblasts and assess functional properties.

Although cell-based techniques might be considered for direct repair of damaged corporal endothelium, therapy for erectile dysfunction with either endothelial or with smooth muscle cells, seems most promising when combined with cell manipulation by gene therapy prior to cell transfer, i.e., genetically engineered cells, as will be discussed below.

At the tissue level, pioneering work by Atala et al. has explored the feasibility of developing corporal tissue (combining human cavernosal smooth muscle and endothelial cells in vivo in athymic mice) using a three-dimensional acellular collagen matrix. Organ bath studies demonstrated cell-seeded corporal tissue matrices responded to electrical field stimulation, whereas unseeded controls did not, demonstrating the formation of well-vascularized corporal tissues derived from donor corpora *(32)*. The possibility of replacing an entire cross-sectional segment of both corporal bodies, as could be required with severe corporal fibrosis, with autologous engineered tissues has also been evaluated using a rabbit model *(33)*. Adequate structural and functional parameters of the neo-corpora were achieved in this proof-of-concept study.

Tissue and biomaterial engineering, although still considered to be in their infancy as areas of research, hold much promise in becoming cell and tissue-specific therapies for ED resulting from pelvic surgeries for malignancy and may develop into effective peri- and post-operative treatment approaches in the not-so-distant future.

4.3   Gene and Stem-Cell Therapies

Gene and stem cell therapies represent the next potential era of advanced therapeutic strategies for genetic or acquired diseases. Future development of these approaches is dependent upon more detailed clarification of the underlying physiology and pharmacology of erectile tissues in both normal and disease states. To date, gene and stem-based therapies remain "treatments of the future" but, as will be detailed below, may become practical successors to today's oral and minimally invasive therapies for ED *(34)*.

The penis is uniquely suited for gene transfer due to its anatomic and ultrastructural features (connexin 43 gap junctions forming allowing rapid communication between cells), and potential targets such as potassium channels. In order for gene therapy to be clinically useful, it needs to fulfill the following criteria: efficacy, safety, extended duration of effectiveness, and patient tolerability *(35)*. Naked DNA has emerged as the transfer vector of choice, due to its lack of chromosomal integration, toxicity, and immune induction, and confirmation of efficacy and lasting duration *(34)*. This plasmid-based vector system (*h*Maxi-k), used to insert the *hSlo* gene which codes for Maxi-k potassium channels, is especially promising for the treatment of cavernous smooth muscle disorders (as seen following penile hypoxia), as corporal smooth muscle relaxation is enhanced. Animal studies have demonstrated a sustained dose-dependent response for 4–6 months and recently reported dose-escalation phase I trial results of intracavernous injection of *h*Maxi-k in demonstrated no adverse events *(36)*. Other potential targets for gene therapy modulation may include eNOS (endothelial nitric oxide synthase), superoxide dismutase (SOD), and RhoA/Rho kinase *(37)*.

Limitations with the use of embryonic stem cells for human disease have led to a focus upon stem cells derived from adult tissues. The potential regeneration of healthy endothelial and smooth muscle tissues in the penis offers enormous promise as a potential treatment for erectile dysfunction, especially should gene-modified ex-vivo expanded adult stem cells prove efficacious and safe in human subjects *(38)*. The action of stem cells is likely multifactorial and includes differentiation into cellular elements of the erectile mechanism, function as substrates for axonal growth, release of neurotrophic factors, and cytokines that inhibit demyelination *(23)*. Experience thus far is limited to animal studies, but has shown that an advantage for functional recovery and increased penile nerve content occurs after bilateral cavernous nerve crush if stem cells are delivered into the major pelvic ganglion and corpora cavernosa *(39)*.

4.4 Next-Generation of Pharmacologic Treatments

Several new pharmacologic treatments hold future promise as primary or adjunctive treatments for ED following pelvic surgeries. These include immunophilin ligands, neurotrophins, erythropoietin, steroid therapy, new PDE-5 inhibitors or ICI agents, and as yet undeveloped, novel molecularmechanism-based agents.

The neurotrophic characteristics of immunophilin ligands, such as tacrolimus (FK506) (see Chapter 12) hold potential for the treatment of many neurological conditions, including spinal cord injury, peripheral neuropathies, and erectile dysfunction. Using a model of cavernous nerve crush injury in the rat, FK506 was found to preserve function, reduce neural degeneration and stimulate axonal regrowth in a variety of neurodegenerative disease models *(40)*. Novel non-immunosuppressant derivatives such as FK1706 may prove more useful in clinical practice, as immunity in the post-cancer treatment patient is not compromised by these agents. Initial pilot studies have demonstrated functional recovery of erectile function and immunohistochemical evidence of neurotrophism and neuroregeneration following 8 weeks of therapy in animal studies *(41)*. A second derivative, GPI-1485 (Guildford Pharmaceuticals, Baltimore, Maryland) is currently the focus of a phase II, multi-center, randomized trial in approximately 200 men following RP.

Neurotrophins have been reviewed in detail in Chapter 12. Although it is likely that one or more of these molecules will eventually attain clinical use, this group is equally valuable for identifying molecular signaling targets for enhanced penile neurogenesis. Through discovery of novel pathways involved in neurotrophin-enhanced recovery after nerve injury, neurotrophins may also serve as the foundation for the next generation of target-specific pharmaceuticals *(42)*.

Intracavernous injection also continues to hold great promise as several novel vasoactive substances that, alone or in combination, target multiple physiologic sites and relax cavernous smooth muscle and/or modify vascular function are in development. Gastrointestinal hydrogen sulfide, potassium-channel openers, calcitonin gene-related peptides, gaunylate cyclase activators, and rho/kinase inhibitors are among agents currently investigated and may represent the next generation of ICI mono- or combination therapies *(43)*.

5 Conclusion

Nerve-sparing radical prostatectomy ushered in a new era of thought focused upon achieving optimal cancer control while minimizing the impact of surgery on patient quality of life. A rapid growth in basic science understanding, specifically the response of tissues to injury on a molecular level, promises to fuel further advances for treatment strategies minimizing erectile compromise following radical pelvic surgeries. Exciting developments in the fields of tissue engineering, neuromodulation, stem-cell and gene-based therapies are examples of the continued evolution of treatments for erectile dysfunction. Although optimistic, it is feasible that one or more of these novel approaches may successfully translate from the lab bench to clinical use in the near future, resulting in an increased likelihood of erectile preservation and improved quality of life.

References

1. Walsh, P.C., and Donker, P.C. (1982) Impotence following radical prostatectomy: insight into etiology and prevention. *J. Urol.* **128,** 492–497.
2. Seftel, A.D. (2006) Erectile dysfunction a decade later: another paradigm shift. *J. Urol.* **176,** 10–11.
3. Mulhall, J., Land, S., Parker, M., Waters, W.B., and Flanigan, R.C. (2005) The use of an erectogenic pharmacotherapy regimen following radical prostatectomy improves recovery of spontaneous erectile function. *J. Sex. Med.* **2,** 532–540.
4. Rozet, F., Galiano, M., Cathelineau, X., Barret, E., Cathala, N., and Vallancien, G. (2005) Extraperitoneal laparoscopic radical prostatectomy: a prospective evaluation of 600 cases. *J. Urol.* **174,** 908–911.
5. Menon, M., Tewari, A., Peabody, J.O., Shrivastava, A., Kaul, S., Bhandari, A., and Hemal, A. (2004) Vattikuti Institute prostatectomy, a technique of robotic radical prostatectomy for management of localized carcinoma of the prostate: experience of over 1100 cases. *Urol. Clin. N. Am.* **31,** 701–717.
6. Dubbelman, Y.D., Dohle, G.R., and Schroder, F.H. (2008) Sexual function before and after radical retropubic prostatectomy: a systematic review of prognostic indicators for a successful outcome. *Eur. Urol.* **50,** 711–718.
7. Kendirci, M., Bejma, J., and Hellstrom, W.J.G. (2006) Update on erectile dysfunction in prostate cancer patients. *Curr. Opin. Urol.* **16,** 186–195.
8. Donohoe, J.F., Mullerad, M., Paduch, D.A., Kobylarz, K.A., Li, P.S., Scardino, P.T., and Mulhall, J.P. (2006) The functional and structural consequences of cavernous nerve injury in the rat model are ameliorated by sildenafil citrate. *J. Urol.* [abstract 1050].

9. Lin, G., Hayashi, N., Carrion, R., Chang, L.J., and Lue, T.F. (2005) Improving erectile function by silencing phosphodiesterase-5. *J. Urol.* **174**, 1142–1148.
10. Bella, A., Lin, G., Tantiwongse, K., Garcia, M., Lin, C.S., Brant, W., and Lue, T. (2006) Brain-derived neurotrophic factor (BDNF) acts primarily via the JAK/STAT pathway to promote neurite growth in the major pelvic ganglion of the rat: Part 1. *J. Sex. Med.* **3**, 815–820.
11. Burnett, A.L., Musicki, B., Jin, L., and Bivalacque, T.L. (2006) Nitric oxide/redox-based signalling as a therapeutic target for penile disorders. *Expert Opin. Ther. Targets* **10**, 445–457.
12. Saad, F., Finelli, A., Dranitsaris, G., Goldenberg, L., Bagnell, S., Gleave, M., Fleshner, N., Canadian surgical wait times (SWAT) initiative. (2006) Does prolonging the time to prostate cancer surgery impact long-term cancer control: a systematic review of the literature. *Can. J. Urol.* **13**(Suppl 3), 16–24.
13. Klotz, L. (2006) Active surveillance versus radical treatment for favorable-risk localized prostate cancer. *Curr. Treat. Options Oncol.* **7**, 355–362.
14. Esposito, K., Ciotola, M., Giugliano, F., De Sio, M., Giugliano, G., D'Armiento, M., and Giugliano, D. (2006) Mediterranean diet improves erectile function in subjects with the metabolic syndrome. *Int. J. Impot. Res.* **18**, 405–410.
15. Polsky, J.Y., Aronson, K.J., Heaton, J.P., and Adams, M.A. (2005) Smoking and other lifestyle factors in relation to erectile dysfunction. *BJU Int.* **96**, 1355–1359.
16. Esposito, K., Giugliano, F., Di Palo, C., Giugliano, G., Marfella, R., D'Andrea, F., D'Armiento, M., and Giugliano, D. (2004) Effect of lifestyle changes on erectile dysfunction in obese men: a randomized controlled trial. *JAMA* **291**, 2978–2984.
17. Bacon, C.G., Mittleman, M.A., Kawachi, I., Giovannucci, E., Glasser, D.B., and Rimm, E.B. (2006) A prospective study of risk factors for erectile dysfunction. *J. Urol.* **176**, 217–221.
18. Kundu, S.D., Roehl, K.A., Eggener, S.E., Antenor, J.A., Han, M., and Catalona, W.J. (2006) Potency, continence, and complications in 3 477 consecutive radical retropubic prostatectomies. *J. Urol.* **172**, 2227–2231.
19. Borchers, H., Brehmer, B., Kirschner-Hermanns, R., Reineke, T., Tietze, L., and Jakse, G. (2006) Erectile dysfunction after non-nerve-sparing radical prostatectomy. Fact or fiction? *Urol. Int.* **76**, 213–216.
20. Kendirci, M., Bejma, J., and Hellstrom, W.J.G. (2006) Update on erectile dysfunction in prostate cancer patients. *Curr. Opin. Urol.* **16**, 186–195.
21. Nomura, H., Tator, C.H., and Shoichet, M.S. (2006) Bioengineered strategies for spinal cord repair. *J. Neurotrauma.* **23**, 496–507.
22. May, F., Weidner, N., Matiasek, K., Caspers, C., Mrva, T., Vroemen, M., et al. (2004) Schwann cell seeded guidance tubes restore erectile function after ablation of cavernous nerves in rats. *J. Urol.* **172**, 374.
23. Burnett, A.L., and Lue, T.F. (2006) Neuromodulatory therapy to improve erectile function outcomes after pelvic surgery. *J. Urol.* **176**, 882–887.
24. Syme, D.B.Y., Corcoran, N.M., Bouchier-Hayes, D.M., and Costello, A.J. (2006) Hope springs eternal: cavernosal nerve regeneration. *BJU Int.* **97**, 17–21.
25. Bannowsky, A., Schulze, H., van der Horst, C., Seif, C., Braun, P.M., and Junesmann, K.-P. (2006) Nocturnal tumescence: a parameter for postoperative erectile integrity after nerve sparing radical prostatectomy. *J. Urol.* **175**, 2214–2217.
26. Mulhall, J.P., Slovick, R., Hotaling, J., Aviv, N., Valenzuela, R., Waters, W.B., and Flanigan, R.C. (2002) Erectile dysfunction after radical prostatectomy: hemodynamic profiles and their correlation with the recovery of erectile function. *J. Urol.* **167**, 1371–1375.
27. Gontero, P., Fontana, F., Bagnasacco, A., Panella, M., Kocjancic, E., Pretti, G., and Frea, B. (2003) Is there an optimal time for intracavernous prostaglandin E1 rehabilitation following nonnerve sparing radical prostatectomy? Results from a hemodynamic prospective study. *J. Urol.* **169**, 2166–2169.
28. Titta, M., Tavolini, I.M., Moro, F.D., Cisternino, A., and Bassi, P. (2006 Mar) Sexual counseling improved erectile rehabilitation after non-nerve-sparing radical retropubic prostatectomy or cystectomy-results of a randomized prospective study. *J. Sex. Med.* **3**(2), 267–273.

29. Fandel, T., Bella, A.J., Tantiwongse, K., Garcia, M., Nunes, L., Thuroff, J.W., Tanagho, E.A., and Lue, T.F. (2006) The effect of intracavernous growth differentiation factor-5 in a rat model of cavernous nerve injury. *BJU Int.* [*epub ahead of print*].

30. Vignozzi, L., Filippi, S., Morelli, A., Ambrosini, S., Luconi, M., Vanneli, G.B., Donati, S., Crescioli, C., Zhang, X.H., Mirone, V., Forti, G., and Maggi, M. (2006) Effect of chronic tadalafil administration on penile hypoxia induced by cavernous neurotomy in the rat. *J. Sex. Med.* **3,** 419–431.

31. Pilatz, A., Schultheiss, D., Gabouev, A.I., Schlote, N., Mertsching, H., Jonas, U., and Stief, C.G. (2005) Isolation of primary endothelial and stromal cell cultures of the corpus cavernosum penis for basic research and tissue engineering. *Eur. Urol.* **47,** 710–718.

32. Falke, G., Yoo, J.J., Kwon, T.G., Moreland, R., and Atala, A. (2003 Oct) Formation of corporal tissue architecture in vivo using human cavernosal muscle and endothelial cells seeded on collagen matrices. *Tissue Eng.* **9**(5), 871–879.

33. Kwon, T.G., Yo, J.J., and Atala, A. (2002 Oct) Autologous penile corpora cavernosa replacement using tissue engineering techniques. *J. Urol.* **168**(4 Pt 2), 1754–1758.

34. Melman, A. (2006) Gene transfer for the therapy of erectile dysfunction: progress in the 21st century. *Int. J. Impot. Res.* **18,** 19–25.

35. Schiff, J.D., and Melman, A. (2006) Ion channel gene therapy for smooth muscle disorders: relaxing smooth muscles to treat erectile dysfunction. *Assay Drug Dev. Technol.* **4,** 89–95.

36. Melman, A., Bar-Chama, N., McCullough, A., Davies, K., and Christ, G. (2005) The first human trial for gene transfer therapy for the treatment of erectile dysfunction: preliminary results. *Eur. Urol.* **48,** 314–318.

37. Deng, W., Bivalacqua, T.J., Hellstrom, W.J.G., and Kadowitz, P.J. (2005) Gene and stem cell therapy for erectile dysfunction. *Int. J. Impot. Res.* **17,** S57–S63.

38. Bunnell, B.A., Deng, W., Robinson, C.M., Waldron, P.R., Bivalaqua, T.J., Baber, S.R., Hymann, A.L., and Kadowitz, P.J. (2005) Potential application for mesenchymal stem cells in the treatment of cardiovascular disease. *Can. J. Physiol. Pharmacol.* **83,** 529–539.

39. Bochinski, D., Lin, G.T., Nunes, L., Carrion, R., Rahman, N., Lin C.-S., and Lue, T.F. (2004) The effect of neural embryonic stem cell therapy in a rat model of cavernosal nerve injury. *BJU Int.* **94,** 904–909.

40. Poulter, M.O., Payne, K.B., and Steiner, J.P. (2004) Neuroimmunophilins: a novel drug therapy for the reversal of neurodegenerative disease? *Neuroscience* **128,** 1–6.

41. Hayashi, N., Minor, T.X., Carrion, R., Price, R., Nunes, L., and Lue, T.F. (2006) The effect of FK1706 on erectile function following bilateral cavernous nerve crush injury in a rat model. *J. Urol.* **176,** 824–829.

42. Lin, G., Bella, A.J., Lue, T.F., and Lin, C.S. (2006) Brain-derived neurotrophic factor (BDNF) acts primarily via the JAK/STAT pathway to promote neurite growth in the major pelvic ganglion of the rat: Part 2. *J. Sex. Med.* **3,** 821–829.

43. Bella, A.J., Brant, W.O., and Brock, G.B. (2006) Contemporary intracavernous pharmacotherapy for erectile dysfunction in the aging male. *Aging Health* **2,** 559–570.

Index

Printed in the United States of America

Color Plates

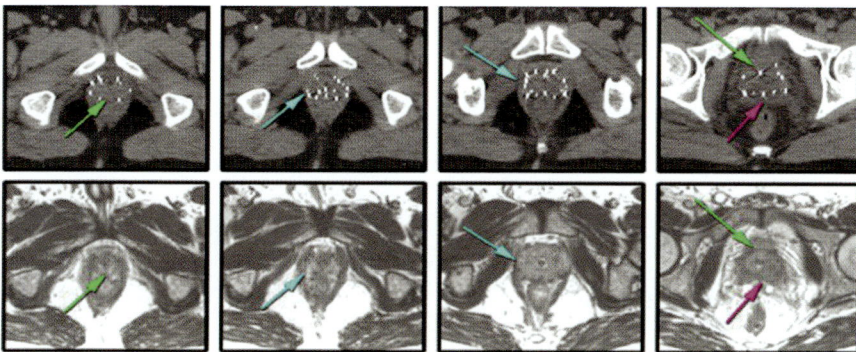

Color Plate 1 Comparison of prostate interface clarity at different levels within the prostate. *Arrow* represents an interface with the prostate clarified by MRI, unclear on CT. *Left to right panels*: Genitourinary diaphragm, apex, mid-prostate, and base (Chapter 7, Fig. 2; *see* discussion on p. 100)

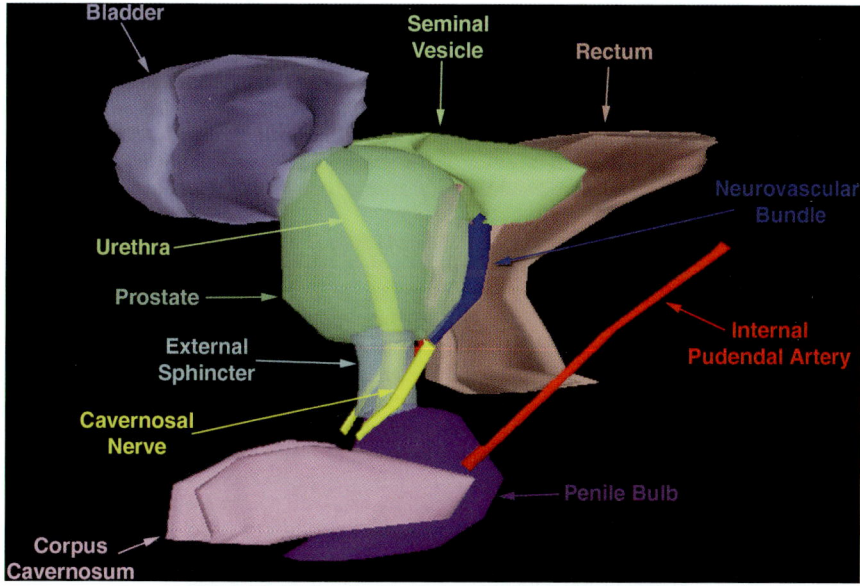

Color Plate 2 Prostate and CES defined by fusion of CT and MRI (Chapter 7, Fig. 4; *see* discussion on p. 101)

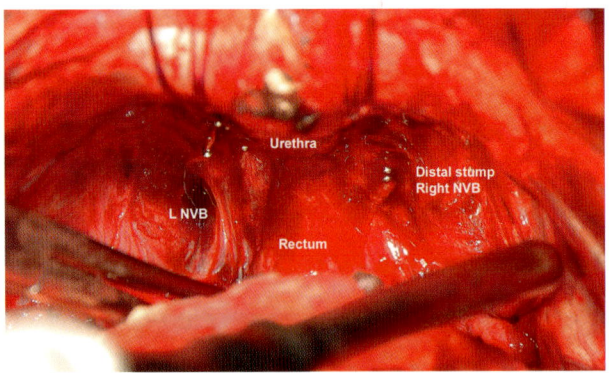

Color Plate 3 Intraoperative photograph showing the right distal neurovascular bundle stump with double clips to distinguish it from a bleeding vessel. These are removed at the time of neural anastomosis (Chapter 9, Fig. 1; *see* discussion on p. 132)

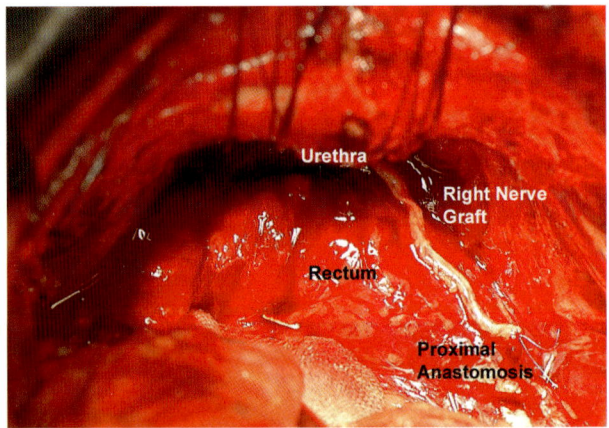

Color Plate 4 Intraoperative photograph showing the completed right cavernous nerve graft (Chapter 9, Fig. 2; *see* discussion on p. 133)

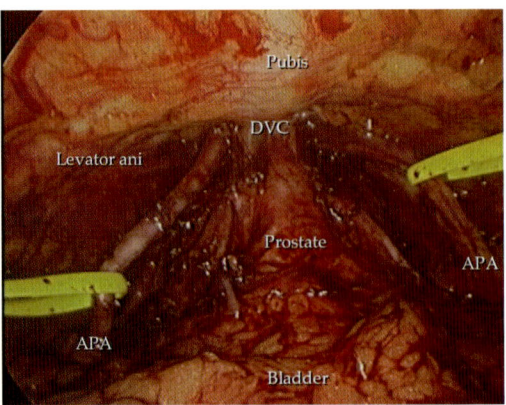

Color Plate 5 Intra-operative photograph taken during laparoscopic radical prostatectomy demonstrating bilateral accessory pudendal arteries (Chapter 10, Fig. 1; *see* discussion on p. 143)